Disability and Equity at Work

DISABILITY AND EQUITY AT WORK

Edited by Jody Heymann, Michael Ashley Stein, and Gonzalo Moreno

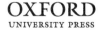
OXFORD
UNIVERSITY PRESS

OXFORD
UNIVERSITY PRESS

Oxford University Press is a department of the University of Oxford.
It furthers the University's objective of excellence in research, scholarship,
and education by publishing worldwide.

Oxford   New York
Auckland   Cape Town   Dar es Salaam   Hong Kong   Karachi
Kuala Lumpur   Madrid   Melbourne   Mexico City   Nairobi
New Delhi   Shanghai   Taipei   Toronto

With offices in
Argentina   Austria   Brazil   Chile   Czech Republic   France   Greece
Guatemala   Hungary   Italy   Japan   Poland   Portugal   Singapore
South Korea   Switzerland   Thailand   Turkey   Ukraine   Vietnam

Oxford is a registered trademark of Oxford University Press
in the UK and certain other countries.

Published in the United States of America by
Oxford University Press
198 Madison Avenue, New York, NY 10016

© Oxford University Press 2014

Library of Congress Cataloging-in-Publication Data
Disability and equity at work / edited by Jody Heymann, Michael A. Stein,
and Gonzalo Moreno.
   p. ; cm.
Includes bibliographical references.
ISBN 978-0-19-998121-2 (alk. paper)
1. People with disabilities—Employment.   2. Discrimination against people with
disabilities.   3. Discrimination in employment.   I. Heymann, Jody, 1959– editor
of compilation.   II. Stein, Michael Ashley, editor of compilation.   III. Moreno, Gonzalo,
(Moreno Ruiz de Elvira), editor of compilation.
[DNLM: 1. Disabled Persons.   2. Employment—legislation & jurisprudence.
3. Prejudice. HD 7255.A3]
HD7255.D54 2013
331.5'9—dc23
2013019022

9 8 7 6 5 4 3 2 1
Printed in the United States of America
on acid-free paper

To Steve

To Irving and Miriam

To Malen and Gonzalo

ACKNOWLEDGMENTS

Disability and Equity at Work represents a collaboration between the Institute for Health and Social Policy at McGill University, the Harvard Law School Project on Disability, and the UCLA Fielding School of Public Health. With the generous support of the Max Bell Foundation, we were able to bring together top researchers, policymakers, and civil society leaders to address pressing health and social policy issues, and to send dedicated fellows to study successful organizations around the globe. This initiative, and the cohort and conference focused on disability and equity at work, would not have been possible if Allan Northcott, David Elton, and Ralph Strother at the Max Bell Foundation had not shared our conviction that sound, evidence-based public policy offers tremendous opportunities to address population health, well-being, and equity.

Putting together *Disability and Equity at Work* was truly a team effort. We are forever indebted to Jennifer Proudfoot, who helped us reach out to experts on disability and employment in every region of the world, and then led the organization of a two-day international conference to bring this exceptional group of experts together. Before Institute Policy Fellows could go into the field to conduct their case studies of top organizations working on improving employment rates and conditions for persons with disabilities, Magda Barrera led a months-long search of hundreds of noteworthy programs. Talia Bronstein and Sheena Melwani worked tirelessly to help organize the conference that first brought together this group of contributing authors and ultimately planted the seeds for this volume. Denise Maines and Kristen McNeill provided immensely helpful insights and suggestions to early chapter drafts. Institute interns Brittany Carson, Keiko Shikako-Thomas, Phoebe Spencer, Jason Tan de Bibiana, and Vicky Tobianah provided invaluable background research.

Edited volumes such as this one rarely occur unless editors and authors believe deeply in the importance of the subject matter. Jody has had the privilege of working for decades with people around the world whose daily lives demonstrate with grit, pain, humor, courage, frustration, quiet and vocal tenacity, aspirations, and accomplishments, the ability to live remarkable lives and leave an indelible mark on all our communities—not only with significant physical health, mental health, and cognitive obstacles, but also with the far greater obstacles of discrimination, incomprehension, neglect, and needless societal barriers.

She would like to dedicate this book to all of these colleagues and to Steve Heymann, who went after his elementary school teacher with his crutches when she thought it would be "better for him" to always be at the back of the line, who was the first one to inspire Jody to study overseas and to go camping in remote areas, whose polio didn't get in the way of him being on the judo team or flipping Jody on her back, who has helped bring accessibility to the US Department of Justice and the world wide web, whom she's never heard use the term "disabled" in reference to himself, but only in terms of equal rights, and whose life for more than five decades has made clear in every way how much disability is constructed by societies, their beliefs, and the barriers they erect that we all need to tear down.

For Michael, who has worked on disability human rights issues in over three dozen countries, ensuring equal access to education for children with disabilities and enabling their transition as adults into the workplace are among the challenges to which he devotes academic time and advocacy skill. Michael is very cognizant of the efforts parents of children with disabilities expend daily to empower their children, and so dedicates this book to his own parents in gratitude for the many battles they fought on his behalf.

Gonzalo grew up in a family of journalists, and he picked up early on that questions that are easy to answer are not worth asking. When you have limited airtime, page space, and attention spans, it is preferable—and much more interesting—to go straight to the thorny issues. This book grapples with such issues, and although it may not provide every possible question with a neat answer, it does provide every difficult question with a good answer. Gonzalo would like to dedicate this book to his parents, Gonzalo and Malen, for giving him the freedom and support to figure out what questions to ask. It is still a work in progress.

TABLE OF CONTENTS

ABOUT THE EDITORS

Jody Heymann is Dean and Distinguished Professor of Epidemiology at the Fielding School of Public Health, Distinguished Professor of Public Policy at the Luskin School of Public Affairs, and Distinguished Professor of Medicine at the Geffen School of Medicine, UCLA. Before becoming dean at UCLA, Heymann served as founding director of McGill University's Institute for Health and Social Policy and held a Canada Research Chair in Global Health and Social Policy. Her research focuses on issues of social equity. She has led large global studies examining working conditions. These studies include examining public policies relevant to work in 190 UN countries, examining private firms in 15 countries that have sought to improve working conditions for marginalized populations while economically succeeding, and interviewing working families in North America, Europe, Latin America, Africa, Asia, and the Pacific.

Heymann has authored and edited more than 200 publications, including 15 books. Among others, these include: *Children's Chances* (Harvard University Press, 2013), *Making Equal Rights Real* (Cambridge University Press, 2012), *Lessons in Educational Equality* (Oxford University Press, 2012), *Protecting Childhood in the AIDS Pandemic* (Oxford University Press, 2012), *Profit at the Bottom of the Ladder* (Harvard Business Press, 2010), *Raising the Global Floor* (Stanford University Press, 2010), *Forgotten Families* (Oxford University Press, 2006), *Healthier Societies* (Oxford University Press, 2006), *Unfinished Work* (New Press, 2005), *Global Inequalities at Work* (Oxford University Press, 2003), and *The Widening Gap* (Basic Books, 2000).

Deeply committed to translating research into policies and programs that will improve individual and population health, Heymann has worked with leaders in North American, European, African, and Latin American governments as well as a wide range of intergovernmental organizations including the World Health Organization, the International Labour Organization, UNICEF, UNESCO, and UNDESA. She has served as chair of the World Economic Forum's Global Agenda Council on Education Systems and vice-chair of the Global Agenda Council on Education and Skills. Her research has been presented to heads of state and senior policymakers around the world.

Michael Ashley Stein holds a JD from Harvard Law School and a PhD from Cambridge University. Co-founder and executive director of the Harvard Law School Project on Disability as well as Cabell Professor at William & Mary Law School, he has taught at Harvard, New York University, and Stanford law schools. Previously, Stein clerked for United States Supreme Court Justice Samuel A. Alito Jr. (while on the Third Circuit Court of Appeals), and practiced law with Sullivan & Cromwell in New York. During that time, he served as president of the National Disabled Bar Association, and pro bono counsel for the United States Department of Justice's Environmental Division and the Legal Aid Society's Juvenile Rights Division.

An internationally recognized expert on disability rights, Stein participated in the drafting of the United Nations Convention on the Rights of Persons with Disabilities, and actively consults with international governments on their disability laws and policies. He serves on disability rights advisory boards and blue ribbon research panels, and was an American Bar Association Commissioner on Mental and Physical Disability Law. Stein has also acted as legal counsel to Rehabilitation International, Disabled Peoples' International, and to Special Olympics International, and has filed amici briefs with the European Court of Human Rights, national-level supreme and constitutional courts, and the Committee on the Rights of Persons with Disabilities on behalf of individuals with disabilities. He works with disabled persons' organizations around the world, and advises a number of United Nations bodies, such as UNDESA, UNICEF, and UNOHCHR, as well as individual national human rights institutions.

Stein is the recipient of numerous awards from global disability rights groups (most recently, the inaugural Henry Viscardi Achievement Award), national-level disability rights organizations that he has been honored to serve, and was recognized by the Boston Globe Magazine as a "Bostonian Changing the World." Academically, Stein has been awarded an American Council of Learned Societies Andrew W. Mellon Faculty Fellowship, a Mark DeWolfe Howe Fund Grant, a National Endowment for the Humanities Summer Stipend, and a National Institute on Disability and Rehabilitation Research Merit Fellowship. He has been a fellow in both the East Asian Legal Studies Program and the Human Rights Program at Harvard Law School. In 2012, President Barack Obama appointed Stein to the United States Holocaust Council.

Gonzalo Moreno is the Disability and Equity Initiative Director at McGill University's Institute for Health and Social Policy. The initiative examines which policies and programs can lead to labor market improvements for persons with disabilities, with a specific focus on equitable, integrated, and sustainable employment. At McGill he is also the project coordinator of MACHE (Maternal and Child Health Equity), a large-scale research project funded by the Canadian Institutes for Health Research that seeks to understand how social policy affects infant, child, and maternal health outcomes primarily in low- and middle-income countries. Moreno holds undergraduate degrees in International Development and Translation, and is a graduate of Carleton University's Norman Paterson School of International Affairs, where he was a La Caixa scholar and specialized in human security and development.

ABOUT THE AUTHORS

Leif Atle Beisland is an associate professor at the University of Agder in Norway. He holds a PhD in capital market-based accounting research from the Norwegian School of Economics. His research covers both general accounting research and more specific research on financial reporting in the microfinance industry. He has researched the use of microfinance services among persons with disabilities.

Susanne M. Bruyère is the Associate Dean of Outreach and Director of the Employment and Disability Institute, at the Cornell University ILR School. She has a doctorate in Rehabilitation Counseling Psychology from the University of Wisconsin-Madison, is a Fellow in the American Psychological Association, executive board member and past president of the American Psychological Association Division of Rehabilitation Psychology, past-chair of GLADNET (the Global Applied Disability Research and Information Network on Employment and Training), past-chair of the CARF (Rehabilitation Accreditation) Board of Directors, and past president of the American Rehabilitation Counseling Association and the National Council on Rehabilitation Education.

John Dattilo is a professor in the Department of Recreation, Park and Tourism Management in the College of Health and Human Development at Pennsylvania State University, where he teaches about inclusive leisure services from an applied, philosophical, and ethical perspective. The overarching purpose of his research is to examine effects of services designed to empower individuals who are experiencing constraints to their leisure so that their lives become more meaningful and enjoyable. Professor Dattilo has published extensively on interventions to increase the community integration of persons with disabilities.

Megan Galeucia is a McGill University graduate and is currently working toward her Master of Public Health at Columbia University in New York. She is interested in the intersections between social justice issues and health inequalities and conducting community-based participatory research. Galeucia was a fellow at the Institute for Health and Social Policy, where she researched employment barriers and opportunities experienced by people with disabilities and worked in London conducting a case study on the Business Forum on Disability.

Laurie Gutmann Kahn is currently a doctoral candidate in Special Education at the University of Oregon focusing on secondary special education and post-secondary transitions. Once a special education teacher in the Bronx, her experiences in the classroom contributed to her interest in equal access for youth with disabilities during transition from high school, as well as in culture and disability and teacher education. She is currently working on her dissertation examining the experiences and beliefs about the future for young adults with disabilities who identify as lesbian, gay, bisexual, transgender, or intersex (LGBTQI.)

Anna Lawson is a senior lecturer in the School of Law at the University of Leeds and deputy director of the University's Centre for Disability Studies. Her research focuses on disability equality and human rights and her publications include *Disability Equality in Britain* (Hart Publishing, 2008), *EU Non-Discrimination Law and Intersectionality* (Ashgate, 2011, co-edited with Dagmar Schiek), and *Disability Rights in Europe* (Hart Publishing, 2005, co-edited with Caroline Gooding). She plays a lead role in a number of research groups, including the Academic Network of European Disability Experts, for which she is part of the international research coordination team. In addition, Lawson is actively involved in the work of various disability and human rights organizations—she is a current trustee of the Budapest Mental Disability Advocacy Centre and the Leeds Society for Deaf and Blind People, and a former trustee of the Royal National Institute of Blind and Partially Sighted People.

Lauren Lindstrom is an associate professor and currently serves as Associate Dean of Research and Outreach for the College of Education at the University of Oregon. Over the last 12 years, Dr Lindstrom has directed or co-directed 10 externally funded projects to develop innovative transition programs and improve post school employment outcomes for students with disabilities. She currently serves as project director for the Oregon Youth Transition Program, a collaborative program that serves 115 high schools and more than 1,400 youth, and as principal investigator for a research study designed to improve educational and career outcomes for young women with disabilities. Dr Lindstrom has published numerous curricula, training materials, and peer-reviewed journal articles focused on topics of career development, post school employment outcomes, and transition services.

Stanislao Maldonado is PhD candidate in development economics from the Department of Agricultural Economics at the University of California at Berkeley and a visiting researcher with the Center of Development and Participation in Peru. He holds master's degrees in Economics from the Universidad de San Andres (Argentina) and in Agricultural and Resource Economics from the University of California at Berkeley. Before moving to California, he was a junior economist with the World Bank in Washington, DC, where he was working with the Department of Human Development for Latin America and the Caribbean on poverty, inequality, pension, and labor market issues. In Peru, he was consultant with the Special Commission in Disabilities Studies at the Congress of Peru and examined labor market issues for people with disabilities.

David R. Mann is a researcher at Mathematica Policy Research. His primary research interests include the labor force participation and benefit receipt of youth and adults with disabilities. Mann has worked on the designs and evaluations for several Social Security Administration initiatives, including Ticket to Work, the Benefit Offset National Demonstration, and the Work Incentive Simplification Pilot. Other ongoing projects include examination of the human capital and labor market outcomes of transition age youth with disabilities and evaluating three Medicaid managed care programs that primarily serve adults with disabilities for evidence of cost savings. He holds a PhD in Economics from the University of Pennsylvania.

Roy Mersland is associate professor at the University of Agder in Norway. He has extensive international management, consulting, and research experience in more than 20 countries in Latin America, Asia, Africa, and Europe. He is member of the Centre for European Research in Microfinance at Solvay Brussels School of Economics and Management and he is the director of the Norwegian Centre for Microfinance Research. He has published extensively in journals such as *World Development, Journal of Banking and Finance, Journal of Development Studies,* and *Journal of Management Studies.*

Sophie Mitra is an associate professor in the Department of Economics at Fordham University with research interests in applied microeconomics, including in the following fields: development, employment, disability and health, and agricultural commodity markets. Mitra is also the director of the Social Justice and Policy Research Unit of the Center for International Policy Studies at Fordham. Mitra earned an MA in development economics and a doctorate in Economics from the University of Paris I Panthéon-Sorbonne in France. Before earning her doctorate, she was a development practitioner and worked for the Overseas Development Institute in Fiji. Recently, Mitra has been studying the association between disability and poverty and the economic impact of disability onset.

Daniel Mont is currently a principal researcher at the Leonard Cheshire Disability and Inclusive Development Centre at University College London. He has worked extensively on disability measurement and inclusive policies in developing countries, in particular in the areas of poverty, social protection, employment, and education. He was a senior economist at the World Bank for 10 years, both in the disability and development unit in Washington, DC and in Vietnam, where he also worked on rural antipoverty programs, statistical system capacity building, and gender issues. He served as the chair of the Analytical Working Group of the UN Statistical Commission's Washington Group on Disability Statistics and has published widely on disability and development issues. Daniel was a Joseph P. Kennedy Foundation Public Policy Fellow in 2003, and currently works as an independent consultant for UNICEF, The World Bank, AusAid, IDA, and others. He received his PhD in Economics from the University of Wisconsin-Madison and his BA from Swarthmore College.

Joyojeet Pal is an assistant professor at the School of Information at the University of Michigan, Ann Arbor. His research covers a range of topics within the broad field of Information and Communications Technology and Development. His ethnographic research on children's computer-sharing behavior in rural South India in 2007 led to the development of multi-mouse technology by Microsoft Research, a product for group-setting learning using multiple input devices. Since 2009, Joyojeet's work has been primarily focused on assistive technology and employability in low- and middle-income countries, including India, Jordan, Peru, and Sierra Leone. His research looks at the impact of access to desktop and mobile assistive technology to the workplace aspirations of people with vision impairments, and contrasts this with the attitudes of employers toward hiring people with disabilities. He received his bachelor's degree at the University of Mumbai and his PhD in City and Regional Planning at the University of California, Berkeley.

Anthony J. Plotner is an assistant professor in the Department of Educational Studies at the University of South Carolina. His primary research interests include community inclusion of individuals with significant disabilities: specifically, transition to college, supported employment, and collaboration across systems to promote positive student outcomes. He directs *Carolina Life, an* innovative, two-to-four year, post-secondary program for students with intellectual or cognitive disabilities, and also teaches a range of courses including courses that focus on individuals with intellectual disabilities.

Rienk Prins is a senior researcher/consultant at AStri Policy Research and Consultancy Group in Leiden, The Netherlands. Prins has coordinated various comparative studies in the field of social security, disability policy, and labor reintegration. He was the scientific coordinator for the project *Who Returns to Work and Why? A Six-Country Study on Work Incapacity and Reintegration*. He has carried out comparative studies in the areas of sickness and disability for the Dutch, Swedish, and Norwegian governments, as well for labor markets and social security agencies in various countries. He has operated as a "thematic expert" in the EU Peer Review Programme on Social Protection and Social Inclusion, and has extensive international consultancy experience, mainly for the World Bank, on reviewing benefit programs and reforming sickness absence management, disability pension programs, and labor (re-) integration services.

Frank R. Rusch, professor emeritus at the University of Illinois, is known internationally for his research related to transition from school to work. Over the past 30 years, Rusch has been studying how to utilize social capital to support individuals with disabilities after graduation from high school, how to structure transition services to promote meaningful outcomes, how to promote individual autonomy as a result of learning to direct one's own behavior, and how to utilize diverse methodologies in the study of socially relevant outcomes. Considered one of the leading researchers in school-to-work transition, Rusch was the founding director of the Transition Research Institute at the University of Illinois and has authored more than 200 publications including books, chapters, and articles on topics associated with transition.

Ryoko Sakuraba is an associate professor at Kobe University in Japan. A graduate of the University of Tokyo (LLB, LLM, PhD), she lectures on labor law. She was also a visiting fellow at University of Cambridge (2010–2012), where she researched employment discrimination laws from a comparative perspective. She has written broadly on Japanese labor law issues, including, extensive work on discrimination issues on different grounds, such as sex, age, and disability.

David C. Stapleton is a senior fellow at Mathematica Policy Research, where he directs the Center for Studying Disability Policy. For more than 20 years his research has focused on the impacts of public policy on the employment and income of people with disabilities. He currently leads Mathematica's Disability Research Consortium cooperative agreement with the Social Security Administration (SSA) and is a senior investigator or advisor on numerous disability research projects, including: SSA's Benefit Offset National Demonstration; SSA's Ticket to Work Evaluation; and projects sponsored by the National Institute for Disability and Rehabilitation Research under three

Rehabilitation Research and Training Centers. Stapleton joined Mathematica in 2007. He holds a PhD in Economics from the University of Wisconsin.

Robert Stodden is the Director of the Center on Disability Studies, University of Hawai'i at Mānoa, and the past president of the Association of University Centers on Disabilities (AUCD). Professionally trained in Psychology, Special Education, and Rehabilitation, Stodden has served more than 25 years as a national leader in the fields of special education, school to adult transition, postsecondary education, and employment for persons with disabilities. Since 1988, he has served as the founding director of the Center on Disability Studies (a University Center for Excellence) and professor of special education at the University of Hawai'i at Mānoa. He also serves as the originator and director of the National Center for the Study of Postsecondary Educational Supports and the National Technical Assistance Center for the Employment of Asian Americans & Pacific Islanders with Disabilities at the University of Hawai'i at Mānoa.

Kali Stull is a McGill University graduate interested in social justice and public health, particularly in work related to food sovereignty. As a fellow of the Institute for Health and Social Policy, she worked in São Paulo examining disabilities and employment in Brazil and reviewing the experience of Serasa Experian's program for workers with disabilities. She is currently conducting research in Mexico.

Sara A. Van Looy is a research assistant with the Employment and Disability Institute in the Extension Division of Cornell ILR school, where she has been providing research and writing support for more than 12 years. She is currently working with the EDI *Rehabilitation Research and Training Center on Employer Practices Related to the Employment Outcomes Among Individuals with Disabilities*, as well as on a study of the role of social networks in the employment experiences of people with disabilities.

CHAPTER 1

Disability, Employment, and Inclusion Worldwide

JODY HEYMANN, MICHAEL ASHLEY STEIN, AND
GONZALO MORENO

1. DISABILITY WORLDWIDE

Few groups experience as much discrimination as people living with disabilities. Together, bias and needless barriers, both of them pervasive, prevent women and men with disabilities from participating fully in society—whether through the labor force, political life, or community engagement. These same obstacles mean that the challenges experienced by adults and children with disabilities are often unseen or ignored.

Yet the group deeply affected is not small. Approximately a billion adults worldwide live with some kind of disability – between 15 and 20 out of every 100 people over the age of 15.[1] Between 100 and 200 million of these adults have a severe disability that – in interaction with socially constructed environmental barriers – poses a significant difficulty to their everyday functioning.[2]

Many of these difficulties could be dramatically reduced if work and community environments were designed to facilitate maximum participation by all people. The current shortage of investment in universal designs of the built and social environment in low- and high-income countries alike that could make everything from schools to workplaces to public facilities readily accessible to all has left the majority of people with disabilities unnecessarily excluded from equal participation in society.

Among the greatest barriers faced by adults with disabilities is the lack of opportunities for fulfilling career trajectories consistent with their full capacity. Drawing on experience from around the world, this volume's contributors describe feasible solutions that would transform the lives of hundreds of millions of people and the economies in which they live.

2. THE IMPORTANCE OF WORK

This book focuses on work because of its centrality to social integration, remaining out of poverty, the realization of rights, and other elements of life. Gainful and freely chosen employment, whether within the boundaries of a labor market or through self-employment or other informal initiatives, provides benefits that are both instrumental means and ends in themselves.

Employment can form a conduit to a spectrum of civil and human rights. Work provides the material means through which to acquire adequate food, clothing, and shelter; access education, health care, and support services; and participate in the cultural, recreational, and social life of one's community. Earning income also creates the opportunity for persons with disabilities to address many of their own needs and increase possibilities for participation. For example, a wage earner can more easily pay for accessible transportation or purchase useful accommodations such as a screen reader than can a similar individual lacking a job.

Labor market inclusion of persons with disabilities also contributes to the realization of equity by reducing stigma and promoting inclusion. Workplace participation has long been considered one of the most effective means of breaking down deeply entrenched stereotypes that act as formidable barriers to social equity. People spend long periods on the job, where they have no choice but to interact with and rely upon individuals who possess identity characteristics with which they might otherwise not come into contact, because of personal bias or societal marginalization. In doing so, prejudices are revealed and eroded, professional and personal attachments created, and greater diversity and tolerance engendered. Even if relationships built on the job are originally mandated, these required interactions can be powerful vehicles for wider social transformation.

In addition to its value as a means to rights and goods, both paid and unpaid work have their own intrinsic value. Productive work, as Judith Shklar argued, creates the means for being considered a viable and active part of the citizenry, whereas lack of productive work can lead to invisibility and irrelevance in a society—whether or not it should.[3] As succinctly noted by labor scholar Vicki Schultz, work is "constitutive of citizenship, community, and even personal identity."[4] Workplaces can give people a place to join physically and now, electronically, an entity with which to identify and strive collectively toward larger goals, a sense of being needed and purpose, and the feeling that they are members of a community. In short, a sense of worth. Conversely, psychological studies evidence the sense of loss, demoralization, and isolation from broader society experienced by persons who lose their jobs.[5] Among individuals with disabilities, as for others, gainful employment has consistently been reported to have a significant positive impact on feelings of worth, ability, and self-determination, all the while increasing social and civic interaction beyond the job site.[6]

Just as persons with disabilities experience work-related challenges because they are discriminated against, they are also discriminated against when they cannot find work. Getting employment right in this context is therefore doubly important. The right to work, and the right to work in just and equitable conditions, are recognized in the Universal Declaration of Human Rights[7] and the International Covenant on Economic and Social Rights,[8] as well as in the United Nations Convention on the Rights of Persons with Disabilities (CRPD).

3. EXITING POVERTY, BENEFITING ECONOMIES

Ensuring equity in the labor market can help break the vicious circle that connects poverty and disability. The poor are more likely to have or develop a disability because of greater exposure to risks such as poor living conditions, insufficient nutrition, hazardous work environments, and other inadequacies.[9] These conditions increase the likelihood of individuals having health conditions underlying disability, and insufficient access to health care makes addressable health issues more likely to become disabling.[10] Persons with disabilities who started off poor are less likely to be able to earn their way out of poverty because of the work- and education-related barriers they face. If not already living in poverty, persons with disabilities are more likely to fall into it because of reduced earning potential and greater expenditures required to meet their health and other needs. These combined effects mean that in countries at every income level, disability prevalence is highest in the poorest income quintile and progressively diminishes until it becomes lowest in the richest income quintile.[11]

A survey-based study of 27 high-income countries showed that persons with disabilities are more likely to live under the poverty threshold in 24 of these countries;[12] in some of these countries, such as Australia, the United States, or the Republic of Korea, persons with disabilities are two and sometimes almost three times as likely to be poor as persons without disabilities.[13] These results have been replicated in low- and middle-income countries, with a study of countries in sub-Saharan Africa, Latin America, and Asia revealing significantly worse economic well-being in 14 out of 15 countries studied. This study also showed significantly higher rates of multidimensional poverty in 11 countries, meaning that persons with disabilities are more likely to have fewer assets, less capacity to spend, and worse utilities in their homes.[14] In high-income countries, where there are more statistical data available to measure the relationship between poverty and disability over time, the trend over the last 20 years is for these disadvantages to deepen or remain unchanged, instead of improving.[15] This is likely due both to the inadequacy of the policy responses and to the fact that, because of higher unemployment and under-employment, persons with disabilities and their families are less able to accumulate assets and thus lack resources to invest in education and business to help exit poverty, as well as personal and societal safety nets when faced with health and economic threats.

Beyond benefiting persons with disabilities, improving employment outcomes for these individuals benefits national economies. Increasing productivity as well as the number of people with disposable income will have positive effects on GDP and the economic recovery. Some estimates put the foregone income of having people with disabilities outside the labor market at between 5% and 7% of a given country's GDP.[16] Additionally, by reducing the proportion of the population relying on public financial support and increasing the economically active population, supporting the employment of persons with disabilities can reduce a nation's dependency ratio. Organisation for Economic Development and Co-operation (OECD) countries, as a whole, spend about 10% of their total social spending on disability benefits.[17] Reducing these expenditures by increasing spending on labor market integration and other work-related benefits can be ultimately less costly and more effective.

4. DISABILITY AND EMPLOYMENT

Given the importance of work, what are the circumstances currently faced by persons with disabilities in the world of work?

Throughout the world, hundreds of millions of working-age adults with disabilities consistently experience far worse employment outcomes than their nondisabled peers—they are far more likely to be unemployed, work worse jobs, be paid less, and encounter barriers to advancement in their careers. In high-income countries in the late 2000s, the employment rate[18] of persons with disabilities was just over 40%, compared with 75% for persons without a disability,[19] and as low as 12% in some low- and middle-income countries.[20] An analysis of 51 countries surveyed by the World Health Organization shows very similar results: an average 44% employment rate for persons with disabilities versus 75% for those without.[21] Although there is great variability among countries,[22] the bottom line is that, all over the world, a person with a disability is invariably less likely to be employed than a person without a disability, often much less so. In a worrying trend, this gap has been widening rather than closing.[23]

Women with disabilities can find themselves doubly disadvantaged. Disability does not manifest itself equitably across populations, and women are a group disproportionately at risk. Throughout the world women of working age are about 10% more likely to be disabled than men in the same age group; in the case of African countries, this difference can be as much as 30%.[24] In a World Bank study, 15 out of 15 developing countries showed higher prevalence of disability in women than men; this disparity was greatest in Bangladesh, where women are twice as likely as men to have a disability.[25] This gap also exists in wealthier economies, although it is somewhat smaller.[26] The range of ratios across countries suggests that social factors play a large role in these disparities. There is also some evidence that women with disabilities have worse outcomes than disabled men in the labor market both in terms of employment rates and wages,[27] and that legislation to close the economic gap between persons with and without disabilities has less of an effect for women than men.[28]

Even when persons with disabilities are employed, they continue to encounter labor market barriers, which are reflected in their employment patterns. Studies in high-income countries consistently show that workers with disabilities are much more likely to be in part-time positions.[29] The OECD reports that one in four employees with disabilities work part-time, compared with one in six or one in seven in the general worker population.[30] Although there is some suggestion that part-time is an option that workers with disabilities themselves select to be able to better manage their disability, this does not account for the entirety of these full-time/part-time differences. To note just one example, research in California has shown that workers with disabilities are involuntarily in part-time employment to greater degrees than workers without disabilities.[31] Moreover, as discussed by contributors to this volume, policy approaches such as facilitating remote work or not removing government benefits when a person with a disability is employed can reduce the preference for part-time work and improve the economic well-being of workers with disabilities at the same time. In addition to part-time work, there is some evidence that workers with disabilities may disproportionately tend to be self-employed, especially in low and middle-income countries with high degrees of informality,[32] which also means that they are less likely to be able to access benefits.

Compounding the employment gap, there is evidence in countries at every income level that employees with disabilities earn lower wages than their comparable colleagues without disabilities. This has been measured in 27 industrialized economies, finding an average earnings gap of 15%.[33] Contributors to this volume have found similar gaps in lower-income countries like India[34] (8%) and Peru (22%).[35] As with employment rates, the tendency is for this salary gap to widen, not narrow.[36] Although as with any employees, productivity- and training-related differences can explain wage disparities, research in the United Kingdom has determined that fully half of this wage gap cannot be explained by differences in productivity and human capital,[37] and research in the United States shows that 44% of the per-hour pay difference experienced by workers with disabilities cannot be explained by observable differences in human capital, training, and experience.[38] Discrimination in pay is com-pounded by discrimination in other areas, such as career advancement,[39] although more research is needed in this particular area.

5. CONTRIBUTORS TO DISADVANTAGE

Clearly, work-related disadvantages faced by persons with disabilities are sub-stantial, and need to be addressed. The problems described in the preceding pages are not set in stone, but are rather the reflection of a myriad of obstacles encountered by persons with disabilities in the labor market. There are many factors that contribute, from discrimination stemming from underestimation of ability to inequitable access to resources.

5.1 Discrimination, Underestimation of Ability, and Overestimation of Costs

Many people implicitly discriminate against persons with disabilities, often without realizing that they do. A Harvard study of more than 2 million implicit association tests found disability and age (with its perceived associa-tion with disability) to be the top reasons for implicit bias, surpassing gen-der and race/ethnicity.[40] In many areas of the world, this discrimination has solidified into cultural stigmatization; a World Bank working paper concluded that "[p]ersons with disabilities constitute the most marginalized group in the Asian and Pacific region," and identified stigma as the first barrier to their social integration.[41]

Much of the employment and income disadvantage faced by persons with disabilities can be attributed to discrimination, either open or implicit. In the case of the earnings gaps described in the preceding section, there is evidence that discrimination and bias based on the employee's disability is a major cause of these discrepancies. In the United States, for example, although the wage difference between employees with and without disabilities in general is 33%, this gap is a vastly smaller—some 6%—for workers with non–visibly discernible disabilities.[42]

Employers also tend to incorrectly estimate the effects that disability has on work capacity. In the United Kingdom and elsewhere, employers tend to underestimate the productivity of a worker with a disability[43] and overesti-mate the cost of alternative work arrangements for them.[44] In a US survey of employer perspectives, 64% of respondent companies cited uncertainty about the cost of accommodations as an obstacle to hiring workers with dis-abilities;[45] however, a separate survey found that 56% of accommodations for workers with disabilities in US companies cost absolutely nothing, and a further 38% only involve a one-time cost of around US $500.[46] Furthermore, employers are frequently unaware of public policies and programs designed to address potential challenges. In a study of local businesses in the southern United Kingdom, the most widely used government support for the employment of adults with disabilities, a system of Disabled Employment Advisors, had been used by just 6% of respondents.[47] Similarly, a study by the United States General Accounting Office found that only a "very small proportion" of businesses utilized either the two available federal tax credits for hiring disabled workers or the barrier removal deduction.[48]

All of these factors can lead to anything from reluctance to hire workers with disabilities to offering wages that do not reflect their real costs and productivity. Affected by societal values, persons with disabilities may also limit their interaction with the labor market in response to inequitable treatment.[49]

5.2 Access to Inputs

As the World Health Organization has observed, persons with disabilities encounter barriers related to inputs such as credit and funding, as well as literal access to buildings and transportation, all of which contribute to their social and labor market exclusion.[50] Access to credit is particularly important in contexts of high informal and self-employment. Four out of five workers with disabilities in low- and middle-income countries are self-employed, often in the informal sector.[51] Workers with disabilities require access to credit, but many are perceived as a loan risk with little collateral or income-generating potential to repay the loan—contrary to evidence[52]—and are consequently excluded from microfinance schemes.[53] These barriers frequently go unrecognized; for example, only 47% of microfinance officials in a Ugandan study think persons with disabilities have specific problems accessing credit, compared with 95% of persons with disabilities themselves.[54]

As the world moves toward technology-intensive occupations, access to information and communication technologies (ICTs) for persons with disabilities is a growing concern. Even tools that are sometimes taken for granted in high-income countries can come with the obstacle of hefty price tags in lower-income countries: US $300 for a Braille keyboard or US $1,000 for a screen reader program is a substantial expenditure for many. Various forms of technology, provided at increasingly affordable prices, can help persons with disabilities obtain and retain employment, but the effective use of ICTs requires access to appropriate technologies and training; for example, text-to-speech programs are critical for a visually impaired worker, but educational and other barriers may prevent access to them.[55]

5.3 Education

Although discrimination and barriers to access affect work experiences, so too do educational barriers. For example, in a study of 15 low- and middle-income countries, in 14 countries persons with disabilities are significantly less likely to have completed even primary school.[56] Educational disparities are also significant in higher-income countries. In a study of 25 OECD countries, persons with disabilities in every country are more likely to have abandoned school at the lower-secondary level or below; whereas an average of about 22% of students without disabilities drop out at that point, almost 40% of students with disabilities do so.[57] The foundation for these gaps is laid early; US students who perform poorly in reading or math by grade three are very unlikely to graduate from secondary school with their cohort.[58] What is worse, the gap is widening: In countries such as Australia or Denmark, a person with a disability between the ages of 20 and 29 is more likely to have left school early than was the case in earlier generations.[59]

6. DISABILITY AND EQUITY AT WORK: PATHS TOWARD IMPROVEMENTS

The common characteristic of all the contributing factors described in the preceding sections is that they are not inevitable, nor will addressing them disadvantage workers without disabilities. This volume brings together lessons from worldwide experts on what policies and programs work best to improve the employment rates and conditions of persons with disabilities. The book identifies successful strategies for workers in different types of work, at different stages of their career, and in different socioeconomic environments, providing a systematic way for policymakers to begin to think about the full range of issues that must be included if one is to successfully address disability and equity at work.

Bringing together evidence-based recommendations and in-depth case studies of successful policies and programs around the world, this edited volume examines innovative and effective solutions to the challenges faced by persons with disabilities in the job market, with a specific focus on integrated, successful employment. The book covers the different stages in the career of a worker with a disability, from the school-to-work transition and finding a job to career advancement to retention in employment when experiencing a late-onset disability. The volume combines this thematic approach with in-depth analyses of what representative countries and organizations worldwide are doing to successfully achieve equity in employment for persons with disabilities. *Disability and Equity at Work* combines insights from fields as diverse as law, economics, sociology, and information and communication technology to analyze what has been done on all six continents to ensure that workers with disabilities can participate in the labor market on an equal footing, focusing on those instances with proven and sustained evidence of success.

Tackling a problem of this magnitude, especially on a global scale, requires as many feasible solutions as possible. The labor market barriers experienced by persons with disabilities are diverse and multifaceted, and cannot be overcome with one silver bullet.[60] To review as full a range of effective approaches as possible, the book takes a multisectoral approach. Contributors to this volume include current and former leaders from international organizations such as the World Bank, national and regional government experts, those working with businesses, advocacy and research professionals from civil society, and senior academics in the field. *Disability and Equity at Work* is structured around the roles and effectiveness of both public sector and private sector actors.

6.1 Employers and Multisectoral Actors

In resource-constrained settings, multisectoral approaches can be indispensable. In chapter 2, Daniel Mont creates a typology of policies that can be applied to improve the labor market situation of persons with disabilities, and examines their applicability in low- and middle-income countries. Mont also provides examples of how multisectoral teams of actors, including aid agencies, civil society organizations, governments, and businesses have created initiatives that work, and recommends guidelines to ensure that employment programs can be effective.

The formulation of nondiscrimination legislation and policies has been a common response around the world to enduring inequity for persons with disabilities in many areas, not only in employment. Landmark legislation and policy in this area includes the American with Disabilities Act (United States, 1990), the Disability Discrimination Act (United Kingdom, 1995),[61] the Employment Equity Directive (European Commission, 2000), and the CRPD, all of which contain strong nondiscrimination language and provisions. However, nondiscrimination legislation and policies are only a start, as attested to by the enduring unemployment and underemployment rates of workers with disabilities even in countries with these measures in place.[62] Actions taken by employers ultimately often shape the experience of persons with disabilities at work. In chapter 3, Susanne M. Bruyère and Sara A. Van Looy discuss tools for evaluating and improving the role of workplaces, including by examining existing workplace policies, organizational data, filed employment discrimination claims, and reports on workplace climate. They place these tools in the context of interviewing and working with human resources professionals, supervisors, and employees with disabilities.

In the United Kingdom, the Business Disability Forum (BDF) is an innovative organization that works with its members to make it easier to hire and conduct business with disabled individuals.[63] It is a nonprofit organization with a membership base consisting of nearly 400 employers from the private and public sectors across all industries. Together its members employ approximately 20% of the UK workforce.[64] In chapter 4, Megan Galeucia describes how the BDF has led to businesses improving their practices in the employment, promotion, and provision of services to persons with disabilities, including the involvement of senior management and the creation of dedicated teams.

As Kali Stull describes in chapter 5, individual employers can also make great strides in closing the employment gap. In Brazil, despite existing quota legislation, the national census and other studies reveal that 54% of Brazilians with disabilities are unemployed,[65] and 30% of employed persons with disabilities receive less than the minimum wage.[66] Stull describes how the credit bureau Serasa-Experian has created an Employment Program for Persons with Disabilities, which has trained and helped employ persons with disabilities over the past 10 years, leading to increased employment and salary equity.

The availability of resources that increase accessibility can shape access to quality education, good first jobs, and return to work after disability. In the context of increasingly technology-intensive occupations, ICTs offer both an obstacle and an opportunity for workers with disabilities. Increasingly inexpensive technology can be used to help persons with disabilities obtain and retain employment; for example, text-to-speech programs for a visually impaired worker. However, the use of ICTs requires access to appropriate technologies and training, and educational and other barriers may prevent some from gaining access to the required training and experience.[67] In chapter 6, Joyojeet Pal reviews how the adoption of ICT tools in low- and middle-income countries is both realistic and productive, focusing on specific examples for workers with visual impairments. New approaches can cut access costs dramatically compared with existing technologies; a five-fold growth in open source programs and the increasing ubiquity of smart phones offer promising avenues among many.

It is estimated that four out of five workers with disabilities in low- and middle-income countries are self-employed, whereas the vast majority of workers with disabilities in industrialized countries work for pay in the formal sector.[68] Self-employment requires access to credit for anything from buying supplies to start up an operation to renting workspace to expand it. In addition to the income it yields, self-employment is a source of agency, and many individuals become better integrated into their own communities following a successful self-employment experience.[69] In chapter 7, Leif Atle Beisland and Roy Mersland discuss the challenges that persons with disabilities face in accessing credit in low- and middle-income countries. In a Ugandan micro-finance institution, sensitization of staff and outreach led to doubling the number of clients with disabilities served, and in Ecuador marketing products tailored to customers with disabilities tripled the number of these customers.

6.2 A Life Course Approach and Beyond

Beginning with education and the transition from school to work, there are a range of paths to improvement. Education has been called a "buffer" against the depression of wages that is normally experienced by workers with disabilities.[70] In the OECD, persons with disabilities who have attained substantial education are much more likely to be employed and to be earning a salary comparable to that of a worker without a disability.[71] In chapter 8, Frank R. Rusch and coauthors argue that elementary schools must prepare students with disabilities to meet general requirements in core subjects so that they do not fall behind their nondisabled peers; middle schools must engage students with disabilities in determining their own postsecondary school goals—including employment and postsecondary education—and designing a curriculum that can help attain them; and high schools must be the coordinating point for services and resources for these students to make a successful transition into their self-determined goals.

Although career advancement is central to equal rights and features prominently in article 27 of the CRPD,[72] there is comparatively little research on how workers with disabilities can fare better in their careers once they have managed to secure employment. There is little doubt that the career advancement of workers with disabilities is often reduced compared with their nondisabled peers,[73] but very few authors have tackled how to do something about these inequities. In chapter 9, Lauren Lindstrom and Laurie Guttman Kahn compellingly make the case that success during early work experiences sets the trajectory for later career advancement. They delineate what can be done during early career stages to lay the foundation for more successful trajectories, including strengthening skills through postsecondary education; increasing access to workplaces through laws, policies, and employer incentives; facilitating a good first job through labor market insertion measures; providing individual support on the job; and enhancing career adaptability.

With rising rates of disability, governments around the world are trying to come to grips with workers that are developing disabilities later in their professional lives because there is an increase in the number of people of working age leaving the labor force as a consequence of a disability and subsequently relying on disability benefits for subsistence, often permanently. In many OECD countries where this number is on the rise, the majority (in some countries, more than 90%) of disability benefit recipients start receiving them after a period of sick leave, which means they were employed before becoming disabled.[74] In addition, the OECD noted a decade ago that there was virtually no outflow from disability benefits into the job market,[75] and confirmed it with more recent data that show that in most high-income economies, only 1% to 2% of workers who are receiving disability benefits stop receiving them for reasons other than retirement or death.[76] In chapter 10, Rienk Prins reviews policy approaches that are important for disabilities with a later onset, including early intervention during initial sick leaves, employer involvement in sickness and disability management, and job protection legislation. For example, Prins reports how, in the Netherlands, a better follow-up program for employees on short- and long-term sickness leave, based on shared responsibility between employer and employee, increased return to employment and reduced outflow into disability benefits.

6.3 The Role of Government

Governments have the ability to markedly help to transform equity at work for people with disabilities, and the 133 States Parties that have ratified the Convention on the Rights of Persons with Disabilities also have the legal responsibility to do so.[77]

In some low- and middle-income countries, however, legal requirements for employers are less likely to be as effective at increasing employment, given the size of the informal economy and limited legal implementation capacity. In chapter 11, Sophie Mitra analyzes the specific constraints faced by low- and middle-income countries, whether within the labor market—lack of labor demand by employers and lack of labor supply by persons with disabilities themselves—or outside of it, through educational, environmental, and other barriers, further advocating for careful analyses of particular challenges in each country, from skills that are insufficient or mismatched with the labor market to discrimination and stigma. Mitra argues that programs targeted to the specific challenges identified in each context are more likely to be successful in improving employment rates. For example, peer training for entrepreneurship to overcome skills shortages and mismatches in South Africa has led to a 90% survival rate for businesses and increased income-generating capacity.

In chapter 12, Stanislao Maldonado looks in detail at approaches taken to labor market inclusion in Peru, a country with a large informal economy and, historically, low levels of education for persons with disabilities, which still need to be addressed. Maldonado thoroughly evaluates the strengths and limitations of government responses in this context, including antidiscrimination laws, quotas, training and special labor programs, and government incentive policies. Within these areas, Maldonado examines schemes such as the creation of specific coordinating bodies and penalty systems, the funding of local projects, youth employment and labor intermediation services, the implementation of quota systems and affirmative action in public employment, and the use of tax and government procurement incentives to promote hiring of workers with disabilities.

In 1990, the United States passed the ADA, a wide-ranging law prohibiting discrimination against persons with disabilities that includes provisions relevant to hiring, retention, and advancement. The ADA was in many ways landmark legislation and served as a model for similar legislation in countries like the United Kingdom and Australia, and a blueprint for action for disabled peoples' organizations working in countries in which legislation for the employment of persons with disabilities is not yet rights-based. Yet, although strong nondiscrimination legislation is crucial to improving the employment rate and conditions of persons with disabilities, it is often not sufficient. In the United States, the passage of the ADA has not markedly increased employment rates,[78] although it may have contributed to improving working conditions.[79] In chapter 13, David C. Stapleton and David R. Mann provide possible mechanisms for improving success in this area, and propose a radical reform of disability benefits in the United States, focusing on evaluating and complementing work capacity rather than on establishing the inability to work to obtain social insurance.

As an alternative to nondiscrimination, a number of countries use quota schemes to reserve a certain proportion of jobs for persons with disabilities. In particular, Asian countries such as Japan are using employment quotas in an attempt to overcome high levels of marginalization and stigma,[80] an approach in contrast to the use of nondiscrimination legislation in countries such as the United States and the United Kingdom. In chapter 14, Ryoko Sakuraba examines how Japan's approach, which centers on the use of employment quotas, would not be as effective without an environment that values corporate social responsibility and provides a framework of complementary legislation and policy, including government guidance, subsidies for training and accommodation, and a public system of vocational rehabilitation. This is further complemented by a labor contracts doctrine, which in some ways functions as nondiscrimination legislation and mandates reassignments and reductions of workloads in response to disability onset while penalizing dismissal.

Through supranational institutions such as the European Commission, the European Parliament, and the European Court of Justice, the European Union (EU) has the power to develop legislation and policy that will apply to 28 member states. This approach has translated into considerable success at increasing equality for persons with disabilities, but also presents unique challenges. Member states implement EU policy in different ways, which has led persons with disabilities in some states to benefit more than in others. For example, the employment rate of persons with disabilities is greater than 60% in Sweden, but less than 40% in Belgium and Ireland.[81] In chapter 15, Anna Lawson reviews disability and employment policymaking in the European Union, and describes how EU directives have accomplished positive legislative change in 24 countries and can involve governments and civil society organizations in innovative policy development initiatives.

7. GAPS IN KNOWLEDGE

Leading to and since the passage of the CRPD, the disability rights movement has become a global phenomenon, with groups working together for results across borders and cutting across age and types of disability. We hope this book can help identify what approaches work best and discuss how they can be implemented to improve the employment rates and conditions of persons with disabilities around the world.

Not all workers with disabilities face the same hurdles. The needs and capacities of a student with a disability who is about to graduate from high school or university and enter the workforce are very different from those of a 60-year-old worker who goes on temporary disability leave, and the concerns of a long-term unemployed job seeker with disabilities are different from those of a long-term employed worker with disabilities.

Finding a job, although crucial given the employment rate for persons with disabilities, is only the first step toward realizing true equity in employment; workers with disabilities have the right to nondiscrimination during recruitment, hiring and employment; to equal pay for equal work; to equal working conditions; to access continuing education and training whilst in employment; to advance in their careers; and to be able to start their own business—an avenue that is explored by workers with disabilities disproportionately compared to workers without disabilities in both rich and poor countries[82]—on equal footing.

Although this volume offers an overview of what policies and programs are having the greatest effect, there are still areas related to the employment of persons with disabilities in which far more research is needed. For example, career advancement is central to equal rights and features prominently in the CRPD, but there is comparatively little research on how people with disabilities can fare better in their careers once they have managed to secure employment.

The lessons contributors bring to *Disability and Equity at Work* are relevant to the work of employers, local and national governments, international institutions, public and private service delivery organizations, and individuals in fields as diverse as business, public policy, labor relations, human rights, and law. We all need to work together to achieve equity at work.

For all of us, from the nearly one billion people currently with disabilities to those who will one day face a disability, to their many friends and family members, for governments and employers worldwide, finding out what works—learning the best information on approaches to augmenting and improving the quality of employment—is essential.

NOTES

1. World Health Organization & World Bank (2011). *World Report on Disability*. Geneva, Switzerland: World Health Organization, 29.
2. Ibid.
3. Shklar, J. N. (1991). *American Citizenship: The Quest for Inclusion*. Cambridge, MA: Harvard University Press.
4. Schultz, V. (2000). Life's work. Columbia Law Review 100(7), 1886.
5. Goldsmith, A. H., Veum, J. R., & Darity, W. Jr. (1996). The psychological impact of unemployment and joblessness. Journal of Socio-Economics 25(3), 333–358.
6. See for example Wehmeyer, M.L., & Bolding, N. (2001). Enhanced self-determination of adults with intellectual disability as an outcome of moving to community-based work or living environments. Journal of Intellectual Disability Research 45(5), 371–383; also Eggleton, I., et al. (1999). The impact of employment on the quality of life of people with an intellectual disability. Journal of Vocational Rehabilitation 13(2), 95–107.
7. UN General Assembly (1948). *Universal Declaration of Human Rights*, 217 A (III), art. 23. Retrieved January 14, 2013, from http://www.unhcr.org/refworld/docid/3ae6b3712c.html
8. UN General Assembly (1966). *International Covenant on Economic, Social and Cultural Rights. United Nations*, Treaty Series 993(3), arts. 6–7. Retrieved January 14, 2013 from http://www.unhcr.org/refworld/docid/3ae6b36c0.html
9. Emmett, T., & Alant, E. (2006). Women and disability: Exploring the interface of multiple disadvantage. Development Southern Africa 23(4), 445–460.
10. Dudzik, P., Elwan, A., & Metts, R. (2002). *Disability Policies, Statistics, and Strategies in Latin America and the Caribbean: A Review*. Washington, DC: Inter-American Development Bank; Yeo, R., & Moore, K. (2003). Including disabled people in poverty reduction work: "Nothing about us, without us." World Development 31(3), 571–590.
11. World Health Organization & World Bank (2011). *World Report on Disability*, 28.
12. The exceptions are Norway, Sweden, and Slovakia; see Organization for Economic Co-operation and Development (2010). *Sickness, Disability and Work: Breaking the Barriers*. Paris: OECD, 55–56.
13. Organization for Economic Co-operation and Development (2010). *Sickness, Disability and Work*.
14. Mitra, S., Posarac, A., & Vick, B. (2011). *Disability and Poverty in Developing Countries: A Snapshot from the World Health Survey*. Washington, DC: World Bank.
15. Organization for Economic Co-operation and Development (2010). *Sickness, Disability and Work*, 55–56.
16. Handicap International (2006). Good Practices for the Economic Inclusion of People with Disabilities in Developing Countries: Funding Mechanisms for Self-Employment. Lyon, France: Handicap International.

17. Organization for Economic Co-operation and Development (2010). *Sickness, Disability and Work.*
18. The use of employment rates instead of unemployment rates to measure employment integration of persons with disabilities is an important distinction because many persons with disabilities may feel discouraged from looking for work and therefore do not count as unemployed when calculating unemployment rates.
19. Organization for Economic Co-operation and Development (2010). *Sickness, Disability and Work.*
20. World Health Organization & World Bank (2011). *World Report on Disability.*
21. Ibid., 237–238.
22. Ibid.
23. Organization for Economic Co-operation and Development (2010). *Sickness, Disability and Work.*
24. World Health Organization and World Bank (2011). *World Report on Disability.*
25. Mitra, Posarac, & Vick (2011). *Disability and Poverty.*
26. World Health Organization & World Bank (2011). *Report on Disability*; Organization for Economic Co-operation and Development (2003). *Transforming Disability into Ability.* Paris: OECD.
27. Randolph, D.S. (2004). Predicting the effect of disability on employment status and income. Work 23(3), 257-66.
28. Jones, M. K., Latreille, P. L., & Sloane. P. J. (2006). Disability, gender, and the British labor market. *Oxford Economic Papers 58,* 407–449.
29. Organization for Economic Co-operation and Development (2010). *Sickness, Disability and Work*; Jones, M. K. (2007). Does part-time employment provide a way of accommodating a disability? *The Manchester School 75*(6), 695–716; Schur, L. (2002). Dead end jobs or a path to economic well being? The consequences of non-standard work for people with disabilities. *Behavioral Sciences and the Law 20,* 601–620.
30. Organization for Economic Co-operation and Development (2010). *Sickness, Disability and Work.*
31. Jones (2007). Does part-time employment; Schur, L. (2003). Barriers or opportunities? The causes of contingent and part-time work among people with disabilities. Industrial Relations 42(4): 589–622; Yelln, E. H., & Trupin, L. (2003). Disability and the characteristics of employment. *Monthly Labor Review 126*(5), 20–31.
32. Mitra, S., & Sambamoorthi, U. (2006). Employment of persons with disabilities: Evidence from the national sample survey. *Economic and Political Weekly 41*(3), 199–203; Mizunoya, S., & Mitra, S. (2012). Is there a disability gap in employment rates in developing countries? World Development 42, 28–43; see also Organization for Economic Co-operation and Development (2010). *Sickness, Disability and Work.*
33. Organization for Economic Co-operation and Development (2010). *Sickness, Disability and Work.*
34. Mitra, S., & Sambamoorthi, U. (2009). Wage differential by disability status in an agrarian labor market in India. Applied Economics Letters 16(14), 1393–1398.
35. Maldonado, S. (2006). Trabajo y Discapacidad en el Perú: Mercado Laboral, Políticas Públicas e Inclusión Social. Lima, Peru: Fondo Editorial del Congreso del Perú and Programa de Naciones Unidas para el Desarrollo.
36. Organization for Economic Co-operation and Development (2010). *Sickness, Disability and Work*, 55.

37. Kidd, M. P., Sloane, P. J., & Ferko, I. (2000). Disability and the labor market: An analysis of British males. Journal of Health Economics 19, 961–981; Jones, Latreille, & Sloane (2006). *Disability, gender.*

38. Baldwin, M., & Johnson, W. G. (1994). Labor market discrimination against men with disabilities. Journal of Human Resources 29(1), 1–19.

39. Wilson-Kovacs, D., Ryan, M. K., Haslam, S. A., & Rabinovich, A. (2008). "Just because you can get a wheelchair in the building doesn't necessarily mean that you can still participate": Barriers to the career advancement of disabled professionals. Disability & Society 23(17), 705–717.

40. Nosek, B. A., et al. (2007). Pervasiveness and correlates of implicit attitudes and stereotypes. *European Review of Social Psychology* 18, 36–88.

41. Takamine, Y. (2004). *Disability Issues in East Asia: Review and Ways Forward.* In Working Paper Series, edited by World Bank. Washington, DC: World Bank, 5.

42. Baldwin & Johnson (1994). *Labor market discrimination.*

43. World Health Organization & World Bank (2011). *World Report on Disability*; Kidd, Sloane, & Ferko (2000). Disability and the labor market; Jones, Latreille, & Sloane (2006). *Disability, gender.*

44. Stuart, N., Watson, A., Williams, J., Meager, N., & Lain, D. (2002). *How Employers and Service Providers Are Responding to the Disability Discrimination Act of 1995.* London: UK Department of Work and Pensions.

45. Domzal, C., Houtenville, A., & Sharma, R. (2008). *Survey of Employer Perspectives on the Employment of People with Disabilities.* McLean, VA: CESSI.

46. Job Accommodation Network. *Workplace Accommodations: Low Cost, High Impact.* Retrieved May 7, 2012, from http://AskJAN.org/media/LowCostHighImpact.do

47. Stevens, G. R. (2002). Employers' perceptions and practice in the employability of disabled people: A survey of companies in south east UK. Disability & Society 17(7), 779–796.

48. United States General Accounting Office (2002). Business Tax Incentives: Incentives to Employ Workers with Disabilities Receive Limited Use and Have an Uncertain Impact. Washington, DC: GAO.

49. Wilson-Kovacs, Ryan, Haslam, & Rabinovich (2008). "Just because you can get a wheelchair."

50. World Health Organization & World Bank (2011). *World Report on Disability.*

51. Handicap International (2006). *Good Practices.*

52. Braithwaite, J., & Mont, D. (2008). A survey of World Bank poverty assessments and implications. In Social Protection and Labor, edited by W. Bank. Washington, DC: World Bank; Mitra, Posarac, & Vick (2011). *Disability and Poverty.*

53. Cramm, J. M., & Finkelflügel, H. (2008). Exclusion of disabled people from microcredit in Africa and Asia: A literature study. Asia Pacific Disability Rehabilitation Journal 19(2), 15–33.

54. Handicap International (2006). *Good practices.*

55. Molina, A. (2003). The digital divide: The need for a global e-inclusion movement. Technology *Analysis & Strategic Management* 15(1), 137–152.

56. Mitra, Posarac, & Vick (2011). *Disability and Poverty.*

57. Organization for Economic Co-operation and Development (2010). *Sickness, Disability and Work.*

58. Hernandez, D. J. (2011). *Double Jeopardy: How Third-Grade Reading Skills and Poverty Influence High School Graduation.* Baltimore: The Annie E. Casey Foundation.

59. Organization for Economic Co-operation and Development (2010). *Sickness, Disability and Work*.
60. World Health Organization & World Bank (2011). *World Report on Disability*; Organization for Economic Co-operation and Development (2010). *Sickness, Disability and Work*.
61. In 2010, the Disability Discrimination Act was combined with several other identity-specific antidiscrimination statutes into the Equality Act.
62. Burkhauser & Stapleton (2003). Introduction; Jones, Latreille, & Sloane (2006). *Disability, Gender*.
63. Employers' Forum on Disability (2012). About Us. Retrieved April 19, 2012, from http://www.efd.org.uk/about-us
64. Ibid.
65. Fundação Getúlio Vargas & Instituto Brasileiro de Economia (c2003). Retratos da deficiência no Brasil. Retrieved September 15, 2011 from: http://www.fgv.br/cps/Retratos_Deficiencia_Brasil.asp
66. International Disability Rights Monitor (2004). Regional Report of the Americas Retrieved March 8, 2012, from: http://www.ideanet.org/idrm_reports.cfm
67. Molina (2003). *The Digital Divide*.
68. Handicap International (2006). *Good Practices*.
69. De Klerk, T. (2008). Funding for self-employment of people with disabilities. Grants, loans, revolving funds or linkage with microfinance programmes. *Leprosy Review* 79, 92–109.
70. Hollenbeck, K., & Kimmel, J. (2008). Differences in the Returns to Education for Males by Disability Status and Age of Disability Onset. *Southern Economic Journal* 74(3), 707–724.
71. Organization for Economic Co-operation and Development (2010). *Sickness, Disability and Work*.
72. UN General Assembly (2007). Convention on the Rights of Persons with Disabilities: Resolution Adopted by the General Assembly, 24 January, A/RES/61/106. Retrieved January 14, 2013, from http://www.unhcr.org/refworld/docid/45f973632.html
73. See, for example, Wilson-Kovacs, Ryan, Haslam, & Rabinovich (2008). "Just because you can get a wheelchair."
74. Organization for Economic Co-operation and Development (2010). *Sickness, Disability and Work*.
75. Organization for Economic Co-operation and Development (2003). *Transforming Disability into Ability*.
76. Organization for Economic Co-operation and Development (2010). *Sickness, Disability and Work*.
77. United Nations Enable (2013). *Convention and Optional Protocol Signatures and Ratifications*. Retrieved January 13, 2013, from http://www.un.org/disabilities/countries.asp?navid=12&pid=166
78. Burkhauser, R., & Stapleton, D. (2003). Introduction. In *The Decline in Employment of People with Disabilities: a Policy Puzzle*, edited by D. Stapleton & R. Burkhauser. Kalamazoo, MI: W.E. Upjohn Institute for Employment Research; Daly, M. C., & Houtenville, A. J. (2002). *Employment Declines Among People with Disabilities: Population Movements, Isolated Experience, or Broad Policy Concern?* In FRBSF Working Paper series. San Francisco: Federal Reserve Bank of San Francisco.

79. Acemoglu, D., & Angrist, J. D. (2001). Consequences of employment protection? The case of the Americans with Disabilities Act. *Journal of Political Economy* 109(5), 915–957; Thompkins, A. V. (2011). Essays on Disability and Employment. Cambridge, MA: Massachusetts Institute of Technology.
80. United Nations Economic and Social Commission for Asia and the Pacific (2009). *Disability at a Glance 2009: A Profile of 36 Countries and Regions in Asia and the Pacific. Bangkok, Thailand.* United Nations.
81. Organization for Economic Co-operation and Development (2010). *Sickness, Disability and Work.*
82. Mitra & Sambamoorthi (2006). Employment of persons with disabilities: Evidence from the national sample survey. Economic and Political Weekly 41(3), 199–203; Pagán, R. (2009). Self-employment among people with disabilities: evidence for Europe. Disability & Society 24(2), 217–229.

Employers and Multisectoral Actors

CHAPTER 2

Employment Policy Approaches and Multisectoral Implementation in Low- and Middle-Income Countries

DANIEL MONT

1. INTRODUCTION

The UN Convention on the Rights of Persons with Disabilities maintains that all people, regardless of disability, should have the same opportunities for finding employment. Sadly, this is not the case. In both high- and low-income countries people with disabilities are significantly less likely to be in the labor market, and more likely to be unemployed. According to the World Health Survey administered in 51 countries, men with disabilities have an employment rate of 52.8% compared with 64.9% for men without disabilities. For women, those percentages are respectively, 19.6% and 29.9%.[1]

At first glance, this disparity might seem less than expected. After all, in the United States the employment ratio of people with disabilities to those without disabilities is roughly half. But an employment ratio, in and of itself, does not tell the whole story. What is the quality of that employment? What is the remuneration? Are people working as many hours as they would like? Are they being treated with dignity?

A recent examination of data on disability and socioeconomic outcomes in 15 countries shows a mixed picture but, generally speaking, households that have disabled members tend to be poorer using both consumption indicators and multiple index measures.[2] In the United States, disabled people are largely overrepresented among the chronically poor. About 65% of those in poverty for at least 36 out of 48 months have a disability.[3]

Focusing attention on disability and employment in low- and middle-income countries, though, can be challenging. Many of these countries have high poverty rates and other challenging issues. Delivery of quality education and the availability of decent employment can be problematic for large sectors of the population. These challenges, coupled with limited resources and capacity, can make a government particularly eager to prioritize issues. Arguing for the rights of people with disabilities is essential and appropriate, but to garner resources and get on the budgetary agenda a case must be made for the economic benefits—in terms of poverty reduction and economic growth—that can result from promoting and enabling people with disabilities to achieve their full potential in the workplace.

Unfortunately, until recently data have not been generally available to examine the link between disability and poverty in low- and middle-income countries. And what is emerging from recent work depicts a complicated landscape.[4] Although disability and poverty are often linked, that link can differ significantly depending on how disability is defined, the type of disability, and the age of onset. Still, estimates of the macroeconomic costs of disability run in the range of 3% to 7% of GDP.[5]

People with disabilities in low- and middle-income countries can face even larger challenges than their counterparts in high-income countries for a number of reasons. First, attitudes toward people with disabilities can be more extreme. The degree of stigma and shame can be higher. In fact, in some cultures the presence of a disability can be considered evidence of transgressions in a past life. Therefore, people with disabilities and their families are more likely to remove themselves from societal interactions, thus limiting their ability to acquire skills and use them in the marketplace. On the other hand, when people are faced with poverty—and without a social safety net to fall back on—not being employed may not be an option. That employment, however, could be own-account work, with low returns and a high degree of vulnerability.

The lower level of accessibility, be it inaccessible transportation or school systems that do not accommodate children with disabilities, creates another barrier to quality employment. In fact, according to Filmer, who undertook a study across 11 low- and middle-income countries, disability had a more pronounced impact on school enrolment than either social class or gender.[6] Globally, disabled children are significantly less likely to attend school.[7]

The phenomenon of disability, however, is complex, and care must be taken not to treat the population as a homogenous group. For example, disability does not necessarily have any effect on primary or secondary education if the onset of disability occurs later in life. And this, of course, will have an impact on the effect of disability on employment, because disability can arise at any age. Some people are disabled from birth, some after they have already obtained an education and employment experience, and some when they are at the end of their working years. Therefore, general comparisons of disabled versus nondisabled people can sometimes mask important differences in the types of problems people face and the most appropriate policies. A recent study in Vietnam showed that the impact of disability in childhood had a more profound impact on employment and poverty than the onset of a disability in adulthood.[8] Looking at overall rates of employment for disabled and nondisabled people will mask this effect.

Moreover, people with disabilities may have difficulties in a wide range of functional domains; for example, physical, cognitive, sensory, and psychosocial, and the degree of their difficulties can range from mild to extreme. Depending on their situation, different types of policies may be more relevant. For example, as discussed in the following, supported employment programs seem to be particularly beneficial for people with mental disabilities.

The reasons underlying employment and wage gaps are multifaceted. One possible explanation is that disabled people are victims of direct labor market discrimination. A second explanation is that barriers in the environment that limit participation undermine their productivity, so they are hired less frequently and for lower remuneration. And although that lower productivity may result from myriad factors beyond their control, including less schooling and training because of non-inclusive school systems, inaccessible workplaces, more difficulty accessing information (e.g., for people with hearing and visual difficulties), and/or more difficulty obtaining credit, it is still true from the employer's point of view that they are less productive and so less likely to be hired. A final reason for lower rates of employment could be that disabled people are less likely to search for work, so there is a lower supply of people with disabilities to the labor market. This could result from the higher costs associated with work that disabled people face, for example, transportation. Or it could be due to anti-work incentives built into disability benefit programs. Finally, it may flow from their own low expectations and lack of confidence stemming from the attitudes toward people with disabilities that they have encountered throughout their lifetime.

When examining employment issues in low- and middle-income countries, it is important to keep in mind the structure of the labor market. In high-income countries the large majority of people are employed in the formal labor market where they are covered by labor contracts, an extensive set of labor laws, and, in general, a system of social insurance. The same is not the case in low- and middle-income countries, in which the majority of people—especially those with low skills—are in the informal labor market, or even in informal employment within the formal sector. They are also more likely to be own account workers, people working at home without pay, or starting small businesses. This chapter focuses on disability and employment in low- and middle-income countries, where the labor arrangements are more often tentative and less subject to regulation.

Before reviewing some examples of employment programs for people with disabilities in low- and middle-income countries, it is important to point out the lack of rigorous impact evaluations in this area. Many programs have been implemented, and most have been evaluated in some sense. By and large, however, these evaluations are not suitable for measuring the economic costs and benefits of the program. This is unfortunate, because a strong "business case" for disability employment programs could go a long way to convincing governments with limited funds to invest in this endeavor. By business case, it is meant that the economic benefits exceed the costs to a significant enough degree to warrant adoption and scaling up of these programs for the sake of overall economic development.

This leads us to another important distinction between high-income countries and low- and middle-income countries when it comes to examining the impact of disability employment programs, namely, the role of cash benefits as a work disincentive. This is a major focus of disability research in high-income countries, in which benefits for disabled people are large enough, especially if combined with health insurance, to dissuade people from looking for work, and a significant benefit of getting beneficiaries to work is the reduction in government outlays. This is generally not the case in low- and middle-income countries, in which benefits, when they exist, are often small. This will change, though, as these countries move into middle-income status. For example, recently expanded disability benefits in South Africa have been linked to a decline in employment among people with disabilities.[9] As these countries develop cash benefit programs for disabled people, it will be important that they do not repeat some of the same anti-work mistakes previously found in other countries, notably the Netherlands and Poland.[10]

Disability employment program evaluations, when they are undertaken at all, generally only evaluate the participants' experiences and whether the program operated as intended. These reports often list the number of people who obtained jobs or whose income increased. However, there are generally no comparison or control groups that can account for selection bias. Nor is there often a well-established baseline against which to evaluate progress. In other words, it may be that the people recruited to these programs and who are willing to participate have attitudes and resources that would have made them more successful than their disabled peers who did not participate regardless of the program. To what extent were their positive outcomes a function of what they brought to the program versus what the program helped them attain? Without a proper comparison group it is not possible to say.

Nevertheless, there is still a lot to be gained by looking at these programs and their various approaches. A substantial amount of information is suggestive of their benefits, and the attributes that may make them successful.

2. A BRIEF POLICY TYPOLOGY

Policies can be grouped into three categories—regulations, counterbalances, and substitutions.[11] Different views on the causes behind the disability employment gap point toward different policy approaches, but they are not mutually exclusive.

2.1 Regulations

Regulations mandate conditions under which employers must hire people with disabilities or suffer specific penalties. Policies that fall into this category include quotas (often accompanied by fines for noncompliance), requiring disabled people to be included on government contracts, and antidiscrimination laws. All of these follow a purely human rights–based approach to the issues of disability.

Antidiscrimination laws basically assume that disabled people are capable of competing for jobs in the labor market, as long as they are not discriminated against and reasonable accommodations are made. However, to the extent that disabled people do not want to compete for jobs or are not as productive as nondisabled people an antidiscrimination law will not, in and of itself, close the employment gap.

Quotas can force the hiring of disabled people, but they can be interpreted as admitting there are extra costs of hiring disabled people. To the extent those extra costs are real, or even just perceived through misinformation, employers could opt for paying fines instead, which is unfortunately often the case. Some argue that the existence of quotas also allows policymakers and employers to "tick off" their responsibilities in this area by setting what they see as an acceptable floor for hiring disabled people, and might unintentionally undermine efforts to strive for a more fully inclusive work environment.[12]

2.1.1 Regulations in Low- and Middle-Income Countries

Regulations may not be as effective in low- and middle-income countries as they are in high-income countries, because of the structure of the society. First, many jobs are in the informal sector, in which quotas are irrelevant. Second, in many countries the legal structures that can allow people to sue for damages are not in place. Third, self-employment is a bigger share of the economy. In that case the issue is not hiring but credit, and discriminatory processes in microfinance are hard to combat.

This is not an argument against antidiscrimination laws. They are necessary to secure disabled people's rights to the greatest extent possible, and they send a strong signal that hopefully can start changing discriminatory attitudes. And of course, antidiscrimination laws can also begin to break down other barriers to employment by increasing the education of disabled children, improving access to public transportation and other public facilities, and other factors. Nevertheless, giving someone a legal right to employment in an economy that is more informal and less bound by the rule of law will be less effective, in and of itself, in achieving more employment for people with disabilities.

2.2 Counterbalances

Counterbalances, the second group of policies, aim to offset the extra costs of employing disabled people—either to the disabled person himself or herself, or to the employer.

2.2.1 Vocational Rehabilitation

One of the leading policies in this area is vocational rehabilitation, which aims to close the productivity gap between disabled and nondisabled people that may have arisen because of a prior lack of access to training, or because that training did not address the particular needs of people with disabilities.

2.2.2 Microfinance

In a similar vein, microfinance programs for disabled people try to give them the resources needed to start their own businesses that are otherwise unavailable or would come at a higher cost. This approach has proved effective in low- and middle-income countries—especially among women—allowing recipients the flexibility to circumvent problems in the labor market and start businesses suited to their family situation and the local economy.

2.2.3 Supported Employment

Supported employment is another approach that is similar to vocational training. Several methods exist (e.g., job coaching), but the basic idea is to provide training and assistance on the job to help with the transition to work. Supported employment is sometimes referred to as "place and train," whereas vocational training is "train and place."

2.2.4 *Offsetting Additional Costs*

An alternative counterbalancing approach is to offset the higher costs of hiring a disabled person. On the employer side, this includes policies such as wage subsidies and funds to cover workplace accommodations. On the worker side, it includes changing the structure of disability benefits to penalize workers less for finding employment, and subsidizing additional expenses, such as transportation costs.

2.3 Substitutions

The final category of policies is substitutions. This approach assumes that disabled workers cannot compete successfully in the general labor market. Instead, they need a special setting or arrangement. This includes sheltered employment, enclave employment (basically a segregated environment within a regular company), and specialized work crews of disabled people. Typically, the more segregated the setting, the more significant are the workers' disabilities, but sometimes with the aim of "graduating" to regular employment.

Most disability advocates are very skeptical of the substitution approach, particularly sheltered workshops, which are the most highly segregated variety. Lack of access to the general labor market could preclude the development of life and job skills that are necessary for integration into the general labor market. By segregating disabled people, they also allow misperceptions of disabled people's abilities among nondisabled people to go unchallenged. Finally, pay scales and the ability to "graduate" can potentially be manipulated for the economic advantage of the people running the workshop instead of for the benefit of the disabled workers.

3. EXAMPLES OF EMPLOYMENT PROGRAMS

Most recent efforts to promote employment for people with disabilities in low- and middle-income countries fall into the counterbalancing category—primarily vocational training, supported employment, microfinance, and also employer-oriented programs designed to increase the demand for disabled workers and overcome the resistance (or feelings of uncertainty) to hiring them.

3.1 Vocational Training

Many employment programs aimed at people with disabilities are of the "train and place" vocational training variety. They may include not only job skills, but also training and assistance with job search activities, as well as life skills. In many countries, these are run by nongovernmental organizations (NGOs) or are special development projects. The advantage of this approach is that it can address the particular needs of disabled people and it ensures that the training program reaches out to them. However, the disadvantage is that it can create segregated training programs, which can require additional costs and can be more difficult to sustain and scale-up. The best approach would be able to integrate disabled people into the general educational and vocational training system within the country, but this can be a slow process. A strong argument can be made that to the extent that these special programs can develop best practices and demonstrate the efficacy of training people with disabilities, they can provide an evidence base for integration down the line.

The Centre for Special Education at the Indian Institute of Cerebral Palsy (IICP) runs a program of this type. It conducts classroom training for people with disabilities based on the curricula from mainstream institutions (and trainees include people with all types of disabilities, not just cerebral palsy). In addition to classroom training, the program teaches social skills needed for independent living and for being a responsible consumer. They also address social and psychological needs. In addition to classroom training, they follow up with on-the-job training.[13]

Training does not have to be restricted to low or semiskilled occupations. In Thailand, the Redemptorist Center includes training on computer skills and other high-tech jobs. And successful programs—like IICP and the Redemptorist Center—generally include job placement programs.

One issue in low- and middle-income countries is that many people live in rural, and often remote, areas. Classroom training may be difficult because of transportation issues, but also because a critical mass is needed in order to make a vocational training center worthwhile. One approach to dealing with this taken in rural Cambodia by the International Labour Organization (ILO) Disability Resource Team was to establish a system of peer training, in which trainees were screened, selected, and matched with trainers who were workers already operating in their geographical area.[14] Local trainers got compensated, adding to the local economy, and disabled trainees acquired skills that were already proved worthwhile in the places they lived.

The focus on imparting marketable skills is an important one. The value of training, of course, depends on the market demand for the skills being imparted. Koistinen, writing about similar programs in Zambia, stressed the necessity of undertaking a market analysis of the demand for skills so that trainees would actually have an opportunity to use what they have learned.[15] This had been a problem in the countries that made up the old Soviet Union, where training programs did not adjust their programs to meet market demands. Or, for example, in many places in Asia, where blind people are often slated for training in massage therapy because that work is considered suitable for them, without a careful assessment of whether the market can absorb them.

Both the IICP and the Cambodia project do undertake market analysis and attempt to modify the skills they teach to meet market demand. Of course this is an issue in programs for disabled people because those programs tend to select what training they offer. Nondisabled people who avail themselves of vocational training generally choose among alternatives and so adjust their demand for training to the skills they see demanded in the workplace. To the extent that mainstream vocational training can be offered in an inclusive fashion, disabled people would have that same flexibility.

Another lesson learned from these programs is the value of having disabled people as trainers. Disabled people can be role models and living proof to trainees that people like them are capable of acquiring skills, finding employment, and being successful. They also better understand the challenges that disabled people face. Interestingly, another advantage is that trainers with disabilities often feel more comfortable being hard on students and pushing them to their full potential. They have higher expectations of what their students can achieve.[16]

3.2 Supported Employment

Supported employment—or "place to train"—programs also exist in low- and middle-income countries. A program in Malaysia, supported by the Japan International Cooperation Agency (JICA), trains NGOs and community-based rehabilitation groups on how to provide job coaching services. The Joy Workshop, also in Malaysia, is actually working to transition disabled people from social workshops into a supported employment setting. The focus for supported employment programs is often people with intellectual disabilities, who at times need special assistance in transitioning to a particular workplace and structuring the job around their particular strengths. Evaluations in high-income countries have typically found that supported employment programs are particularly effective for people with cognitive disabilities or mental illness.[17]

Another example is the Ntiro Project for Supported and Inclusive Employment in South Africa. This program focuses on people with intellectual disabilities, again providing them with a supported employment approach to acquiring life and work skills. The program goes further, though, by actively working on awareness-raising activities. These include training local government officials and community organizations on disability and on how to make their own operations more inclusive.

This indicates a need for a holistic approach to disability employment, especially in low- and middle-income countries. Training is necessary, but so are improved public accessibility and more enlightened attitudes among employers and disabled people and their families, who often try to "protect" their disabled relatives from disappointment and hardship, but in actuality prevent them from fully integrating into society. This is true even for people who become disabled later in life. Thailand's Industrial Rehabilitation Center, developed with the Thai government in partnership with JICA and the ILO, focuses on retraining and reintegrating people who become disabled on the job. An important component of that program was family counseling to enlist family members' support in getting the injured worker back into the workplace.[18]

3.3 Microfinance

As stated, self-employment is an important livelihood option for people in low- and middle-income countries—first because people with disabilities generally suffer from discrimination in the labor market, but also because own-account work is much more common in those environments. Unfortunately, disabled people also tend to face discrimination in the credit market. Programs in a number of countries have tried to fill that gap, and have taken a variety of approaches that focus on different aspects of microfinance.[19] Some offer grants, other loans. Some establish separate programs for disabled people, others try to integrate people with disabilities into existing programs—either by incorporating them in their own finance programs or by reaching out to existing programs to be more inclusive.

Microfinance programs sometimes offer small grants to individuals to help start or expand a small business or other activities related to livelihood production, such as tuition for training. One reason for offering grants is so that programs can be targeted to the poorest people with the least collateral or ability to secure a loan. This can cause problems, however. First, the poorest people might not be the ones most able to utilize the funds effectively. Investing money—even small amounts—requires some skill and experience that the most disadvantaged people may not have. Microfinance programs generally try to build the business capacity of the recipients, but still, as any banker will express, some recipients have a higher likelihood of success.

Also, when a person is not risking his or her own money, he or she does not have as much incentive to follow through on plans. Therefore, a program providing grants must generally also include a substantial amount of training and oversight. But maybe the largest disadvantage of a microgrant-based program is the problem of sustainability. A constant infusion of money is needed in order to continue providing grants. One advantage of microfinance programs is that when loans are repaid and capital is raised in the community for the purpose of investment, with an associated return, these programs can be self-sustaining.

Most microfinance programs, therefore, opt for the loan strategy. And they typically form self-help groups (SHGs) that work together as mutual supports in developing capacity, sticking to savings plans, and ensuring loans get repaid. The SHG's approval of a member's business plan and oversight of their activities can be a powerful assurance of repayment when the whole SHG's ability to take out further loans is contingent upon their members' ability to repay.

Indira Kranthi Patham (IKP) is a government antipoverty program run by the Society for the Elimination of Rural Poverty in Andhra Pradesh, a state in southern India. The objective of IKP is to enhance the economic livelihood and social opportunities of the poorest of the poor in rural areas by mobilizing poor women into SHGs and facilitating their access to microcredit, bank credit, government safety nets, and social security programs such as life and health insurance. Supported by the World Bank, the program also includes the establishment of SHGs for disabled people. The groups receive training on saving and developing business plans before obtaining access to microcredit. Disabled members also receive assistance in navigating the procedures to get a disability certificate and the associated government benefits that go along with that certification. Members of disabled SHGs also serve as role models for each other, and can assist each other in thinking through the particular problems that disabled people face in their community.

Disabled people are often denied credit because of the belief that they are poor credit risks. That is, they are presumed to be unable to use their loans effectively to generate income. But in the IKP program, the payback rates of disabled people were equivalent to the nondisabled women who also participated in the broader program, at rates of greater than 95%.[20] However, the proportion of people with mental disabilities in the SHGs was much lower than in the population at large, suggesting that the community organizations forming the SHGs were either not identifying those people or choosing not to enlist them in the SHGs.

The IKP program is not unique. A similar program in Nicaragua, called ProMujer, has also included disabled people. The village banks established by that program loan money to disabled women under the same arrangements as nondisabled women, charging them market rates and providing them with business training and health care services. As in IKP, the disabled borrowers are as successful in paying back their loans as their nondisabled counterparts.

One option that lies between straight microcredit and microgrants is providing subsidized loans. This lessens some of the pitfalls of microgrants while making loans more attractive to potential borrowers. This was the strategy undertaken by the Ethiopian Federation for Persons with

Disabilities (EFPD), financed by the ILO. In that program EFPD subsidized half of the interest rate, as well as providing half of the mandatory savings generally associated with microfinance programs. The mandatory savings was seen as a barrier preventing disabled people from joining the program. Program participants were also provided with business development services to help them draw up and implement their business plans, as well as vocational training.[21]

Another strategy that has been employed is simply to lobby and build capacity of established microfinance programs to be accepting of disabled loan applicants. This has been the approach in Uganda, where a project supported by the Norwegian Association of the Disabled works to both raise awareness and build the capacity of existing microfinance institutions to include disabled people. This effort is marketed as a way for those programs to expand their markets. The project provides data on repayment rates of disabled people and offers awards to the most "disability friendly" microcredit institutions.

Finally, to ameliorate the concerns of financial institutions unfamiliar with dealing with disabled people, programs will sometimes guarantee the loans given to disabled people, thus absorbing the default risk. This strategy has been used by Handicap International's program in Senegal in association with USAID, as well as in the Central African Republic.

One project in Danang, Vietnam, administered by the Vietnam Assistance to the Handicapped (VNAH) and funded by USAID attempts to combine vocational training with access to microfinance. Similar to other vocational programs, it provides training on job skills and soft skills, such as applying for jobs, problem solving, communication, and conflict management. But it also includes business advice and negotiates with microfinance institutions to gain access to credit for disabled people. Although farming is the core activity of participants, one fourth have their own businesses. The program reports increased assets and earnings of members, but again, without a baseline and comparison group it is hard to judge its efficacy. Also, as in some other programs, a screening process is involved that weeds out potential trainees who are not considered viable job candidates. The VNAH program is not unique in this regard, which makes it hard to predict the impact of the program without a detailed understanding of the screening process.

Unfortunately, a full evaluation that can report on the economic costs and benefits of microcredit programs is also not available. However, the repayment rates of disabled people are well documented, and their continual demand for loans is suggestive of the value of this endeavor. However, its success compared with other strategies cannot be measured, nor are there good enough data to give us a clear picture of which groups of disabled people are best served by which programs.

All the strategies mentioned up to this point are focused on the disabled individual, but another approach is to focus on the employers. This strategy, of course, is only relevant to formal sector employment, but it still represents a significant number of jobs in a sector that will hopefully grow in size as the economies of low- and middle-income countries develop. Besides, success in any sector should have spillover effects as both disabled and nondisabled people get accustomed to the productivity of disabled workers in a supportive environment.

In 1999, the Government of Sri Lanka and the Japanese Association for the Employment of Disabled Persons (JAED) helped a group of businesses establish the Employer's Federation of Ceylon (EFC), which, with funding from the ILO, developed an Employer's Network on Disability, which rose to nearly 500 members. The EFC assesses the demand for skills and compares them with the skills found among the disabled population. It also maintains a computer database of disabled people looking for jobs, categorizing them by their skills and training needs, and has various initiatives—such as job fairs, newsletters, and a Web site—that attempts to match job seekers with employers. Employers share their success stories, and many have since developed their own training programs upon becoming convinced of the productivity and reliability of their disabled workers. After being established with ILO funds, the EFC is self-sustaining.

Another organization aimed at employers is the Blue Ribbon Employment Council (BREC) in Vietnam, which was established by VNAH and the Vietnam Chamber of Commerce and Industry (VCCI). The BREC recruits employers to its membership organization and teaches them about disability and disability management. The goal is to convince employers of the benefits of hiring and retaining employees with disabilities. The BREC also provides technical assistance to employers, serves as a forum for sharing experiences, and conducts extensive job fairs. Similar to the EFC, it documents the skills demanded by its members, and attempts to forecast future demand for worker skills to help vocational programs provide needed, marketable skills. It also maintains an employment database. Currently it is funded by USAID, but it is in the process of transitioning to a member-financed organization for longer-term sustainability.

A third example of this model is the Business Advisory Board on Disability (BABD) in Russia, also funded by USAID. Like its counterparts, the BABD works to raise awareness of disability issues in the business community and to promote inclusive workplaces. In addition to workplace interventions like training, internships, and assistance with workplace accommodations, the BABD works on the consumer end of business operations, helping to ensure that companies' services and products are more accessible to disabled customers. It also encourages its members to work with its suppliers and vendors to become more inclusive. This is similar to the employer-led Business Disability Forum in the United Kingdom, which works on inclusiveness not only in hiring practices, but also in reaching disabled consumers.

4. STRATEGIES FOR DEVELOPING EMPLOYMENT POLICIES

As stated, impact evaluations with comparison groups, high-quality data, and consistent definitions of disability are generally not available in low- and middle-income countries. Therefore, it is not really possible to present data in a manner that can help us quantify the impact of what is perceived to be best practices. Nevertheless, the growing participation of employers in various efforts, the high demand and payback rates of disabled people involved in microfinance, and various reports of the number of jobs participants in various vocational training and supported employment programs suggest that these efforts can make a difference. And there is ample evidence of the success of disabled people in the workforce.

Up until now, intergovernmental organizations and other development agencies have not paid a great deal of attention to the issue of employment for people with disabilities. When they have, they have tended to focus on special training programs, or in some cases on microfinance programs.

Segregating employment efforts for people with disabilities, however, could be a mistake. Making separate programs can make them less efficient and less sustainable because there will be a constant battle for funding to operate a parallel system of employment supports. Making ongoing programs more inclusive—for example, those promoting education, training, school-to-work transition, and entrepreneurship—would solidify their presence, and could take advantage of economies of scale in providing services. It also sends a signal that disabled people are part of the mainstream and can demonstrate that inclusion works. It could also be an important step in changing people's attitudes by having disabled and nondisabled people working and learning alongside each other.

The final section of this chapter lays out some recommendations for developing employment programs for people with disabilities in low- and middle-income countries, based on these experiences.

4.1 An Employment Policy for People with Disabilities Must Be Part of a Broader Program of Inclusive Development

Employment is the end product of an involved process that results from matching a worker with the desire and ability to be productive with an employer who needs and recognizes that worker's skills. Therefore, for an employment policy to be effective, many things are required, including:

- *Awareness-raising*: Disabled people must have the confidence to pursue education and employment. Their family members must be supportive of them—believing in them, not being ashamed of them, and not desiring to coddle them. Employers must be convinced that disabled people can be effective workers. As disabled workers enter the workforce and are successful, these attitudes will change, but to expedite the process various awareness-raising or counseling programs may be needed.
- *Education*: Many employment programs aim to impart new skills to people with disabilities, but to the extent that they receive a solid primary, secondary, or even tertiary education, this will be an easier—or maybe even an unnecessary—task. Inclusive education is a must.
- *Inclusive Health Care*: Good health is obviously important for maintaining productivity, or even for avoiding absenteeism. Access to health care and rehabilitative services is thus an important prerequisite for ensuring that disabled people can obtain employment and remain in their jobs.
- *Transportation*: Transportation can be a major barrier to employment, especially for people with physical disabilities. Accessible public transportation, transportation subsidies to cover the extra costs disabled people face, or even just high-quality roads can thus be seen as an important component of an overall disability employment policy.

4.2 Approaches to Promoting Employment Must Take into Account the Diversity of the Disabled Population

There is no one-size-fits-all program for employing people with disabilities. Some disabled people became injured on the job. Their primary needs might be medical rehabilitation or adjustments to the workplace with an employer already familiar with their abilities. Or they might need to be completely retrained, but are still very familiar with the world of work. Some people are disabled at birth and might need more basic and extensive training, including life skills. Some people with physical disabilities might primarily need physical adjustments to the workplace, whereas people with mental disabilities might require job coaching and more extensive help in dealing with employers' concerns. People becoming disabled near the end of their work lives might be best served by cash transfer programs.

Also, disabled people are heterogeneous in ways that do not relate to their disability. People in rural areas might require different interventions, for example, peer training instead of classroom training. They might be members of ethnic minority groups facing language barriers or other forms of discrimination.

4.3 An Employment Strategy Must Recognize That the Majority of Livelihood-Generating Activities Are Not in the Formal Sector

Many policies are aimed at the formal sector. These include antidiscrimination laws, quotas, employer groups, job fairs, and often job placement programs associated with vocational training and supported employment. Even social insurance programs that provide disability benefits are often linked to previous formal employment. These are important, but they do not cover the majority of livelihood-generating activities that people with disabilities have available to them. An employment strategy for people with disabilities must address self-employment and informal sector work. This can be done through microfinance programs and by acknowledging the skills that are demanded in the informal economy.

4.4 Employment Programs Must Be Linked to the Skills Demanded in the Marketplace

The global economy is changing more rapidly than in the past, and is more integrated. Low- and middle-income countries are thus becoming more subjected to positive and negative economic shocks around the world. As countries develop, the skills demanded in their economies will be in flux. Therefore, it is important that vocational training programs not get caught in preparing people with disabilities for jobs stereotypically considered appropriate—or just in continuing to train workers in the same skills—without constantly assessing the needs for skills in the job market.

4.5 Attention Must Be Paid to the Long-Run Sustainability of These Programs

Funding sources come and go, especially in hard economic times, so programs must be designed in a sustainable manner. To the extent that programs for people with disabilities can be integrated into mainstream programs, this will be easier. Microfinance programs that provide loans, not grants, are more sustainable, as are employer organizations that can be member-funded. One important factor that can contribute to their sustainability is demonstrated proof that these programs are cost-effective.

4.6 Monitoring Activities and Impact Evaluations Should Be Undertaken, the Design of Which Should Be Included at the Beginning of the Program

Programs should be designed and implemented with monitoring and evaluation in mind. In terms of monitoring, administrative data should be collected in real time to ensure that activities are being undertaken as anticipated, and to identify problem areas of implementation. As for impact evaluations, they should include control groups or comparison groups and a well-established baseline. Thought should be put into what type of evidence would be most important to identify best practices and convince policymakers and other stakeholders that these activities are cost-effective and beneficial to both disabled people and the general society.

4.7 As Countries Expand Their Social Protection Programs, They Should Minimize Antiwork Incentives in Their Benefit Programs

Many high-income countries have experienced notable antiwork effects from their disability benefit programs, and have made major modifications in an attempt to rectify that situation.[22] As countries become more developed, they will no doubt establish more extensive social protection programs, including programs for people with disabilities. These are important programs and essential to the support of people who are not capable of work. Nevertheless, care must be taken to design them in the most pro-work way that is consistent with the program's social protection goal. As noted, South Africa has already experienced a decline in work among people with disabilities as a result of its new social protection program.

People with disabilities make up a substantial proportion of the world's population. And the numbers are greater in terms of people who are directly affected in their households. For example, in Vietnam the disability rate is 7.5% by a somewhat conservative measure, but the percentage of people living in a household with a disabled member is greater than 23%.[23] If their household members cannot work or are dependent on them, this will have a direct impact on their lives as well.

In terms of both human rights and economic development, it is essential that people with disabilities be included in the world of employment. In low- and middle-income countries, efforts to do this confront special challenges. But the wide range of efforts, some of which are reported in this chapter, demonstrate that it is definitely possible.

NOTES

1. World Bank & World Health Organization (2011). *World Report on Disability*. Geneva, Switzerland: World Health Organization.
2. Mitra, S., Posarac, A., & Vick, B. (2011). Disability and Poverty in Developing Countries: A Snapshot from the World Health Survey. Social Protection Discussion Paper 1109. Washington, D.C.: World Bank.
3. She, P., & Livermore, G. (2009). Long-Term Poverty and Disability Among Working Age Adults. Journal of Disability Policy Studies *19*(4): 244–256.
4. Trani, J.-F., & Loeb, M. (2012). Poverty and Disability: A vicious circle? Evidence from Afghanistan and Zambia. *Journal of International Development 24*(S1), S19–S52; Mete, C. (Ed.)(2008). *Economic Implications of Chronic Illness and Disability in Eastern Europe*. Washington, D.C.: World Bank; World Bank & World Health Organization (2011), *World Report on Disability*.
5. Buckup, S. (2009). The Price of Exclusion. Employment Working Paper No. 43. Geneva, Switzerland: International Labour Organization.
6. Filmer, D. (2008). Disability, Poverty, and Schooling in Developing Countries: Results from 11 Household Surveys. *The World Bank Economic Review 22*(1), 141–163.
7. World Bank & World Health Organization (2011), *World Report on Disability*.
8. Mont, D., & Cuong, N.V. (2011). Disability and Poverty in Vietnam. *World Bank Economic Review 25*(2), 323–359.
9. Mitra, S. (2008). The Recent Decline in the Employment of Persons with Disabilities in South Africa, 1998-2006. *South African Journal of Economics 76*(3), 480–492.
10. Mont, D. (2004). Disability and Employment Policy. Social Protection Discussion Paper No. 0413. Washington, D.C.: World Bank.
11. Semlinger, K., & Schmid, G. (1985). Arbeitsmarktpolitik fur Behinderte, Betriebliche Barriaren und Ansatze su ihrer Uberwindung. Basel, Switzerland: Birkhauser Verlag.
12. Mont (2004), Disability and Employment Policy.
13. Tines, J., & Buzducea, D. (2009). *Transitions Towards an Inclusive Future: Vocational Skills Development and Employment Options for Persons with Disabilities in Europe and Eurasia*. Washington, D.C.: USAID.
14. Perry, D.A. (Ed.) (2003). *Moving Forward: Toward Decent Work for People with Disabilities*. Geneva, Switzerland: International Labour Organization.
15. Koistinen, M. (2008). *Understanding experiences of vocational training and employment for persons with learning disabilities in Zambia: Lessons for the future*. Helsinki, Finland: Finnish Association in Developmental Disabilities.
16. Perry (2003), *Moving Forward*.
17. Becker, D.R., Bond, G.R., & Drake, R.E. (2008). Individual placement and support: the evidence-based practice of supported employment. In G. Thornicroft, G. Szmukler, K.T. Mueser, & R.E. Drake (Eds.). *Oxford Textbook of Community Mental Health* (161–166). New York: Oxford University Press; Drake, R.E., and Bond, G.R. (2008). Fidelity of Supported Employment: Lessons Learned from the National Evidence-Based Practice Project. *Psychiatric Rehabilitation Journal 31*(4), 300–305; Perry (2003), *Moving Forward*.
18. Perry (2003). *Moving Forward*.

19. Handicap International (2006). Good Practices for the Economic Inclusion of People with Disabilities in Developing Countries: Funding Mechanisms for Self-Employment. Lyon, France: Handicap International.
20. Mont, D., & Sen, S. (2008). Findings from an Assessment of the Indira Kranthi Pratham Program for Persons with Disabilities. Working Paper.
21. Handicap International (2006). *Good Practices*.
22. Organization for Economic Co-Operation and Development (2010). *Sickness, Disability and Work: Breaking the Barriers* (Paris, France: OECD).
23. Mont & Cuong (2011). Disability and Poverty in Vietnam.

CHAPTER 3

Finding and Maintaining Employment

Lessons from Workplace Nondiscrimination Measures in
High-Income Countries

SUSANNE M. BRUYÈRE WITH SARA A. VAN LOOY

1. GLOBAL CONTEXT FOR WORKPLACE NONDISCRIMINATION

The opportunity to work and use one's talents to contribute to the community around us is a fundamental human need, yet people with disabilities throughout the world continue not to have equitable access to employment. The purpose of this chapter is to identify ways to examine employment disability nondiscrimination policies and practices in the United States and around the world that maximize the likelihood that people with disabilities will be able to enter the labor market (find a job), and keep that job once found. The focus is on workplace policies and practices.

In order to effectively address disability-based discrimination in employment and specific settings, it is necessary to know the degree of discrimination that is occurring and how it might be changing over time. Past research in the rehabilitation and disability field has focused more heavily on personal factors that influence employment outcomes, without paying sufficient attention to workplace factors. This has limited understanding of the factors that affect the employment outcomes of persons with disabilities.[1] The field of rehabilitation has generated research focused on functional characteristics and vocational skills and abilities, and how to best match these to the world of work. Those studies that have concentrated on disability and the workplace have been conducted methodologically either on student samples in laboratories[2] or been based on small samples.[3] Given this, Colella and Stone[4] have urged researchers to conduct field research involving larger samples and to also target work-group inclusion of individuals with disabilities as an employment outcome of interest.

The purpose of this chapter is to provide a broad overview to document the continuing employment and economic disparities for people with disabilities, and explore ways to better measure how workplace policies and practices contribute to individuals with disabilities being able to enter the labor force and subsequently thrive there. Examples of related employer-focused research, the measurement approaches used, key findings, and its implications for future workplace policy and practice are presented.

Although the usefulness of national survey and administrative data to document the employment and economic status of people with disabilities is widely acknowledged, the emphasis in this chapter is on ways to measure the impact of employer actions on employment outcomes for people with disabilities. Included is information on a variety of strategies and mechanisms that can be used to do so, such as analyses of employment disability discrimination charge data statistics; examination of human resources (HR) and workplace policies and practices, including data collection through business and disability advocacy networks; the use of company archival data and analytics; and in-depth company case studies that use measures to assess the workplace culture of inclusion for people with disabilities. Examples of each approach are provided, including a review of the advantages and disadvantages of each, and the evidence of their usefulness, where available. This chapter concludes with a discussion of the implications of these findings for existing and future public policy, service programs advancing employment outcomes for people with disabilities, and research.

To set the context for the overview of workplace measures of discrimination, the importance of work to the economic, social, and personal well-being of all individuals, including individuals with disabilities, is first briefly discussed. Existing significant disparities in workforce participation rates for people with disabilities globally, and their resulting economic impact, are confirmed. This section concludes with the rationale for the need for closer scrutiny of employment disability discrimination in workplace policies and practices.

2. IMPORTANCE OF WORK TO ECONOMIC, SOCIAL, AND PERSONAL WELL-BEING

Given the major role that work plays in human life, the implications of being without meaningful work are significant.[5] Work is an important step toward socioeconomic well-being, and also provides a forum for individuals to use their innate talents and develop skills and thereby contribute to their communities and society more broadly.

In addition to providing a source of income, work holds important social value, creates the opportunity to develop community networks, and contributes to an individual's healthy sense of identity and self-worth. Work is only one part of being valued and respected within society, but it is an important means of social inclusion.[6]

Research in the area of the meaning of work to overall well-being shows that having work provides not only a critical link between an individual and society, but is also an important determining factor in the individual's overall self-esteem.[7] The World Health Organization (WHO) also discusses the fact that mental health professionals agree that the workplace environment can have a significant impact on an individual's mental well-being, although they also conclude that is often difficult to quantify the impact of work alone on personal identity, self-esteem, and social recognition.[8]

People who lose their jobs are reported to also be more prone to developing depression symptoms. For example, Dooley, Catalano, and Wilson found that people who become unemployed have more than twice the risk of depressive symptoms than those who remain employed.[9] Employment for people with disabilities is also a vital route to obtaining affordable health care to access needed treatment for mental health concerns, as well as physical accident and illness issues when they arise, and employment also can assist in providing access to health promotion programs necessary to maintain health and well-being.[10] Sullivan and von Wachter found that job loss leads to a 10% to 15% increase in annual death rates during the subsequent 20 years of the individual's life.[11]

3. WORKFORCE PARTICIPATION DISPARITIES FOR PEOPLE WITH DISABILITIES

To document continuing employment and economic disparities of people with disabilities, research using national survey and administrative data is extremely valuable. In the United States, people with disabilities are a sizable concentration in the population and self-report that they want to work, yet there is a continuing disparity in employment rates of people with disabilities, and the numbers of people collecting Social Security disability benefits continue to rise. The employment rate in 2009 of American working age people (21–64) with disabilities was 36%, as compared with 77% of people without disabilities.[12] These employment disparities lead to significant subsequent economic disparities, with 26% of US people with disabilities in 2009 living below the poverty line, compared with 11% of people without disabilities. There is also a US $21,600 gap in annual median household income for households with a person with a disability (US $39,600/year), compared with households without a person with a disability (US $61,200/year).[13] In addition, it appears that once in the workforce, people with disabilities experience discrimination in terms of wage differentials. Baldwin and Johnson demonstrated that a worker with a visible impairment is paid on average 33.2% less than an average nondisabled worker. Only 55.7% of the wage differential between the average nondisabled worker and the visibly impaired peer can be explained by the differences in the human capital and job-related characteristics, and the rest can be attributed to non-productivity-related differences between these two groups of workers. The wage differential varies considerably across disability types. People with visual impairments have 27% lower salaries than the average of people with other disabilities.[14]

Similarly, people with disabilities in other parts of the world experience disparities in their ability to access training, employment, and full community participation. In both developed and developing countries, households with a person with a disability are more likely to be poor than their nondisabled counterparts.[15] In general, persons with disabilities in the labor market tend to have lower education than others, and are also more likely to be in part-time jobs.[16]

Each country uses different definitions of disability; additionally, the national surveys that collect data on the status of people with disabilities utilize different determinations of disability and what is considered employment, making direct comparisons extremely difficult.[17] Given this, it is generally true in other countries as well that working-age individuals with disabilities have a significantly lower rate of employment than those without disabilities. According to Canada's most recently reported figures from the Health and Activity Limitation Survey (HALS),[18] disabled people make up 12.7% of the non-institutionalized working age (15–64) population. Of these, 48.2% people with disabilities were employed compared with 73% of nondisabled workers.[19] The Australian Bureau of Statistics estimates are quite similar. They estimate that 14.8% of the non-institutionalized working age (15–64) population had a disability. The Bureau reports that just under half (47%) of these individuals were employed verses three fourths (76%) of the nondisabled.[20]

The Organization of Economic Cooperation and Development (OECD) has provided some similar comparative statistics across 27 countries. The OECD reports that the employment situation for working-age persons with disabilities in the late 2000s was that 44% were in employment, compared with 75% of people without disabilities, and that the former figure continues to fall. Also, where one in five people without disabilities was economically inactive in OECD countries, approximately one in two people with disabilities was so. In addition, people with disabilities are more likely to be in short-term and part-time employment, and the employment rate for people with mental health disabilities was particularly low.[21]

People with disabilities represent approximately 10% to 12% of the world's population, or more than 650 million people.[22] Of this number, 80% live in low-income countries. Approximately two-thirds of this group—470 million people with disabilities—are of working age, and yet the majority of them are not employed.[23] In developing countries, labor markets are often largely informal, with many workers being self-employed. When they work, persons with disabilities are more likely to be self-employed than people in the overall working-age population.[24]

4. EXAMINING WHAT IS OCCURRING IN WORKPLACES

Measurement of disability inequalities in labor market outcomes are taken as proxies for disability discrimination. These continuing employment disparities, despite the articulated desire of people with disabilities to work, as well as continued claims of discrimination, point to the need for continued study on how to lessen workplace discrimination for this population. National survey and administrative data provide prevalence rates, workforce participation rates, and household income and poverty rates, in order to identify economic disparities for people with disabilities. These disparities are well documented globally. The focus of this chapter is to examine more closely how employer practices might ameliorate them.

A variety of scholars over the past 20 years have surveyed the global development of international law that provides protections for the civil rights of people with disabilities.[25] Some studies focus on identifying disability nondiscrimination laws and policies in place from a country perspective; examples are reports coming from Finland and Turkey.[26]

Few studies closely examine the efficacy of workplace organizational practices. As a 2010 literature review conducted by the National Centre for Vocational Education in Australia observed: "Most research on employment, equity, and disadvantage has been focused upon the labour "supply" side of the employment equation. That is to say, it examines the barriers, constraints, and challenges from the point of view of people with disabilities seeking employment. The focus tends to be upon what they . . . need to do to break through the perceived barriers."[27] This review failed to find any specific studies in OECD countries that looked at good practices from the employer perspective, and found similar gaps in the North American literature.[28]

A more recent systemic review of the literature on employer behavior in five OECD countries focused on the effectiveness of government policy in changing employer behaviors. This review found 30 potential studies between 1990 and 2008 across Canada, Denmark, Norway, Sweden, and the United Kingdom, but found that few studies provided robust evaluations, many of the potentially most effective programs suffered from low take-up by the targeted employers, and they failed to find any population-level effects of legislation.[29]

Although not research per se, there are also examples of educational efforts in select countries that provide summaries of employer good practices in the employment of people with disabilities.[30] Similarly, some efforts focus on identifying the information needs of employers in a particular part of the employment process. For example, a study funded by the European Union (project partners were Spain, Sweden, Poland, and the United Kingdom) identified and exchanged good practice in the area of employment retention. The key areas identified were: early intervention, educating health practitioners about employment issues, educating employers about state, national, and community supports available in the return-to-work process, and instituting an effective disability leave policy. The review concluded that educational materials were needed in the areas of employment retention, the business case for recruiting and retaining disabled people, and how to best influence policymakers.[31]

There is a significant need for further investigation of workplace anti-discrimination policies and programs, and the purpose of this chapter is to present an overview of a variety of ways by which we can better identify and precisely measure workplace policies and practices, using examples from research conducted to date in the United States and other countries where such research has been identified. This is not meant to be an exhaustive presentation of such efforts, but rather an illustrative one, highlighting the kinds of approaches and informative results to date that can be used to improve our evidenced-based knowledge of workplace good practice in minimizing employment disability discrimination and maximizing inclusion globally.

This chapter provides an overview of the ways in which employment participation at the workplace level for people with disabilities can be documented, including a discussion of the usefulness and limitations of these data, and suggestions for ways in which we might improve our metrics for measuring positive employment outcomes for people with disabilities in all facets of the employment experience. Where these methodologies afford findings with important implications for workplace policies and practices, these are highlighted. Included are the use of employment disability discrimination charges; information which can be gained from organizational/HR policies and practices; organizational data (equity in recruitment, hiring, career advancement/promotion, compensation, coaching/mentoring, leave, and retirement opportunities; accommodation policies, etc.); and workplace climate and bias.

5. WORKPLACE MEASURES AND RELATED FINDINGS

5.1 Employment Discrimination Claims

Discrimination in hiring and in the workplace is one possible reason for the observed disparities in the employment of people with disabilities. To encourage the employment of people with disabilities and prohibit discrimination, many countries have laws prohibiting discrimination on the basis of disability or have set quotas for the employment of persons with disabilities.[32]

Claims or charges of discrimination are a relevant source of information about where discrimination may be occurring in employment settings. This information can be taken from discrimination claims filed with local or national authorities or internal grievance records of employers themselves, if available. Some of the useful information found in such data sources are types of issues occurring, where they occur in the employment process (in the application or lay-off/firing processes, accommodations, or harassment), and the basis upon which the claim was made (age, race/ethnicity, sex, religion, or disability, and possibly further distinctions made by type of disability). In addition, this information may be informative in looking at trends in claims filed over time (perhaps assisting in examination of the possible impact of changes in policies), and trends in claims filed relative to other kinds of employment discrimination claims (comparisons across different protected-group categories).

To illustrate the potential usefulness of such data, numbers from the United States are presented here. In the United States, the Americans with Disabilities Act of 1990 (ADA) employment provisions (Title I) provide protections against employment disability discrimination. The US Equal Employment Opportunity Commission (EEOC) is charged with enforcing the ADA, along with other laws prohibiting employment discrimination. The EEOC maintains a database of discrimination charges filed (including charges filed with state and local Fair Employment Practice Agencies that contract with the EEOC).

Since 2005, McMahon and colleagues have published a series of articles using EEOC charge data to investigate discrimination against people with specific disabilities or in specific industries, as well as taking a more general look at the roots of and nature of discrimination.[33] In addition, Roessler, Hurley, and McMahon describe findings from a study of the prevalent disabling conditions in discharge allegations and found that these conditions included back injuries, nonparalytic/orthopedic conditions, depression, and diabetes.[34] Rumrill and Fitzgerald looked at characteristics of employers where charges of unlawful discharge were filed and found discharge allegations (as compared to allegations involving other issues) more likely to be made against smaller employers (15–200 employees), in the South US Census Tract Region, and in the industries of manufacturing, health care and social assistance, retail, administrative support, and others.[35] Rumrill, Fitzgerald, and McMahon describe findings from a causal comparative study of the characteristics of charging parties who filed allegations related to discharge (unlawful and constructive discharge), finding they were more likely to be male, younger (15–34 years of age), with heart/cardiovascular conditions, cancer, bipolar disorder, epilepsy, HIV/AIDS, alcoholism, drug addiction, and mental retardation.[36]

Figure 3.1, taken from related Cornell University research using the US employment disability discrimination charge data, illustrates how these data can be used to determine the relative number of charges across different protected class characteristics. The figure highlights that people with disabilities in the labor force are perceiving discrimination in the workplace at a much higher rate than other protected classes. Far more labor-force adjusted charges of discrimination are filed under the ADA than any other statute. Over the 15-year period from 1993 to 2007, the average number of ADA charges per 10,000 people with disabilities in the labor force was 81.6. This is four times the number of US Civil Rights Title VII-Nonwhite (race-ethnicity) charges per 10,000 nonwhite people in the labor force (19.5), and compares with 4.3 Age Discrimination in Employment Act (ADEA) charges per 10,000 people aged 40 and over in the labor force, and 5.6 US Civil Rights Title VII-Female charges per 10,000 females in the labor force.

Also informative in this kind of analysis of the perceived workplace disability discrimination experience of persons with disabilities is identifying the

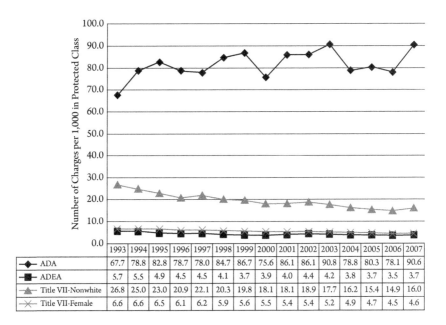

Figure 3.1
Number of ADA, ADEA, Title VII-Nonwhite, and Title VII-Female Charges per 10,000 People in the Labor Force with Protected Class Characteristics, 1993–2007.[37]
Note: The number of charges represents the number of charges filed per 10,000 people in the base population where the ADA was cited (i.e., those charges filed based on the ADA alone or in combination with other statutes) and similarly for ADEA, Title VII-Nonwhite, and Title VII-Female. Estimates of the size of the labor force for each protected class were derived from the Annual Social and Economic Supplement to the Current Population Survey.

most prevalent type of basis (i.e., disability type) and issue (i.e., the reason a charge was filed) upon which ADA charges were filed. Across the years 1993 to 2007, the top five most common specific impairments cited in ADA charges were orthopedic/structural back impairment (12.2%), nonparalytic orthopedic impairment (7.5%), depression (5.8%), diabetes (3.8%), and other psychiatric disorders (3.6%). The most cited issue by far across this 15-year period is discharge, cited on 55.3% of charges—more than twice as many charges as the second most cited issue, failure to reasonably accommodate (24.6%). The three next most often cited issues were discrimination in terms and conditions of employment (18.8%), harassment (12.2%), and discrimination in hiring (8.2%).

As illustrated here, one strength of examining discrimination claims as a source of information about where bias occurs in the workplace is that such an approach can assist in identifying specific issues for attention and vulnerable populations, and in this case also particular disabilities for attention. In addition, such an approach may be useful to illustrate changes in policies and practices over time or in assessing the impact of changes in legislation, policies, and environmental factors in a given geographic area.

These data also have their disadvantages. Data include all charges filed, not only those determined to have merit by the EEOC. These charges represent perceived discrimination in the workplace by the individual filing the charge. In addition, another drawback of using employment discrimination charges filed with a state or federal agency is that many disputes may not rise to the level of a grievance or discrimination charge, and so are not captured through such data. In addition, even if discrimination charges are captured in some way, the data may not consistently be filed across offices or regions, making interpretation and generalization difficult. Last, there may be uneven reporting of discrimination depending on the stage at which it takes place; for example, discrimination in hiring may be less likely to be reported by those who experience it, as it is harder to prove. Federally filed charge data are therefore not a perfect measure of the prevalence of employment discrimination, but do provide useful insights regarding where in the employment process people with disabilities perceive discrimination as occurring.

5.2 Workplace/Human Resource Policies and Practices

Another source of data about employer behavior that can contribute to an understanding of workplace discrimination can be gained from information about workplace or HR policies and practices. Some of the elements of such an inquiry are the following: evidence articulated in top leadership commitment to equal opportunity in hiring and advancement for people with disabilities; evidence of HR policies and practices in the promotion of approaches to minimizing discrimination in recruitment, screening, and hiring processes; evidence in HR policies and practices of efforts to maximize equal opportunity in access to health, retirement, and other benefits of employment; evidence of approaches to maximize equal access to career advancement, training, promotional opportunities, as well as in redeployment, layoff, and termination actions; and other relevant policies to support the employment and advancement of people with disabilities, such as accommodation policies. Such studies may also afford us an opportunity to examine differences in policies and practices across employer size and sectors, and conduct cross-country comparisons.

There are a variety of ways and a number of key informants to gather information on workplace and HR policies and practices. Discussed here are approaches using the following as key informants: HR professionals, supervisors, and individuals with disabilities and disability advocates. The benefits of using research partnerships with national associations representing the interests of HR professionals, employers, and disability advocates, and people with disabilities themselves are also discussed.

5.2.1 Human Resource Professionals' Perspective

Studies have been conducted to examine workplace, policies and practices, particularly in HR, that can minimize employment disability discrimination and heighten the likelihood that individuals with disabilities will be retained and able to advance in their careers. The key informants for these studies have been HR professionals in their respective organizational settings.[38] In the United States, an average of one HR professional for every 100 employees has been considered the standard for some time,[39] but actual numbers vary by industry, organization structure, and organization size.[40] Associations representing HR professionals are an excellent source of information about current practices, if researchers are afforded access to their membership for study purposes.

In the United States, the Society for Human Resource Management (SHRM)[41] offers a comprehensive view into the perspectives and priorities of HR practices related to individuals with disabilities. The SHRM partnered with Cornell University in 1999[42] and again in 2011[43] for a study of workplace practices in support of the employment provisions of the ADA, which provided information about policy and practice differences across employer size. To examine HR policies and practices across different sectors, Cornell also conducted similar research with HR and Equal Employment Opportunity (EEO) professionals in the US public/federal sector.[44] Both of these studies asked organizational informants (more than 1,200 human resources professionals across the private and federal sectors) what their organization does to meet the needs of employees with disabilities in such areas as making physical facilities accessible, modifying workplace policies on work hours and assignments, and making accommodations in equipment, training, transportation, and supervisory methods. Questions were also asked about the respondents' familiarity with making such accommodations and their perception of the difficulty in doing so.

A related survey was done with supervisors in US federal government agencies to afford comparisons of perceptions on accommodations from these different informants.[45] The HR professional survey was also conducted with a comparative sample of HR professionals in the United Kingdom to study their response to the UK Disability Discrimination Act of 1995.[46] The results of these multiple inquiries through survey research were a confirmation of the importance of the role of HR professionals and HR policies and practices in supporting implementation of disability employment nondiscrimination legislation.[47]

Figure 3.2 illustrates how research results from such surveys of HR professionals can inform about policies and practices to accommodate current employees with disabilities, and about how perspectives of these responses may differ by organizational size. Note in Figure 3.2 that, compared with other listed possible accommodation actions, respondents across all employer sizes reported proportionally less activity in accommodations for persons with sensory (visual and hearing) impairments (i.e., percent of respondents reporting having modified training materials or provided readers for persons with visual or cognitive impairments). However, a significantly larger proportion of HR professional respondents from employers of more than 2,500 employees, reported making such accommodations in their workplaces.

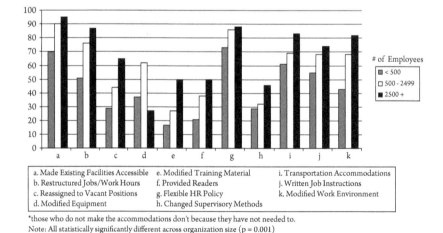

a. Made Existing Facilities Accessible   e. Modified Training Material   i. Transportation Accommodations
b. Restructured Jobs/Work Hours   f. Provided Readers   j. Written Job Instructions
c. Reassigned to Vacant Positions   g. Flexible HR Policy   k. Modified Work Environment
d. Modified Equipment   h. Changed Supervisory Methods

*those who do not make the accommodations don't because they have not needed to.
Note: All statistically significantly different across organization size (p = 0.001)

Figure 3.2
Actions to Meet Needs of Employees with Disabilities, by Organization Size[48]

Respondents in these HR professional survey studies were also asked about their perceived difficulty in making certain accommodations, and comparisons were made across private and federal sectors. Differences between responses in these two sectors were most marked again in the area of accommodations for individuals with visual and hearing impairments, where the private sector respondents reported significantly more difficulty with such accommodations (Figure 3.3).

As the research described in the preceding demonstrates, one of the strengths of using HR professional perspectives on workplace accommodation and disability nondiscrimination policies and practices as a way to learn more about and possibly measure workplace discrimination is that it may afford comparisons across companies on a number of topics. When coupled with reviews of stated policies and more in-depth personal interviews with managers and employees (more fully discussed later), it can provide a much more accurate portrayal of actual practice within organizations than a review of organizational quantitative data alone can provide.

Some of the limitations of this approach are that surveys or interviews of key informants such as HR professionals are really only a proxy for being able to actually observe real policies in practice. Articulated policies are not always implemented in practice, or actual practice may be different than policies suggest. In addition, organizations may sometimes prevent interviews or surveys of employees, access to policies is sometimes precluded, and even if afforded

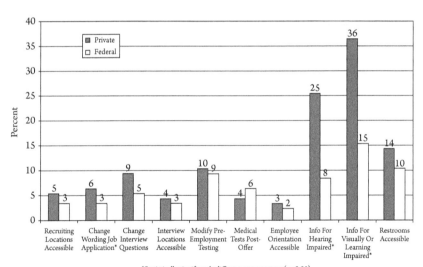

*Statistically significantly different across sectors (p<0.05)
Note: Between 10-60% all organizations did not need to make these changes.
Percentages also do not include those who were not able to make the change.

Figure 3.3
Percent Reporting Difficulty to Make Changes by Federal Private Sectors (of Those Who Made Changes)[49]

direct contact and the opportunity to observe policies in implementation, it may be difficult to observe actual practices that would demonstrate whether discrimination is minimized through the articulated policies.

5.2.2 Employer National Associations as Key Informants

The informational source just discussed, HR professionals perspectives, is made possible by partnerships with the national professional organizations that represent them. An additional and most valuable perspective is also partnerships with national organizations representing employers. In the United States, examples are The Conference Board, the US Chamber of Commerce, and the National Federation of Business. It can also be useful to partner for survey and research purposes with disability-focused employer groups, such as the US Business Leadership Network in the United States, and the Business Disability Forum in the United Kingdom.

An advantage of such alliances is again that perspectives can be gathered across company sizes and industry sectors to examine how employment disability non-discrimination public policies and organizational practices are being implemented and functioning within companies. In addition, such groups offer access to input from high-level company executives on topics in which an in-depth focus is needed on a particularly difficult area. A partnership between The Conference Board and Cornell University in 2011–2012 has afforded an opportunity for in-depth examination from company informants' perspective of such issues as follows: the need to build a business case within the organization and to company leadership for disability inclusion; applicants' and employees' willingness to disclose their disability; factors that improve organizational readiness for increasing hiring and advancement for people with disabilities; and needed company metrics/analytics for measuring the effectiveness of targeted efforts to increase the hiring, retention, and advancement of individuals with disabilities.[50]

The limitation or disadvantage of such an approach is that often with surveys and even in-depth focus groups using national employer associations memberships, the perspectives may come from people at very different levels of the company and in very different positions, making it sometimes difficult to distinguish "the voice" from which the information and perspective is coming. Information from senior managers needs to be complemented by responses from employees at all levels.

5.2.3 Supervisors' Perspective

Another key informant in the workplace, one that can often be very difficult to reach for research purposes, is the direct supervisor. Many of the necessary workplace conditions for a culture inclusive of people with disabilities (e.g., job empowerment, participation in decision making, fair treatment, climate) are under the direct control of managers. The central role and impact of the manager in fostering inclusion, minimizing employment disparities, implementing disability practices, and increasing engagement have been repeatedly affirmed.[51]

Research that has been conducted to date confirms that supervisor behavior is critical for both the implementation of effective workplace practices and the creation of a climate of inclusion for people with disabilities. Research by Gates showed that successful adjustment to work for employees with disabilities was related to the ability to complete job requirements, get along with others at work, see a future at work, and feel good about work.[52] Many supervisor behaviors were associated with these factors, including the extent to which supervisors treat workers fairly, allow workers to participate in decisions related to their work, and utilize workers' skills.

Cornell University, in collaboration with the Presidential Task Force on Employment of People with Disabilities, conducted a study of federal sector supervisors in 17 agencies.[53] The supervisor survey was based on the prior survey of federal sector human resources and EEO representatives previously described. The benefit of this study was not only gaining the perspective of supervisors, a hard-to-reach workplace informant, but it also afforded a comparison of EEO/HR and supervisors' perspectives on accommodations and other employment disability nondiscrimination policies and practices. For example, HR/EEO respondents were significantly more likely than supervisors to identify "costs of accommodations" and "supervisor knowledge of which accommodation to make" as being barriers to the employment and advancement of employees with disabilities in their agencies. HR/EEO respondents were more than twice as likely as supervisors to identify coworker attitudes as being a barrier to the employment and advancement of employees with disabilities in their agencies. Supervisors, however, were slightly less likely to identify lack of related experience as a barrier than the HR/EEO respondents.[54] Not surprisingly, supervisors were slightly less likely to be knowledgeable about the agency's affirmative action employment goals, with about one in ten responding "don't know," when asked whether their agency sets affirmative action employment goals and makes an effort to reach them.[55]

More recent research conducted by our group raises important questions about the effectiveness and consistency with which well-intentioned disability policies are implemented within organizations, and again points to the importance of seeking out supervisors as informants. Nishii and Bruyère found that a vast majority of private sector managers surveyed were unaware of the existence of various policies and practices for individuals with disabilities within their organization.[56] For example, 83% of managers in this sample reported not knowing whether their organization provided central funding for accommodations, 78% did not know about the existence of targeted advancement opportunities, 68% were unaware of targeted recruiting efforts, 65% were unaware of mentoring opportunities, 62% did not know whether education and training on disability issues was offered within their organization, 56% did not know whether their organization offered equal access to training opportunities, 48% did not even know whether their organization had clear accommodation policies in place, and 46% did not know about return-to-work or other disability management services that were available within their organization.[57]

5.3 Persons with Disabilities' Perspective

There is a need for policymakers to have information about the perceptions and experience of people with disabilities directly from people with disabilities, as well as their ideas about what the strategies might be to combat what they experience as discrimination.[58] Because HR managers' reports and the actual experiences of employees can differ,[59] it is critical that research examines experiences of inclusion from the perspective of employees with disabilities. A 2010 study by Kulkarni and Valk explored perceptions of people with physical disabilities and HR managers in the Netherlands, to examine if people with disabilities and HR managers view organizational HR practices in a similar manner or not. The authors used a convenience sampling method resulting in a sample of 24 people with disabilities and 14 HR managers.[60] Data from interviews were analyzed to examine common themes and variation across both employee and HR respondents. The findings overall were that respondents, both people with disabilities and their HR managers reported the same reality. However, the experience of and reasons for that reality were different. One example is in the area of training or job skill development opportunities. More than half of the people with disabilities interviewed reported not having received such training. When the same question was posed to the HR managers, half indicated that they did not offer any specific training to all because people with disabilities received the necessary training when they came to the organization from a disability-focused employment agency, or because they thought that if such training was needed, the employee with the disability or his or her manager would initiate training.

This research, although preliminary, points to the importance of gathering perspectives from people with disabilities as well as from managers and HR professionals. Whenever possible, a survey of employees inside a company should be conducted, to provide needed comparisons of perspectives with those of supervisors, HR professionals, and top-level leadership.

When researchers are unable to directly access employees, another way to get a perspective on the impact of employer/HR employment disability nondiscrimination policies and practices and their impact on employees with disabilities is to work with disability advocacy organizations to solicit perspectives from people with disabilities themselves. Kulkarni and Legnick-Hall conducted an exploratory qualitative study in India, identifying their study subjects through examination of the directory of disability empowerment centers in Bangalore, India (e.g., schools for blind children, training agencies for adults); their final sample consisted of 31 respondents.[61] In their interviews of these subjects, they examined how people with disabilities viewed various aspects of their workplace socialization process. They specifically looked at the role of coworkers, supervisors, organizational practices, and proactive employee behaviors in influencing organizational integration. They found that integration was most influenced by coworkers and supervisors. Results showed that coworkers were seen by these informants as the most influential people in their workplaces in terms of the socialization phase of their getting to know the organization, as well as in understanding and executing work tasks. Supervisors were seen as sources of task-related support as well, and as a source of informal support for personal issues. Regarding organizational practices, the respondents were not aware of specific policies or practices aimed toward them. One of the conclusions drawn and recommendations for managerial good practice was that the socialization processes may be more difficult and require greater attention when people with disabilities are new employees.

A US example of research targeted at persons with disabilities that uses a disability association as the source of key informants is a study we recently conducted in partnership with the American Association of People with Disabilities (AAPD) and The Substance Abuse and Mental Health Services Administration (SAMHSA).[62] Distribution of an online survey was done through a variety of approaches, including: AAPD's general listserv, AAPD Facebook posts, AAPD Twitter posts, articles in AAPD's *Justice for All Newsletter* as well as SAMHSA's network listserv, and an article in SAMHSA/ Center for Mental Health Services Consumer Affairs E-News.

An area that emerged as the most significant issue and has implications across all other issues studied was that of disclosure of disability; survey results provided significant findings regarding factors reported by respondents as ones that may influence the decision to disclose or not disclose their disability to an employer.

About two thirds of the respondents with disabilities rated the *need for accommodation* and *supportive supervisor relationship* as being very important factors in influencing a person to choose to disclose his or her disability. In addition, the context of the workplace was reported as very important, with high ratings for having a *disability-friendly workplace* and *knowing that the employer was actively recruiting people with disabilities*. Persons with a disability rated the importance of belief in new opportunities higher than individuals without a disability, and this response was quite consistent between groups.[63] Nearly three fourths of respondents viewed *risks of being fired/not hired* as being very important factors in choosing not to disclose their disability. This was followed by *employer may focus on disability, fear of limited opportunities*, and *risk of losing health care*. People with a disability rated the *desire for privacy* as less important than those without a disability. People with a disability were more likely to rate the *risk of being fired/not hired, losing health insurance* and *fear of limited opportunities* as very important factors than people without disabilities.[64]

The experiences uncovered in this survey, particularly those around disability disclosure in the application and employment processes, demonstrate how such research can provide a foundation for future public policy development and employer practices around such very critical issues. It illustrates the importance of getting the "voice" of people with disabilities in the public policy and policy evaluation processes. The significant advantage of this approach is that it provides the perspectives of those most directly impacted by the HR policies being considered or actually being implemented at the public policy or organizational level. As happens when one interviews any particular group, the strength and limitation is that survey respondents are viewing the inquiry from their vantage point. In the same way that employers often cannot directly report the experience of employees with disabilities, employees often cannot report on the employers' perspective of regulatory or organizational factors that may impact the formulation of relevant policies.

5.4 Organizational Data

Archived human resource data and related records of individual companies can also be of significant assistance in determining whether discrimination is occurring either in the hiring and/or employment processes. Also useful might be available data on disability accommodations and disability-specific initiatives that the company has. This is not an entirely new idea, as some studies broadly using this methodology were conducted 30 years ago.[65] But HR analytics have moved far along the metrics continuum since that time. Leading-edge companies are increasingly adopting sophisticated methods of analyzing employee data to enhance their competitive advantage.[66] However, not all companies collect data, and in many cases data are not as informative as needed, even for the organization's own strategic purposes,[67] let alone to inform organizational disability inclusion and nondiscrimination policies and practices.

The need of such analytics to examine diversity and disability practices more broadly was further confirmed in a more recent study conducted by SHRM, which found that only slightly more than one third (38%) of respondents are measuring the impact of diversity overall, and that this number had only increased by two percentage points in the last five years. No examples of separate metrics for people with disabilities were identified in this study.[68]

Researchers interested in studying employment disability nondiscrimination policies and practices using organizational data might also consider identifying those employers who might have a higher need for more careful tracking of people with disabilities in the recruitment, hiring, and retention pipeline, based on their sector or receipt of federal funding. For example, in the United States, federal agencies and federal contractors have such affirmative action requirements. Under Executive Order 11246, covered employers who are federal contractors and subcontractors must take "affirmative action" to recruit and advance qualified minorities, women, persons with disabilities, and covered veterans.[69] Federal contractors' affirmative action efforts are enforced by the US Office of Federal Contract Compliance Programs (OFCCP). The OFCCP is currently proposing new regulations that will increase the enforcement of these laws, which historically have not been heavily enforced.[70]

The OFCCP's proposed rule would strengthen the affirmative action requirements established in Section 503 of the Rehabilitation Act of 1973, obligating federal contractors and subcontractors to ensure equal employment opportunities for qualified workers with disabilities. The proposed regulatory changes detail specific actions contractors must take in the areas of recruitment, training, record-keeping, and policy dissemination, similar to those that have long been required to promote workplace equality for women and minorities, perhaps opening the door to increased opportunities to conduct work using organizational data, particularly with US federal contractors. Legislation such as equal employment opportunity protection, health and safety regulations, or workers' compensation programs might necessitate record-keeping that includes disability-related information.

The issue of being able to "count" people with disabilities is also a critical one in countries in which quota systems are in place. The quota is the requirement that an employer is required to hire a minimum percentage of people with disabilities, and the level is country-specific. The quota requirement is often tied to some kind of enforcement sanction, such as fines, levies, or even criminal penalties.[71] The majority of European countries have a quota system, including Austria, Bulgaria, the Czech Republic, France, Germany, Greece, Hungary, Italy, Luxemburg, Malta, Poland, Portugal, Romania, Slovakia, Spain, and the Netherlands.[72] The assumption that quotas correct labor market imperfections to the benefit of persons with disabilities is yet to be documented empirically, however, as no thorough impact evaluation of quotas on the employment of persons with disabilities has been performed.[73] Ideally, in addition to legislation, other factors such as a management that is genuinely concerned for the success of the diversity and inclusion strategy, and an actively encouraging and supportive organizational culture, can also heighten the likelihood that data may be included that will inform disability inclusion strategies.

Still, within workplace practices, progress needs to be made in encouraging employers to keep better metrics on their efforts to minimize workplace discrimination. The advantage of informing workplace discrimination inquiries using organizational data or metrics available is that it can provide very concrete information about the progress of the organization in recruiting, hiring, and retaining people with disabilities, as well as other protected populations, if available. It can also assist in informing about the efficacy of relationships with select community agencies that serve as a pipeline for qualified applicants with a disability, if agency-specific data are kept to document the success of outcomes of applicants coming from each source.

Organizational data and records that might be of assistance in determining the efficacy of these practices are as follows: application and interviewing statistics; data confirming equity in career advancement and training opportunities; data confirming equity in pay, other compensation, and job classification/function; data confirming equity in the application of performance management protocols; data confirming equity in access to health and retirement benefits, leaves, and layoffs; data on sick leave and absences; data on accommodations/adjustments; and grievances relating to disability and accommodation.

Data on sick leave and absence can also be of assistance in improving retention of employees incurring health and disability-related issues, by identifying challenges early on that might be mitigated through earlier intervention and workplace accommodation. This can increase longer-term retention and minimize number of these employees that abandon work and are driven to disability benefits.[74]

Wynne and McAnaney did a 2009 study across seven European Union member states (Finland, Germany, Ireland, Italy, the Netherlands, Sweden, and the United Kingdom) on the factors and services that influence successful return to work.[75] They identified relevant measures and initiatives aimed at achieving a range of outcomes for chronically ill or disabled employees, including: health improvement measures (general medical services and specific post-acute health maintenance interventions); retention measures to ensure that people at work maintain their workability (through health promotion, risk management, and occupational health and safety activities); and measures to facilitate the redeployment of employees to other positions within the same company.

Another area of increasing concern in which closer scrutiny of existing practice might be of assistance is in the use of accessible information and communication technologies in the recruitment and hiring processes.[76] As Internet access becomes more common, businesses are becoming network-intensive. Web applications can pose barriers for those with vision, hearing, or dexterity-related disabilities, and most Web sites are not designed to be accessible to people with disabilities. Therefore, information on the accessibility of the company's online recruitment process, as well as internal e-communications use, must now become a regular part of any self-assessment of compliance with employment disability nondiscrimination requirements.

The strength of the use of organizational reports and related data is that they may contain much more objective and reliable information about the impact of organizational practices than organizational self-report from interviews alone provides. In addition, if kept by multiple organizations, it may make comparisons across organizations possible. This can provide much-needed benchmarks to assist in setting standards and comparisons to help organizations correct their policies and practices that disparately disadvantage people with disabilities and other minority groups.

The drawback of relying on such an approach is that these kinds of records are not consistently available within all organizations, and even if kept, not always reliably documented among units, departments, and divisions of the organization. The most significant impediment is that organizations are often reluctant to share such records and data. Finally, organizational confidentiality considerations and/or national legal personnel record privacy requirements may prevent even those that are willing to share from doing so.

In addition, getting sufficient data on disability employment nondiscrimination and inclusion can be challenging. At the heart of the disability inclusion strategy are the organizational ability, willingness, and comfort to gather disability-related data from employees and link it to the employee who reports it in varying levels of specificity (e.g., whether to link information to individual employees or simply report metrics in the aggregate, such as by department). It is important for both employers and researchers to be aware of the regulatory requirements that govern workplace disability and confidentiality issues. This interplay between the incentives and challenges of implementing, and furthering a disability inclusion strategy has produced a continuum of organizations that contains, on the one hand, organizations that do not collect any data and, on the other, organizations that have successfully—and skillfully—collected and used it to develop and advance their disability inclusion strategies.

6. MEASUREMENTS OF WORKPLACE CLIMATE

6.1 Workplace Climate and Disability Inclusion

How does a company's "culture"—values, norms, policies, and practices— facilitate or hinder the employment of people with disabilities? Although it appears that at present disability is still not at the forefront of most organizations' diversity strategy, some gains are being made. In a 2009 study jointly conducted by Linkage and the Novations Group, respondents indicated that age and disability would increase in importance for diversity and inclusion as the aging population expands and organizations advocating for both these groups become more prominent.[77] Respondents reported that disability has been the forgotten diversity issue, but that this will change with the expansion of disability advocacy groups. In addition, because of their sheer numbers, senior citizens were also seen as becoming a force in society.[78] Bjelland and coworkers investigated the nature of employment discrimination charges that cite the ADA or ADEA individually or jointly. They found that claims that originate from older or disabled workers are concentrated within a subset of issues that include reasonable accommodation, retaliation, and termination. Bjelland and coworkers as well as Nafukho, Roessler, and Kacirek emphasize the importance of workplace culture as a critical factor in supporting a diverse workforce, which also includes consideration of various forms of disability.[79]

The focus of this chapter is both hiring and retaining individuals with disabilities in the workforce. Those who do become employed still experience lower pay, less job security and training, fewer opportunities for advancement, and lower levels of participation in decision making than do non-disabled employees.[80] Post-hire engagement and employment success are critical factors in continued employment and the ability of persons with disabilities to be economically self-sufficient. Yet globally, research examining within-organization, post-hire factors that impact the employment outcomes of persons with disabilities has been limited. Research has more often focused on identifying organizational policies and practices that should be implemented to improve these outcomes, but relatively little is yet known about their effectiveness, or about the more informal, non-policy factors that determine the employment outcomes of persons with disabilities. The limited research that has been conducted to date addressing the role of corporate culture has primarily been based on laboratory studies and employer surveys.[81] Sometimes proxy job applicants are used to study bias—individuals who enter into the application process declaring their minority status either by appearance or demographic information presented in resumes.

Two nationally representative employer surveys in the United States on disability issues found that one fifth of employers report that attitudes are a major barrier to the employment of people with disabilities.[82] These figures likely are understated due to social desirability bias in responding to surveys; that is, there are frequently discrepancies between attitudes that employers express toward people with disabilities on surveys and their actual hiring practices.[83] As previously described, research results from a prior study on climate and inclusion for people with disabilities suggested that although policies are indeed critical, other factors within the organization play a significant role in determining the employment outcomes.[84]

Research conducted by a consortium led by Syracuse University carried out in-depth case studies of six organizations in an effort to identify how company policies and practices, climate, managerial attitudes and styles, coworker attitudes, and group processes influence the experiences and engagement of persons with disabilities. The companies were part of a larger group that volunteered to participate in focus groups and interviews to inform the creation of a rigorous method of conducting and benchmarking case studies. The companies selected for the actual case studies were picked from this larger group to ensure variation in characteristics such as sector and size. Results showed that organizational climate and culture, inclusive managerial behaviors, and the biases or attitudes of supervisors and coworkers are key factors affecting the employment of people with disabilities. Compared with employees without disabilities, persons with disabilities experience the organization as being less inclusive, perceive HR practices as being less fair, suffer from lower-quality relationships with their managers, experience lower levels of fit between their skills and the demands of the job, and are overall less satisfied and more likely to turn over.[85] However, the research also confirmed that the experiences of people with disabilities are significantly enhanced when their work climates are inclusive and their managers are also inclusive in their supervisory tactics. People with disabilities involved in high-quality relationships with their managers are more likely to feel fairly treated during the accommodation process, feel psychologically empowered, experience greater subjective fit between the demands of the job and their skills, and experience lower levels of harassment from coworkers and supervisors, thereby suggesting that managers confer "safe passages" to individuals with disabilities by establishing high-quality relationships with them.[86]

As a result, measurement of organizational culture or climate may be another source of information of how and where discrimination is occurring in a work environment. This information might be captured by gaining access to the results of surveys previously conducted by the company, if access to such data is afforded for external research purposes. An alternative would be that the external researchers, working in partnership with the business, conduct a workplace climate survey more broadly, and/or a survey or interviews of selected organizational informants regarding their own attitudes toward persons with disabilities, whether organizational leadership, HR professionals, supervisors/managers, or coworkers. If people with disabilities can be identified in such surveys, comparisons between the perspectives of employees with and without disabilities can also be made by such a survey. Interviews or focus groups can also be conducted with those who self-identify as employees with disabilities.

The strength of such an approach is that it offers complementary qualitative data not available from other sources, and may assist in pinpointing specific areas for intervention. In such an approach, data can be gathered from a variety of sources and informants. Using multiple means of data collection and analysis afford an opportunity to triangulate across different sources of data, thereby compensating for the limitations of any one method. The limitations of such an approach are that feedback is reliant on self-report. In addition, real issues may be understated due to social desirability bias.

7. IMPLICATIONS

It is important to assess how workplace practices may contribute to employment disparities, as well as to understand which parts of the employment process and which disability-related issues give rise to the most significant challenges. Further research on workplace policies and practices that enhance the hiring, retention, advancement, and inclusion of people with disabilities is needed. Preliminary effort in the study of workplace climate factors that enhance or impede inclusion of people with disabilities has only begun.

There is a growing consensus globally that there is a need for more research and reporting related to prevention of discrimination and the promotion of equality for people with disabilities.[87] With an increasingly global economy, a critical next step in understanding where employment disability discrimination is occurring and how to address such discrimination will be to gather such data globally. This means working to create consistent disability measures in national census data that will afford us cross-country comparisons on prevalence rates, employment participation rates, poverty and household incomes, equity in wages, and so forth. This also means having a common definition of disability across countries and cultures that will provide comparable items that will afford such comparisons.

Another area in which increased national attention to more consistent and refined data collection is needed is in employer analytics. Our ability to understand how people with disabilities fare in the employment process compared with their nondisabled peers is significantly compromised by the lack of data for this population kept by organizations about their recruitment, hiring, retention, and advancement efforts. The presence of such employer analytics will make cross-country and across-industry comparisons possible, thereby greatly improving our understanding of how cultural context, including differing regulatory environments, affects the prevalence and nature of workplace disability discrimination. Although disability disclosure is a complicating factor in this process, it is imperative for policymakers to work to find a way to create alternatives that incent companies to better self-assess their progress on increasing workforce participation and promotion of people with disabilities. And, hopefully, in this process, as workplace cultures become truly more inclusive, individuals will rightfully experience the confidence needed to openly disclose the presence of a disability, without the fear of bias and discrimination that has historically inhibited such disclosure.

ACKNOWLEDGMENT

This work was supported in part by a grant to Cornell University for a Rehabilitation Research and Training Center (RRTC) on Employer Practices Related to Employment Outcomes among Individuals with Disabilities (Grant No. H133B100017).

NOTES

1. Butterworth, J., & Strauch, J. (1994). The Relationship Between Social Competence and Success in the Competitive Work Place for Persons with Mental Retardation. *Education and Training in Mental Retardation* 29(2), 118–133.
2. Koser, D.A., Matsuyama, M., & Kopelman, R.E. (1999). Comparison of a Physical and a Mental Disability in Employee Selection: An Experimental Examination of Direct and Moderated Effects. *North American Journal of Psychology* 1, 213–222.
3. Chima, F.O. (1998). Workplace and Disabilities: Opinions on Work, Interpersonal, and Intrapersonal Factors. *Journal of Applied Rehabilitation Counseling* 29(3), 31–37; Duckett, P.S. (2000). Disabling Employment Interviews: Warfare to Work. *Disability & Society* 15(7), 1019–1039.
4. Colella, A., & Stone, D.L. (2005). Workplace Discrimination Toward Persons with Disabilities: A Call for Some New Research Directions. In R.L. Dipboye & A. Colella (Eds.). *Discrimination at Work: The Psychological and Organizational Bases* (Mahwah, NJ: Lawrence Erlbaum Associates), 221–246.
5. Waters, L.E., & Moore, K.A. (2002). Self-esteem, Appraisal, and Coping: A Comparision of Unemployed and Reemployed People. *Journal of Organizational Behaviour* 23(5), 593–604.
6. Evans, J., & Repper, J. (2000). Employment, Social Inclusion and Mental Health. *Journal of Psychiatric and Mental Health* 7(1), 15–24.
7. Doyle, C., Kavanagh, P., Metcalfe, O., & Lavin, T. (2005). *Health Impacts of Employment: A Review* (Dublin, Ireland: Institute of Public Health in Ireland).
8. Harnois, G., & Gabriel, P. (2000). *Mental Health and Work: Impact, Issues, and Good Practices* (Geneva, Switzerland: World Health Organization and International Labour Organization).
9. Dooley, D., Catalano, R., & Wilson, G. (1994). Depression and Unemployment: Panel Findings from the Epidemiologic Catchment Area Study. *American Journal of Community Psychology* 22(6), 745–765.
10. Karpur, A., Bjelland, M.J., & Bruyere, S.M. (2010). Public Health Considerations of People with Disabilities. In M. Finkel (Ed.). *Public Health in the 21st Century, Vol 1: Global Issues in Public Health.*, (Santa Barbara, CA: Praeger Press), 181–208.
11. Sullivan, D., & Von Wachter, T. (2009). Job displacement and mortality: an analysis using administrative data. *Quarterly Journal of Economics* 124(3), 1265–1306.
12. Erickson, W., Lee, C., & von Schrader, S. (2011). *Disability Statistics from the 2009 American Community Survey (ACS)* (Ithaca, NY: Cornell University).

13. Ibid.
14. Baldwin, M.L., & Johnson, W.G. (1994). Labor Market Discrimination Against Men with Disabilities. *Journal of Human Resources* 29(1), 1–19.
15. She P., & Livermore, G.A. (2009). Long-Term Poverty and Disability Among Working-Age Adults. Journal of Disability Policy Studies 19(4), 244–256.
16. O'Reilly, A. (2003). The Right to Decent Work of Persons with Disabilities. Skills Working Paper No. 14 (Geneva, Switzerland: International Labour Organization).
17. National Science Foundation (1998). *Women, Minorities, and Persons with Disabilities in Science and Engineering* (Arlington, VA: National Science Foundation).
18. Statistics Canada (1991). *Health and Activity Limitations Survey* (Ottawa, Canada: Statistics Canada).
19. Human Resources Development Canada (1996). *Living with Disability in Canada—An Economic Portrait* (Ottawa, Canada: Human Resources Development Canada).
20. Australian Bureau of Statistics (1997). *Australian Social Trends 1997: Work— Paid Work: Employment of People with a Handicap*. 1997 (Canberra, Australia: Australian Bureau of Statistics).
21. Organisation for Economic Co-Operation and Development (2010). *Sickness, Disability, and Work* (Paris, France: OECD).
22. Mont, D. (2007). Measuring disability prevalence. Discussion Paper No. 0706 Washington, D.C.: World Bank.
23. World Health Organization, 58th Assembly (2005). Resolution WHA 58.23. May 25. Retrieved on February 15, 2013, from: http://www.who.int/disabilities/WHA5823_resolution_en.pdf
24. Mitra S., & Sambamoorthi, U. (2006). Employment of Persons with Disabilities: Evidence from the National Sample Survey. *Economic and Political Weekly* 41(3), 199–203.
25. Centre for Strategy and Evaluation Services (2007). *Non-discrimination Mainstreaming: Instruments, Case Studies and Way Forwards* (Kent, United Kingdom: Centre for Strategy and Evaluation Services); Degener, T., & Quinn, G. (2002). *A Survey of International Comparative, and Regional Law Reform*. Human Rights and Disability (New York: United Nations); Dixon, J., & Hyde, M. (2010). Legislation (Disability Rights in a Global Setting). In Center for International Rehabilitation Research Information and Exchange (Ed.), *International Encyclopedia of Rehabilitation*. Retrieved on February 15, 2013, from: http://cirrie.buffalo.edu/encyclopedia/en/article/24; Kanter, A. (2003). The Globalization of Disability Rights Law. *Syracuse Journal of International Law and Commerce* 30, 241–269; Waddington, L., & Diller, M. (2000). Tensions and Coherence in Disability Policy: The Uneasy Relationship Between Social Welfare and Civil Rights Models of Disability in American, European, and International Employment Law. In M. Breslin & S. Yee (Eds.). Disability Rights Law and Policy: International and National Perspectives (Ardsley, NY: Transnational Publishers), 241–256; Meyerson, A., & Yee, S. (2001). The ADA and Models of Equality. *Ohio State Law Journal* 62, 535–554.
26. Green, E. (2007). *How to Measure Progress in Combating Discrimination and Promoting Equality: Country Report on Finland* (Brussels, Belgium: BPI); Turkish Prime Ministry (2010). *The Research on Measurement of Disability Discrimination* (Ankara, Turkey: Government of Turkey).

27. Waterhouse, P., Kimberley, H., Jonas, P., and Glover, J. (2010). *What Would It Take? Employer Perspectives on Employing People with a Disability* (Adelaide, Australia: National Centre for Vocational Education Research), p. 3.
28. Ibid.
29. Clayton, S. (2012). Effectiveness of Return-to-work Interventions for Disabled People: a Systematic Review of Government Initiatives Focused on Changing the Behaviour of Employers. *European Journal of Public Health* 22(3), 434–439.
30. Confederation of Indian Industries (2009). *A Values Route to Business Success: The Why and How of Employing Persons with Disabilities* (Bangalore, India: Confederation of Indian Industries); Employers Forum on Disability (n.d.). *Catalog of Publications* (London, United Kingdom: Employers' Forum on Disability).
31. Simkiss, P. (2005). Will I Keep My job?—Disability Management for Employment Retention. *International Congress Series* 1282, 1186–1190.
32. World Health Organization & World Bank (2011). *World Report on Disability* (Geneva, Switzerland: World Health Organization); Quinn, G., & Degener, T. (2002). *The Current Use and Future Potential of the United Nations Rights Instruments in the Context of Disability* (Geneva, Switzerland, and New York: United Nations).
33. McMahon, B., Edwards, R., Rumrill, P.D., & Hursh, N. (2005). An Overview of the National EEOC ADA Research Project. *Work* 25(1), 1–7.
34. Roessler, R.T., Hurley, J.E., & McMahon, B.T. (2010). A Comparison of Allegations and Resolutions Involving Issues of Discharge Versus Constructive Discharge: Implications for Diversity Management. *Advances in Developing Human Resources* 12 (4), 407–428.
35. Rumrill P.D., & Fitzgerald, S.M. (2010). Employer Characteristics and Discharge-Related Discrimination Against People With Disabilities Under the Americans With Disabilities Act. *Advances in Developing Human Resources* 12(4), 448–465.
36. Rumrill, P.D., Fitzgerald, S.M., & McMahon, B.T. (2010). ADA Title I Allegations Related to Unlawful Discharge: Characteristics of Charging Parties. *Advances in Developing Human Resources* 12(4), 429–447.
37. Bruyère, S., von Schrader, S., Coduti, W., & Bjelland, M.J. (2010) United States employment disability discrimination charges: Implications for disability management practice. *International Journal of Disability Management* 5(2), 48–58. © 2010 Cambridge University Press. Reprinted with permission.
38. Bruyere, S.M., Erickson, W.A., & VanLooy, S.A. (2000). HR's Role in Managing Disability in the Workplace. *Employment Relations Today* Autumn, 27(3) 47–66.
39. Flood, K. (n.d.). Poll: HR-to-staff Ratios Holding Steady. *BLR.com News*. Retrieved February 15, 2013, from http://hr.blr.com/whitepapers/HR-Administration/HR-Management/Poll-HR-to-Staff-Ratios-Holding-Steady; Dooney, J., and Smith, N. (2005). *SHRM Human Capital Benchmarking Study. Executive Summary* (Alexandria, VA: Society for Human Resource Management).
40. See Society for Human Resource Management (2011). Staffing the Human Resource Function. SHRM Templates and Toolkits. Retrieved on February 15, 2013, from http://www.shrm.org/TemplatesTools/Toolkits/Pages/StaffingHRFunction.aspx; Wexler, S. (2010). How Many Employees Do You Have—and Should You Have—in Your Organization? *I4CP. com Newsletter*. Retrieved on February 15, 2013, from www.i4cp.com/productivity-blog/2010/05/21/how-many-hr-employees.

41. SHRM was founded in 1948, currently has 575 affiliated chapters representing more than 250,000 members in over 140 countries, and as such is the world's largest association devoted to HR management SHRM's membership covers the full range of HR professionals from HR Vice Presidents and Directors to HR managers and staff. Further information can be found at the SHRM website at www.shrm.org.
42. Bruyère, S., Erickson, W., & Ferrentino, J. (2003). Identity and Disability in the Workplace. *William and Mary Law Review* 44(3), 1173–1196.
43. Erickson, W., von Schrader, S., Bruyere, S., Esen, R., & Boyd, R. (2012). Leading HR Practices in Improving Outcomes for Individuals with Disabilities. Working paper.
44. Federal sector organizations are covered under the Rehabilitation Act of 1973. Bruyere, S.M., & Horne, R. (1999). *Disability Employment Policies and Practices in U.S. Federal Government Agencies. Report by the Presidential Task Force on Employment of Adults with Disabilities* (Ithaca, NY: Cornell University); Bruyère, S., Erickson, W., & Horne, R. (2002). *Disability Employment Policies and Practices in U.S. Federal Government Agencies: EEO/HR and Supervisor Perspectives. Report by the Presidential Task Force on Employment of Adults with Disabilities* (Ithaca, NY: Cornell University).
45. Bruyère, Erickson, & Horne (2002). Disability Employment Policies and Practices.
46. The HR membership organizational partner for this study was the Chartered Institute of Personnel Development (CIPD), in London, United Kingdom; for further information, see http://www.cipd.co.uk/
47. Bruyere, S.M., Erickson, W.A., & VanLooy, S. (2004). Comparative Study of Workplace Policy and Practices Contributing to Disability Nondiscrimination. *Rehabilitation Psychology* 49(1), 28–38.
48. Bruyère, S. Erickson, E., & VanLooy, S. (2006). The impact of business size on employer ADA response. *Rehabilitation Counseling Bulletin* 49(4), 194–206. © 2006 Sage publications. Reprinted with permission.
49. Bruyère, S.M. (2000). Disability Employment Policies and Practices in Private and Federal Sector Organizations (Ithaca, NY: Cornell University). Reprinted with permission.
50. Linkow, P., Barrington, L., Bruyère, S., Figueroa, Y., & Wright, M. (2013). Leveling the playing field: Attracting, engaging, and advancing people with disabilities. New York: The Conference Board. Retrieved from http://digitalcommons.ilr.cornell.edu/edicollect/1292/
51. The Conference Board (2007) *Middle Managers: Engaging and Enrolling the Biggest Roadblock to Diversity and Inclusion* (New York: The Conference Board).
52. Gates, L. (1993). The Role of the Supervisor in Successful Adjustment to Work with a Disabling Condition: Issues for Disability Policy and Practice. *Journal of Occupational Rehabilitation* 3(4), 179–190.
53. Bruyère, Erickson, & Horne (2002). Disability Employment Policies and Practices.
54. Ibid.
55. Ibid.
56. Nishii, L., & Bruyère, S. (2009). Protecting Employees with Disabilities from Discrimination on the Job: The Role of Unit Managers from Workpalce Policies and Practices Minimizing Disability Discrimination: Implications for Psychology. Presented at the 117th Annual Convention of the American Psychological Association (Toronto, Canada), August 6-9.

57. Nishii, L.H., Bruyere, S.M., & VanLooy, S.A. (2009). *Organizational Policies and Practices for People with Disabilities: Summary of Survey Results, Interviews, and Focus Groups* (Ithaca, NY: Cornell University).
58. Turkish Prime Ministry (2010). *The Research on Measurement of Disability Discrimination.*
59. Nishii, L.H., & Wright, P. (2008). Variability at Multiple Levels of Analysis: Implications for Strategic Human Resource Management. In D.B. Smith (Ed.). *The People Make the Place* (Mahwah, NJ: Lawrence Erlbaum Associates), 225–248.
60. Kulkarni, M., &Valk, R. (2010). Don't Ask, Don't Tell: Two Views on Human Resource Practices for People with Disabilities. *IIMB Management Review* 22(4), 137–146.
61. Kulkarni, M., & Lengnick-Hall, M.L. (2011). Socialization of People with Disabilities in the Workplace. *Human Resource Management* 50(4), 521–540.
62. von Schrader, S., Malzer, V., & Bruyere, S.M. (2011). Perspectives on disability disclosure: The importance of employer practices and workplace climate. *Employee Responsibilities and Rights Journal.Doi 10.1007/s10672-013-9227-9. Retrieved from http://link.springer.com/content/pdf/10.1007%2Fs10672-013-9227-9.pdf*
63. Ibid.
64. Ibid. p. 18
65. Bressler, R.B., & Lacy, A.W. (1980). An Analysis of the Relative Job Progression of the Perceptibly Physically Handicapped. *The Academy of Management Journal* 23(1), 132–143.
66. Davenport, T.H., Harris, J., & Shapiro, J. (2010). Competing on talent analytics. *Harvard Business Review* 88(10), 52–58.
67. Lawler, E.E. III, Levenson, A., & Boudreau, J.W. (2004). HR Metrics and Analytics: Use and Impact. *Human Resource Planning* 27(4), 27–35.
68. Society for Human Resource Management (2010). *Workplace Diversity Practices: How Has Diversity and Inclusion Changed over Time?* (Alexandria, VA: Society for Human Resource Management).
69. U.S. Department of Labor (n.d.). Hiring: Affirmative Action. *U.S. Department of Labor*. Retrieved on February 15, 2013, from http://www.dol.gov/dol/topic/hiring/affirmativeact.htm.
70. Notice of Proposed Rulemaking (n.d.). *Affirmative Action and Nondiscrimination Obligations of Contractors and Subcontractors Regarding Individuals with Disabilities.* 76 Fed. Reg. 77056 (2011).
71. Stein, M., & Stein, P. (2007). Beyond Disability Civil Rights. *Hastings Law Journal* 58, 1203–1240.
72. Eichhors, W., et al. (2010). *The Mobility and Integration of People with Disabilities into the Labour Market* (Brussels, Belgium: European Parliament).
73. World Health Organization & World Bank (2011). *World Report on Disability.*
74. Burkhauser, R.V., Butler, J., & Kim, Y. (1995). The Importance of Employer Accommodation on the Job Duration of Workers with Disabilities: A Hazard Model Approach. *Labour Economics* 3(1): 1–22; Wynne, R. & Mcananey, D. (2004). *Employment and Disability : Back to Work Strategies* (Dublin, Ireland: Eurofound).
75. Wynne, R., & McAnaney, D. (2009). Preventing Social Exclusion Through Illness or Disability: Models of Good Practice. *Work* 32(1), 95–103.
76. Bruyère, S.M., Erickson, W., & VanLooy, S. (2006). Information technology (IT) accessibility: Implications for employment of people with disabilities. *Work* 27(4), 397–405.

77. Novations Group and Linkage (2009). *The Changing Face of Diversity and Inclusion: Then, Now, and Tomorrow* (Boston, MA: Novations Group and Linkage).
78. Ibid.
79. Bjelland, M.J., et al. (2010). Age and disability employment discrimination: Occupational rehabilitation implications. *Journal of Occupational Rehabilitation* 20(4), 456–471; Nafukho, F.M., Roessler, R.T., and Kacirek, K. (2010). Disability as a diversity factor: Implications for human resource practices. *Advances in Developing Human Resources* 12(4), 395–406.
80. Schur, L., Kruse, D., & Blanck, P. (2005). Corporate culture and the employment of persons with disabilities. *Behavioral Sciences and the Law* 23(1), 3–20.
81. Blanck, P., & Schartz, H. (2005). Special issue: Corporate culture and disability. *Behavioral Sciences and the Law* 23(1), 1–2; Schur, Kruse, & Blanck (2005). Corporate culture and the employment of persons with disabilities.
82. Bruyere, S.M. (2000). *Disability Employment Policies and Practices*; Dixon, K.A., Kruse, D., & Van Horn, C.E. (2003). *Restricted Access: A Survey of Employers About People with Disabilities and Lowering Barriers to Work.* (New Brunswick, NJ: Rutgers University Heldrich Center for Workforce Development).
83. Wilgosh, L.R., & Skaret, D. (1987). Employer attitudes toward hiring individuals with disabilities: A review of the recent literature. *Canadian Journal of Rehabilitation* 1(2), 89–98.
84. Nishii, Bruyere, & VanLooy (2009). Organizational Policies and Practices for People with Disabilities.
85. Disability Case Study Research Consortium (2008). *Conducting and benchmarking inclusive employment policies, practices, and culture* (Washington, D.C.: Disability Case Study Research Consortium).
86. Nishii & Bruyère (2009). Protecting Employees with Disabilities; Nishii, L. (2009). *The inclusion and engagement of employees: The role of climate for inclusion.* (Ithaca, NY: Cornell University).
87. Green (2007). *How to Measure Progress*; Turkish Prime Ministry (2010). The Research on Measurement of Disability Discrimination.

CHAPTER 4

Working with Employers to Improve "Disability Confidence"

The Business Disability Forum

MEGAN GALEUCIA

1. INTRODUCTION

The Business Disability Forum (BDF),[1] a non-profit organization located in London, offers a unique model for promoting more equitable employment for persons with disabilities that involves providing services to a membership base of nearly 400 employers in the private and public sectors and across all industries. According to the organization its members, which include United Kingdom-based as well as global corporations, together employ approximately 20% of the UK workforce.[2]

The BDF's strategy centers on involving employers and leveraging the influence of high-profile executives to implement more equitable employment practices. Although the BDF's success has been in many ways dependent on the particular historical and legal context and business culture of the United Kingdom, its model can arguably be replicated in other contexts because it is not dependent on having specific public policies in place. Businesses that have joined the BDF and maintained their membership have improved their overall performance over time. Some businesses' advancements have been especially significant, and an exceptional few organizations have emerged as exemplary leaders on disability as it affects businesses, acting as role models in the business community.

This report is a case study on the Business Disability Forum and aims to understand how the organization achieves its goal of making it easier for businesses[3] to promote equal employment opportunities for people with disabilities and serve disabled customers.

1.2 Context: Disability and Employment in the United Kingdom

Of the more than 10 million people living with disabilities in the United Kingdom, 5.1 million are working age.[4] Yet, as of 2011 the employment rate of people with disabilities remains only 48.8%, compared with 77.5% for non-disabled people.[5] According to the Sayce Report, a report on employment support for people with disabilities in the United Kingdom, disabled people are twice as likely to live in poverty than nondisabled people.[6]

In 1995, the Disability Discrimination Act (DDA), the first piece of rights-based legislation protecting people with disabilities in the United Kingdom, was passed. The DDA makes it unlawful to discriminate against people with disabilities. Furthermore, employers and service providers are required by the Act to make reasonable adjustments for disabled individuals;[7] adjustments may include reconstructing premises, reallocating duties, modifying working hours, providing equipment, and offering support services.[8] In 2010, the Equality Act came into effect; it aimed to simplify the existing legislation by bringing several pieces of nondiscrimination law together under a single act. As part of the new legislation, in April 2011, an updated general Public Sector Equality Duty came into force, replacing the previously separate race, disability, and gender equality duties.[9]

Despite these legislative advancements, the present is not without its challenges. The Conservative-Liberal Democrat coalition government, formed after the 2010 UK general election, vowed to cut back on public expenditure accompanying the global recession and a prevailing uncertain economic climate. This resulted in major changes to spending and programs, including those for disabled people.[10] According to the Sayce Report on disability and employment in the United Kingdom, current research illustrates that "existing programs do not provide a clear continuum of support" for disabled people.[11]

In terms of employment, funding for the Employment and Support Allowance has been tightened significantly.[12] Claimants are being re-interviewed, and those deemed able to work are given less public support when looking for work and receive a reduction of their benefits after 12 months. Funding for the Access to Work scheme, which provides employers with funds to make reasonable adjustments for disabled employees, has also been reduced.[13] In addition to a lack of adequate support programs, UK employers are arguably not equipped with adept knowledge of the legal and benefits system. The Sayce Report calls for employment support to "make it as easy as possible for employers to employ disabled people. This means that employers must know where to go for help, and support should be delivered quickly and with as little cost to employers as possible."[14]

The prevailing situation provides essential context to the Business Disability Forum, affecting how its work unfolds in the face of benefit cuts and funding squeezes.

2. METHODOLOGY

2.1 Analytical Framework

There is no universally accepted definition of disability in the United Kingdom. The Equality Act (2010) states that a disabled person is someone with "a physical or mental impairment, which has a substantial and long-term adverse effect on his ability to carry out normal day-to-day activities."[15] It is furthermore important to note that "people are 'disabled' by barriers to participation—from low expectations to inaccessible IT or the built environment."[16] In line with the social model of disability and the language used by user-controlled organizations, the term "disabled people" is generally used in the United Kingdom when referring to disabled people as a group, irrespective of specific impairment.[17] Both the terms "disabled" and "people with disabilities" are used in this report with the acknowledgement that people living with disability or long-term health conditions have a diversity of experiences and define their own experience in various ways.

2.2 Data Collection

This case study was conducted using qualitative research methods to describe and analyze the selected organization and its influence on employers' performance on disability. Forty-five semi-structured interviews were conducted with board members, senior executives, managerial staff, colleagues, representatives from the Forum's members, and Disabled Associates of the Forum. Interviews were also conducted with representatives from disability charities and other stakeholders to provide a contextualized understanding of the Forum's external functions and influence. All interviews were voluntary and participants were asked for their oral consent. Data from the interviews was transcribed, systematically coded, and analyzed.

In addition to interviews, publications, reports, and evaluations provided by the Forum, employers, and other stakeholders were reviewed and analyzed. Participant observation and direct observation of meetings and events, where available and appropriate, provided two complementary data collection methods.

2.3 Participants

The BDF staff provided information about their members and oftentimes facilitated contact with primary and secondary contacts from member organizations. A particular effort was made to interview a cross-section of members representing both the public and private sectors as well as all areas of industry. When possible, more than one representative from member organizations was interviewed.

2.4 Limitations

During the summer of 2011, the BDF had between 350 and 400 members. Given the sheer multitude of members and the relatively small size of the interview sample, it is important to note that the views of member representatives and data about member organizations in this report are not truly representative of all businesses or BDF members in any particular sector or industry.

3. THE BUSINESS DISABILITY FORUM

3.1 Background

The Forum was founded by its current chief executive, Susan Scott-Parker, in 1980, with the support of business-led charity Business in the Community and the Prince of Wales Advisory Group. Before the establishment of the Forum, Canadian-born Scott-Parker had been commissioned by the Alberta government to design a campaign to persuade employers to hire disabled individuals. Scott-Parker insisted that employers be consulted and involved in developing this campaign. She recounted that at the time it was unprecedented to ask "a target audience to comment on messages that were designed to influence them."[18]

Scott-Parker argues that, "[E]mployers who wanted to do well didn't know where to find the candidates; the candidates didn't actually appear at the right time, with the right skills, for the right jobs" and "secondly, employers don't know where to go for employer-relevant information. . . . There isn't anywhere to go for help if something goes wrong after they have hired the individual."[19] This led Scott-Parker to establish an employer-centered forum: "I suggested to a small group of senior executives... 'why don't we set up an employers' organization that will focus on making it easier for the employer, the well-intentioned employer, to employ disabled people and keep people who have become disabled?' "[20] What ensued from this discussion was the creation of the Business Disability Forum.

Originally consisting of just five original UK-based employers—the first members—and a small core staff team, the BDF has evolved significantly in size and reach over the years. Today the organization has a staff team of about 35 employees and a current membership list that includes more than

350 employers, representing a variety of private and public industries and sectors. Employers join the Forum to improve their performance on disability and gain access to expert advice and knowledge. Through their annual membership fees, the members fund the Forum's activities almost in their entirety.

3.2 Mission, Objectives, and Values

The Forum's primary aim is to make it easier for employers to recruit and retain disabled employees and conduct business with disabled customers. The Forum carries out its mission by offering comprehensive advice, publications, training, support, and assessments to businesses that join as members.

Underlying the Forum's mission is this crucial component: All of its activities are designed to mutually benefit employers and people with disabilities. As Scott-Parker affirms, "The entire premise of this organization is mutual benefit. Disabled people must benefit and the business community must benefit."[21]

Scott-Parker emphasizes the Engage-Equip-Deliver model as a foundation of the BDF's operations. Engage-Equip-Deliver is based on the idea that employers are involved in a process whereby they must first be persuaded to want to improve their performance on disability; then be given the tools to learn how to improve their business practices; and finally, they reach a point of delivering best practice by reaching out to disabled applicants and effectively reengineering the way they work with intermediary disability organizations that help disabled people into jobs.[22] "Best practice" describes an organizational state that a company attains when it has removed all the barriers for disabled people and provided all reasonable adjustments. The Forum contends that best practice involves exceeding legal compliance in order to create the best experience for their disabled applicants, employees, and customers as well as to minimize the risk of litigation being brought against them.

The BDF believes that two important ideological shifts are integral to fulfilling its vision. One shift concerns reframing negative beliefs about disability and employment. The Forum works to transform business's views from those that relate disability to legal compliance, risk, and incapacity to investment in human potential, capability, and equal opportunities.[23] The other shift entails challenging the common tendency of disability nonprofits, service providers, and the government to frame the employer as avaricious, uneducated, and discriminatory. The Forum believes this negative assumption about employers is widely fallacious and certainly not productive;[24] the Forum aims to reposition the employer from adversary to valued stakeholder and potential partner.

3.3 Funding

The Forum is a not-for-profit registered charity. A unique aspect of the Forum's structure is its revenue model. Since its creation, the Forum has primarily been funded by its members, for about 80% to 85% of its total revenue.[25] Other revenue streams, primarily the sales of publications and licenses and income generated from trainings and events, comprise the remaining funding.[26]

Notably, over the years, the Forum has refrained from seeking government, European Union, or philanthropic funding. Susan Scott-Parker comments on this decision:

> We've avoided government money on the grounds that we're established in order to demonstrate that employers can be trusted to take this issue seriously enough to invest in self-improvement.... The other thing is that we've had some conversations with government in the past and they always wanted us to guarantee that our members would hire 2000 disabled people for the money. [BDF] cannot control what its members do.... [G]overnment money is rarely given to an organization simply so that they can capacity build. They always want peopling jobs as a result.[27]

She adds that although it is a charity, the BDF does not accept charitable donations either:

> We've never gone for charitable donations on the grounds that it's unlikely we'll get a charitable donation when some of the richest companies are on the membership list....I was always concerned and we must remain so with not taking monies that would ordinarily go directly to people with disabilities who need it.[28]

4. STRATEGIES

The Business Disability Forum has pioneered a wide range of strategies that form a distinct approach to increasing the employment opportunities for people with disabilities in the United Kingdom.

4.1 Structural Organization

Before enumerating the Forum's strategies, it is important to note that the structural organization of the Business Disability Forum is an important feature of its capacity to influence businesses. Like many nonprofits, its structure includes a Board of Trustees, Chief Executive, senior management team, and several additional staff members.

4.1.1 Membership

As an employers' organization, the BDF could not exist without the many employers that enroll as members and pay fees to access BDF services and resources. Business Disability Forum membership is not obligatory for employers in the United Kingdom; rather, members join of their own accord. They include employers from both the private and public sectors and across a variety of industries, and range in size and experience. Although the majority of members are UK-based organizations, several operate globally and a few, such as Toronto Dominion Bank Group of Canada, have joined the BDF to access its services and toolkits even though they are located in other countries.

Members are categorized as either Gold or Standard. The distinction between these two categories of membership is purely fiscal, not based on achievement. Gold Members pay higher fees—between $14,000 and $20,000, compared with $2,750 for standard—and receive additional services and benefits such as free admission to many of the BDF's events and trainings.[29]

4.1.2 The Disabled Associates

The BDF has also strategically established a network of more than 30 Disabled Associates, who are individuals with disabilities as well as business professionals and experts in their field. They work with BDF in contributing to events and publications, consulting with members, and providing advice and feedback on the Forum's initiatives. There is no formal recruitment and selection process; rather, outstanding disabled individuals are asked to become associates of the organization typically after interacting with BDF staff at events or collaborating with the organization on various projects and activities.

4.2 The Business Case

First, in order to impact the performance and attitudes of employers, the Forum must persuade employers that disability is an issue that affects all aspects of their business. Kate Nash, a Disabled Associate who also runs her own consultancy specializing in developing disabled employee networks, explains:

> For so many years there's been nothing other than disability charities; however well meaning they are, their existence meant to most of the [United Kingdom]

that disability is a charity issue, an altruistic issue, a philanthropic issue. And the [BDF] have been really able to cut into that to help employers see it as a business issue, whether that's about employing disabled talent or whether it's about making sure services and goods are designed to be accessible . . . it's about recasting it in a completely different angle of disability.[30]

One of the strongest aspects of the business case is the commercial benefits of being an accessible, inclusive business. Not hiring disabled individuals means missing out on a "tremendous talent pool," explains David Goodchild, Director of Business Development at BDF.[31] It also results in higher employee productivity and retention, and thus, reduced costs. Furthermore, if a business produces inaccessible goods and services they will be alienating an entire demographic of potential customers, disabled individuals. When the BDF Business Development team meets with potential members, they will often cite the figure that disabled people in the United Kingdom have £80 billion (US $124 billion) spending power.

Being a disability confident business will also have a positive effect on the company's reputation and legal protection. "Disability confidence" means understanding and thinking ahead about the needs of people with disabilities throughout the process of hiring employees and designing products and services, fostering business-wide inclusion and awareness. Not complying with the law by failing to make reasonable adjustments for employees and customers, for example, may result in significant legal, financial, and reputational costs to a company.

The business case is different for every organization. It depends on how they prioritize what matters to them and how they see people with disabilities figuring into their business: Will training staff to understand disability make their services more accessible? Will ensuring that their company retains disabled employees who have many years of experience save them money? Will developing their reputation as a disability-inclusive business appeal to investors and shareholders? These are all important considerations that a business must make. Developing a tailored business case, with the help of BDF staff, appeals to potential members because it shows that the Forum understands their business. "You have to contextualize it, if that makes sense. What I wouldn't do is simply say to them, 'you've got to employ disabled people, it's a disgrace that you don't'—it never works!" advises Disabled Associate, Rick Williams.[32]

Among interview participants from member organizations a frequent explanation why their businesses joined the BDF was that it was the right thing to do—an ethical rationale—and several expressed their organization's need for assistance and guidance on disability.[33] Interviewees from organizations that recently joined the BDF tended to emphasize wanting to be compliant with the law. It was common among public sector members to refer to the

Public Sector Equality Duty, set out in the Equality Act, which legally obliges public sector bodies to consider the impact of their work and services on disadvantaged groups, including disabled people, and to take action to tackle discrimination. Organizations that deliver public services must demonstrate that they have designed those services and reviewed them while taking into consideration the needs and views and experiences of these groups.[34]

Helen Chipchase, the Disability Care Lead at British Telecom (BT) discusses the telecommunication company's business case:

> The reason we would have joined would have been the reason why we still know this is important is we want to do better business; and we do better business by understanding the needs of all of our customers rather than excluding the needs of a bunch of them, and that's really always been our business case. And we want the best talent, regardless of whether that person has a disability or not.[35]

4.3 Strategic Positioning

In addition to developing the business case for disability equity and confidence, the Forum has situated itself strategically in order to maximize its impact on employers and contribute to social change.

4.3.1 What Is the Business Disability Forum?

Unlike many nonprofits in the disability field, the Business Disability Forum does not directly work with disabled individuals. Instead, by changing employers' and colleagues' attitudes and behaviors concerning disability in the workplace and refuting misconceptions about hiring people with disabilities, the Forum aspires to improve employment for people with disabilities indirectly.

The BDF's positioning is distinctive because it is neither a conventional disability charity nor a business confederation. Susan Scott-Parker calls it a hybrid:

> We are an employers' organization like the Confederation of British Industry in that we are led and funded entirely by the employer community, particularly the private sector.... But our job is to persuade the company to pay to join something that tells them that they've got it wrong on an issue that the[ir] board does not regard as important.[36]

Members are involved and invited to shape the Forum's activities by giving feedback and effectively voting with their dollar by renewing their membership each year. At the same time, however, the Forum continuously challenges its members, which is hardly customary for an employers' confederation.

4.3.2 Working with Employers, Not against Them

Another angle of the Forum's positioning is that employers are neither obliged to join the Forum nor required to deliver any results. It is instead a space where they can learn and share their experience. Scott-Parker adds, "How do you help a blind person fill in the form? How do you welcome a deaf customer, and so on? Very practical things that people find helpful because it gives them permission to talk about the fact that they don't know."[37] Some members, for instance, have been taken to Employment Tribunals for disability claims made against them, yet they were not expelled from the BDF. "We're here to help them be better, which you can't do by chastising them," explains Senior Disability Consultant, Brendan Roach.[38]

Unfortunately, not demanding any results from employers allows some members to be less engaged. Joy Dearden, also a BDF Disability Consultant, explains the downside of this positioning, "Some of them are doing what they think is the right thing, but they just don't seem to want to engage on what is for us a higher level and network with each other."[39] Nevertheless, the membership fee tends to compel the vast majority of members to improve their performance while allowing them to maintain a sense of autonomy, an attribute that businesses tend to value.

4.3.3 Limiting Its Scope to Achieve Mutual Benefit

Although the organization is also involved in accessible technology projects and lobbying, for example, all of its activities can be traced to disability as it affects business. "I have been absolutely obsessed with making sure that we stay in our domain," says Scott-Parker.[40] The BDF strategically refrains from becoming involved in non-employment disability issues, leaving such activities up to activists and other organizations.[41] "We cannot shift every aspect of a society, all we can do is do what we do best, which is to transform a senior business leader from someone who doesn't care and assumes there's no problem ... into someone who thinks, 'oh, there is something I can do, it will benefit my business, it will make me a better person, and it will help an individual,'" Scott-Parker comments.[42]

4.4 Delivering Practical Guidance to Members

A central aim of the BDF is to equip their members with tools and resources so that they can become "disability confident." The Forum describes a disability-confident organization as one that

> understands how disability affects all aspects of their business—people, markets, competitors, suppliers, communities, and key stakeholders; creates a

culture of inclusion and removes barriers for groups of disabled people; makes adjustments that enables specific people to contribute—as employees, customers, partners and valued stakeholders; and does not make assumptions about what people can do on the basis of a label.[43]

The Forum has strategically developed tools and provides specialized services to make the most impact on the members.

4.4.1 Guidance and Publications

The Forum provides a variety of publications for their members. Some of the most popular and best-received publications have been the *Disability Communications* guide and *Welcoming Disabled Customers*. These short guides, around 25 pages long, outline the issues relating to a variety of other topics and provide straightforward advice and address misconceptions based on research conducted by the Forum and external disability organizations. These publications are available to members in accessible formats, in either print or digital form. Some of these guides are included in membership fees, whereas others can be purchased by businesses and distributed to staff and colleagues. They can be useful tools for management (*Line Manager Guide Series*), recruitment (*Recruitment That Works*), and human resources departments (*Monitoring for Change: A Practical Guide for Monitoring Disability in the Workforce*) for training and reference. The BDF also allows businesses to personalize the guides, disseminating them to their staff with their corporate branding on them.

Several interview participants from member organizations commented on the value of the guides and their ability to effect change. One employee from Lloyds Banking Group stresses the Director of Group Operations' positive reaction to one particular publication and the impact it had on the bank:

> He saw the *Invisible Disabilities* guide and was present at the launch, a Gold event, and said 'Right, I want all of my senior managers to get a copy of that.' So we purchased . . . 2,500 copies and sent them out and it had a big impact. It really, really raised the visibility of what we were doing with the disability program.[44]

4.4.2 Training and Events

Employers confront disability-related questions on a daily basis: How can call centers be made fully accessible? How does a business develop a disability network that empowers employees? How do employers recruit people with mental health distress? To help employers find solutions to these commonly faced and often difficult issues, the BDF hosts approximately 100 trainings and events each year.[45] Instructional and practice-based master classes and conferences are held on relevant topics affecting members. Interactive phone-ins and telephone tutorials have become popular in recent times because they allow companies based outside of London to attend while avoiding the time and financial encumbrances of travel. The Forum is well-regarded for its lively, well-organized after-hours dining events—often described as "parties with a purpose"—in which representatives from member organizations attend to network with others; exchange personal experiences and acquired knowledge; and listen to speakers, often including the Disabled Associates and individual members that want to share success stories.[46]

The BDF also helps members in host their own internal events. For example, television station Channel 4 hosted Talent Boutique during the summer of 2011 for "disabled high flyers," a networking event for the professional development of disabled talent interested in working at Channel 4.[47]

4.4.3 Networks

Members represent all sectors of industry, and therefore have different insights into how disability affects their businesses. In order to make it easier for members to share their knowledge, the BDF has facilitated the creation of sector-specific networks. For example, members in the police and emergency services sector belong to the Emergency and Law Enforcement Network (ELEN). A specific BDF disability consultant responds to the needs of these members, holds sector-specific networking events, and develops trainings and workshops on pertinent subject matters that are often challenging these members. An event on nonvisible disabilities was held specifically for ELEN because nonvisible impairments, especially dyslexia, are more prevalent in the police force than physical disabilities.[48]

Members generally commented that the Forum's networks have very pragmatic benefits. For example, when searching to train and hire disabled presenters to cover the 2012 London Paralympic Games, Channel 4 executives met with other employers in BDF's Broadcasting and Creative Industries Disability Network to get assistance in finding interested and talented presenters who have disabilities. The relationships between employers made the search successful and not burdensome.[49]

4.5 Tailored Relationship Management and Services

A significant part of the BDF's offering are its tailored relationship management and services. The BDF recognizes that no two businesses are the same. By tailoring services to the members, it equips employers with specific guidance and resources, enabling them to improve their performance, as opposed to presenting them with general, one-size-fits-all resources.

4.5.1 Disability Directions

For example, a confidential advice telephone line for members known as Disability Directions is one of the BDF's most highly regarded services. It is run by several of the Forum's disability consultants who are trained and experienced in answering complex queries. Staff members log conversations with members so that they can be used for future reference. Marcia Wolfe, Equality and Diversity Officer at NHS Blood and Transplant, provides an example of a recent query her organization received:

> We had somebody who was long-term and had been on the redeployment register for a while and instead of looking at what she was capable of doing, we started looking at incapability and possible termination of employment. We got= some information from [BDF] and actually put our heads to that—we would actually be contravening the law. I think that was tricky and we took advice from them, and we also saved a person from being made unemployed.[50]

One of Channel 4's BDF representatives added, "I definitely use them more than we would use a lawyer, because you get a good service in that respect," and added that Channel 4 was able to save a significant amount of money by calling Disability Directions instead of a lawyer.[51]

Interview participants from member organizations repeatedly highlighted the value of being able to pick up the phone with a question and have it answered either immediately, or within a short period of time if the query was more complex. Several representatives from member organizations emphasized their appreciation for the fact that the advice they receive is tailored to their specific business and personal situations.[52]

Furthermore, each member is provided a relationship or account manager.[53] It is their job to understand the members' businesses, constantly adapt services to members' feedback, and give the BDF's offering a personal touch. Gold members tend to be more involved in shaping the BDF's internal initiatives and external influence on public policy and legislation, and thus the relationship manager usually "works with the member on a more strategic level," a BDF staff member explains.[54] Gold organizations are invited to sponsor events, participate in lobbying activities, and share their success stories at trainings and networking events. Speaking about British Telecom's correspondence with its relationship manager, its Human Resources Disability and Care Lead says, "She's very professional, she understands the issues from our perspective very clearly, and she makes sure that we are kept up to date with all the latest things that we need to be involved in."[55] Monthly engagement reports, which detail everything from the number of times the member calls the Disability Directions line to the number of events the member attended, along with the results from the Disability Standard—the Forum's performance measurement tool—allow managers to keep track of their members' progress and the areas in which they may need help improving.

4.5.2 Performance Measurement

Tracking the performance of members has been a key strategy for the organization. The BDF developed an assessment tool that allows employers to measure their performance on disability, providing feedback about which areas they need to improve in and how they rank against other employers. The assessment, called the Disability Standard, was created by the BDF in 2004 with the help of leading BDF Disabled Associates.[56] Although the assessment is designed to be difficult and to challenge employers, a score of 100% is not made to be an impossible target.

Members submit answers to questions about their business practices and initiatives and supporting evidence on the following areas:

Employment and recruitment
Customer services and e-commerce
Health and safety
The working environment
IT systems
Accessibility of goods and services
Outsourcing and procurement
Corporate responsibility and brand reputation

Trained BDF staff members then analyze the organizations' completed assessments and disseminate individualized diagnostic reports to each employer. Members who choose to enter into the disability benchmark can then compare their results with other organizations of their size or sector. There have been three rounds of the Standard since its creation. In 2009, 106 employers—about one fourth of all members—participated, 77 of which had completed the assessment once or twice before.

Performance measurement is an important strategy because the assessment tool provides employers with a comprehensive report that outlines what the organization needs to do to improve its performance on disability. "It identifies where we are as an organization and where we need to be," says Matthew Thomas of Ernst & Young.[57] The Standard also rewards best practice as "it gives us recognition for the good work that we've done," he continues.

Many businesses compete against each other for high rankings in the benchmark, which likely gets businesses to improve on average. As Tim Taylor of Lloyds Banking Group describes, the Director of Group Operations set the "very, very clear goal that we need to be back into the top 10."[58] Additionally, the results act as evidence of the organization's improvement. This is particularly helpful since the report can be disseminated to senior managers and executives to justify the organization's membership.[59]

4.6 Working with Stakeholders

4.6.1 Government

In addition to working toward shifting the attitudes and behaviors of organizations, the Forum endeavors to achieve macro-level impact in terms of contributing to social change. Although direct credit cannot be assigned entirely to the Forum for these societal shifts, it can effect change and has done so by influencing its stakeholders: government, business, and international bodies. The BDF is involved in several policy-related activities and has built relationships with government and external organizations, such as Business in the Community and the Royal Institute for the Blind. Meetings often take place between disability groups and government bodies, including the Department of Work and Pensions, the Minister of Disabled People, and various Members of Parliament. In 2011, the Forum was involved in four public consultation responses; one concerned policy related to workplace disputes and another concerned the public sector Equality Duty.[60] When proposals were likely to directly affect members and their disabled staff, the BDF asked their members to submit their opinions, which were then included in the consultation responses.

4.6.2 Disabled Associates

As mentioned, the Forum's Disabled Associates are a key feature of the organization. Although the Disabled Associates do not claim to represent all disabled people, the BDF's relationship with these leaders and entrepreneurs who contribute their personal insights as disabled individuals grant the Forum a sense of authority. "The development of Disabled Associates was a brilliant idea in that it gave a sense of credibility of the BDF amongst the disabled community," expressed Stephen Duckworth, a BDF Board member, Disabled Associate, and senior executive at the public service company Serco. He describes how the relationship between the Disabled Associates and the Forum is also advantageous to the disability activist movement because it "enhances and enforces their message to central government."[61]

Although the Disabled Associates are not compensated monetarily and have different backgrounds, jobs, and reasons for undertaking this role, they generally also benefit from this relationship. Rick Williams, a Disabled Associate in addition to being the Managing Director of his own disability and diversity consultancy agency, explains his motivation:

> BDF gives me, if you like, a forum to help me develop my own expertise, give me people to bounce ideas off of, and it just helps networking, all of those sorts of things. And sometimes it puts work my way, which is quite nice as well.[62]

4.6.3 President's Group

The Forum also created the President's Group. Consisting of about 35 chief and senior executives from Gold member organizations, the group meets annually to discuss strategies for getting disability onto the global business agenda. At the time of writing, its president was John Varley, former CEO of Barclays Bank. The chief and senior executives who elect to join the group are asked by the BDF to mention their involvement in their public bio. This is what Scott-Parker describes as "public positioning," saying that disability is so important that "I personally, as chief executive, am prepared to once a year join this thing and be part of this network" [and] to make it easier for their own people [organization] to make progress."[63]

The president's group is not a governing body of the Forum; its function springs from the individual members' reputations and statuses as business leaders. Attaching their name to the message of disability awareness and spreading it from business to business, these individuals "create peer pressure at the chief executive level," says Joanna Wootten, Director of Member Services at BDF.[64]

4.6.4 Disability Organizations

Finally, the Forum has built relationships with an array of other disability organizations. The Policy and Campaigns Manager at Mind, a prominent UK mental health charity, describes the importance of these relationships:

> We don't have all the answers, we have limited resources, so for us to make as much impact as possible I just absolutely think that you need to know others working on this issue, how you can add value to what they're doing, how they can support what you're doing.... It's good to work in partnership, bring all of that expertise together and have that solidarity.[65]

5. FINDINGS

As a result of the wide array of guidance and services described in the preceding, employers all over the United Kingdom (and internationally) have improved their performance on disability, ameliorating the experiences of individuals with disabilities as both workers and customers. However, there are still many areas in need of improvement. The following sections detail findings from the case study in relation to particular areas of business.

5.1 Monitoring Performance: Results from the Disability Standard

Strong evidence of the Forum's impact on its members can be found in the 2009 Standard results, which reveal that member organizations that have repeatedly taken the standard assessment have made clear progress and scored significantly higher across all areas than members who participated for the first time.[66] Such findings also illustrate that employers are taking the results seriously and acting to improve upon them. Fifty organizations participated in the 2007 and 2009 Disability Standards, and 27 organizations participated in all three assessments since the creation of the Standard in 2005. The most recent results reveal that 15 organizations that had benchmarked previously scored exceptionally highly—greater than 80%—on the 2009 Standard. In the BDF's analysis of the results, it posits that members that have entered into the Standard on two or three occasions have scored significantly higher than the average in the following areas: taking a planned approach to achieving disability equality, valuing disabled customers, evaluating the impact of their actions to achieve disability equality, realizing the potential of disabled employees, and investing in disability equality. For example, 30% of first-time Standard participants use staff surveys to compare employee engagement of nondisabled employees to those who reported they had a disability to help identify where changes need to be made, in comparison with 58% of organizations who benchmarked twice and 67% of those who benchmarked three times. An improvement in career development of employees with disabilities can also be detected. Only 5% of organizations that only completed the 2009 Standard encourage known disabled colleagues to seek or apply for promotions, whereas 14% and 26% of two- and three-time benchmarkers, respectively, do so.

This finding underlines the importance of employers' engagement with the Forum. It suggests that merely being a member of the Forum does not endogenously increase a business' disability confidence. Employers must engage in active membership in order to improve their performance.

5.2 Top-Scoring Employers

A total of 21 organizations scored greater than 80% and a small percentage—just four organizations—scored 95% and higher in 2009. This high-scoring group encompasses organizations from both the public and private sector.[67] Some notable actions set high-scoring members apart. These organizations all have disability action plans in place that are related to their core business plans and have a Board member responsible for tracking their progress on disability equality. They also scored highly in terms of meeting the needs of their disabled customers and clients. Providing disability equality training for all employees is another domain in which these organizations excel. Importantly, the organizations that scored 95% and above have all set out a clear vision for what their organization will look like when it has achieved disability equality; they have also created communications strategies that describe to employees how disability relates to specific roles and outline the business case for disability equality.

5.3 Accessibility

Overall employer organizations are improving accessibility. In terms of the built environment, 68% conduct audits on accessibility of the physical workplace, from doorways to ramps. Seventy-two percent—a 14% increase from 2007—now audit the accessibility of equipment, such as desk chairs and special software that employees with disabilities may use. Employers have made notable improvements in their recruitment and selection processes. Eighty-five percent regularly review job descriptions and requirements. For example, having "good communication skills" in order to qualifty should not be specified in an ad if the job does not actually require such skills. In addition, 78% regularly check medical questionnaires and occupational health policies to ensure they do not discriminate. A high total of 90% of employers offer adjustments to candidates at every stage of the selection process. Although the public sector outperforms the private sector on average, more private sector members have recruitment and development programs in place for disabled applicants and employees, and have policies on reasonable adjustments.

Despite significant improvements in accessibility overall, little progress has been made in ensuring that information is accessible to employees and customers. For example, just 43% of organizations guarantee that all communicated information is accessible and meets the differing needs of customers with disabilities; and just 44% have fully accessible Web sites.

5.4 Putting Disability on the Business Agenda

An emerging trend is that most businesses are finally making commitments to disability equality. This is likely a result of many factors, including increased awareness about disability rights and the United Kingdom's new Equality Act. "Disability is high on the agenda and that's a huge change for our organization...To have something written and for it to become part of our strategy, the organization's strategy, is huge," explains the NHS Blood and Transplant's Diversity and Equality officer.[68] Almost all organizations that participated in the 2009 Standard Assessment (97%) have publicly stated their commitment to achieving disability equality and have senior management backing this position through some or all of the following approaches: creating action plans across the business, devising policies and guidelines that detail how disability equality will be achieved within their business, and creating a position that is responsible for carrying out these plans. Also, a high percentage of organizations have an individual or team of disability experts (86%).

Just over half of organizations have set clear disability-equality goals and 42% are working toward setting them. Although the number of employers that have disability policies on employment has risen by 19% since 2007, the latest results reveal that the number of employers with such policies is only 60%. More than two thirds of organizations have garnered board-level responsibility for disability equality, which provides supporting evidence that many more businesses are taking a strategic approach on disability equality (up 18% since 2007).

5.5 Training

Training is another area in which members made significant progress. The number of organizations that deliver training on disability equality for every employee as a means of achieving their disability goals has doubled since the 2007 Standard. British Telecom has developed an innovative training program for their engineers: "We train up a number of our engineers locally to go to a disabled customer's premises and make sure they get it right by that customer."[69] However, a large number of all participants (43%) did not have effective training in place when they completed the Standard in 2009. When training exists, it is often not required for all employees.[70] Some organizations provide specialized disability equality training, whereas others incorporate it into employee training on diversity and equality more generally. More could be done to monitor disability awareness training on the whole; the 2009 Standard found that just 56% of members review the quality and impact of training.

5.6 Career Development

Although recruitment and selection processes are improving across the board, little progress in general has been made by employers to improve the career development of employees with disabilities. Only 35% of employers who took the Disability Standard check the format of training and development programs and remove any barriers; and just 13% monitor the take-up of mainstream training by employees who have told their employer about their disability. Although many organizations reported in 2007 that they were working to improve their promotion and appraisal procedures, only 42% are confident that their systems operate on objective and measurable criteria, and that employees are not penalized for needing reasonable adjustments. Just less than one third of organizations take action to encourage known disabled colleagues to seek or apply for promotions. And, very few organizations monitor the proportion of employees gaining promotion with a known disability—a mere 11%.

However, some organizations are taking initiatives on this front. Lloyds Banking Group developed programs on personal and career development for disabled individuals and conducted research that compared 100 disabled individuals who attended the programs with 100 who did not attend. "We found the promotion rate was higher [for those who attended], so we know that that cause has positive impact," explains Diversity and Inclusion Manager Tim Taylor.[71]

Susan Scott-Parker shared information about what some other member companies were doing to promote career advancement.[72] One company paired 250 disabled employees as they were hired with mentors in management positions within the corporation. "This inspires them to raise their personal aspirations," says Scott-Parker.[73]

5.7 Monitoring and Evaluation

In the Disability Standard Benchmark Report, the BDF argues that more organizations need to internally monitor and evaluate their policies and practices. Even many top performing members can improve in this area. Although more senior managers are supporting disability equality agendas, few organizations (only 13% in both 2007 and 2009) incorporate disability equality measures into managers' performance goals. Only 7% of organizations evaluate managers on attaining these disability-related goals. Furthermore, just about half of members monitor the number of disabled people who apply for jobs and their progress throughout the recruitment and selection processes. Fifty-six percent review the quality and impact of disability equality awareness training, which has increased 15% since 2007. Furthermore, more employers are monitoring the impact of actions taken to improve disability equality. For example, 67% monitor the success of actions taken to retain employees who become disabled. Higher retention rates will keep more disabled employees in work throughout their lives and can be advantageous to a business because they will not have to hire and train new, inexperienced employees. Also, several organizations have improved on monitoring complaints from customers who say they have a disability and 43% give employees the option of anonymously telling their employer that they have a disability.

5.8 Customers

Although significant progress has been made in getting businesses to make their products and services accessible to customers with disabilities, there remains a lot of work to be done in the customer domain. More than two thirds of employers provide instructions to their designers, architects, and other consultants to incorporate the fullest possible access for disabled customers and that customer compliant procedures are accessible. Yet 44%—less than half—of organizations have policies or guidelines in place for achieving disability equality in the provision of their product and services (compared with the 60% that have set standards to achieving disability equality in employment).

5.9 General Trends

On the whole, employers are improving their performance. For the 2009 Disability Standard the total average score of employers in 2009 was 63%, an increase from the 57% average achieved in 2007. Although the overall progress is small, it is not insignificant. Almost all employers that took the assessment made improvements.

5.10 Affecting Policy and Social Change

One of the BDF's greatest contributions to policy was its involvement in the legislation of the Disabilities Discrimination Act (1995). "When we first started," the BDF Director of Policy and Public Affairs explains, "the DDA did not exist. There was the quota system and now we've got the equality Act."[74] The Forum's Legal Director adds:

> BDF thought that legislation was needed, it got together a group of corporate businesses who agreed and tried as a result, rather than having legislation that

was drafted on behalf of individuals.... [T]hey managed to be involved in the consultation process and therefore got legislation that Susan [Scott-Parker] would describe as being credible in the eyes of both employers and disabled people.[75]

Although it is difficult to measure the reach and impact of the BDF's contribution to change in the United Kingdom and potentially globally, examples such as this illustrate the strategic role the organization has played in affecting disability antidiscrimination policy and establishing a backdrop of employer involvement in government conversations concerning disability and work.

Furthermore, since 1991, the year the Forum was officially established, the employment rate of people with disabilities in the United Kingdom increased by 8%.[76] While the Forum is only part of a greater web of organizations, policies, and other factors responsible for this increase affecting the 1.3 million disabled people who are currently living in the United Kingdom and are available for and want to work,[77] the organization has certainly played a significant part.

6. CHALLENGES AND LIMITATIONS

A recent government report on disability and employment identifies "confident, well-informed employers" in addition to "confident, well-informed disabled people" and an "enabling state" as an essential factor in creating equal access to and opportunities in the labor market for disabled people.[78] Despite success of the BDF in improving its members' performance and contributing to social change, the organization still faces a range of challenges in both these areas of work. Although some members excel, scoring highly on the Standard and implementing progressive and innovative disability policies and programs, others have only improved slowly—or barely at all. Taking a step back to look at the bigger picture, most businesses in the United Kingdom are not members of the Forum, so it is likely that the organizations that are most engaged are not a random sample of UK businesses, but those who place a greater value on diversity and corporate responsibility in the first place.

6.1 Internal Challenges

6.1.1 Monitoring Statistics

Many factors contribute to the difficulty of measuring the Forum's members' improvements in the area of disability. The United Kingdom does not have quotas and employees are not required to tell their employer about their disability; therefore, it is difficult to collect quantitative data on the number of disabled employees in a company. Several interviewees report that their businesses conduct employee surveys that are filled out anonymously, but this does not guarantee that an employee will report his or her disability. Of course, many individuals have nonvisible disabilities and people fall in and out of disability over the course of their lives, so using statistics on numbers of disabled staff as evidence of progress is problematic.

There are two predominant opinions on how this monitoring issue can be addressed. Some believe that they can achieve a more accurate representation of the numbers of employees with disabilities if they "create the right perception and send out the right messages about us as an organization so firstly, we attract more people with disabilities, and secondly, that they feel more confident about declaring a disability whilst they're applying for a job."[79] The Forum, however, maintains that this will not necessarily guarantee accuracy, as surveys are very subjective. Scott-Parker says that employers should consider these questions when reviewing their surveys: Is the survey fully accessible? Does it ask if employees have a long-term health condition? Can employers answer, "I prefer not to say"? Who will see the results of the survey? The BDF believes that monitoring employee engagement is important, but it does not provide a full picture.

6.1.2 Limitations of the Standard

Although the standard is a useful tool to monitor performance, it cannot provide a full picture of how businesses are doing on disability. In the three periods the standard has been utilized by members (2005, 2007, 2009), less than one third of members chose to complete it. There could be many reasons for this, including time and financial constraints, lack of interest in obtaining quantitative results, and reluctance to submit results if the organization is not performing highly.

Furthermore, how different organizations complete the assessment is in itself subjective. It is possible that organizations that benchmarked three times ranked higher because they became better at filling out the forms. Perhaps others took a more critical approach to their own initiatives on disability, therefore giving themselves lower marks. And maybe, managers filling out the Standard are not in the position to make executive decisions. In addition, it is obviously difficult to quantify anecdotal evidence and feedback to show where a member organization stands. Finally, other factors such as the merging of two companies and financial constraints may affect performance over time, yet these considerations are not discernible from the results.

Although newer members may feel hesitant about completing the standard if they have yet to implement many disability positive changes, other top performing members do not think the Standard challenges them enough: "Just 3% room to improve.... I don't think the disability standard can help us stretch and understand where we need to go next," comments Helen Chipchase, Human Resources Disability and Care Lead at British Telecom.[80] Furthermore, several interviewees expressed misgivings about the Disability Standard, regarding the length of time it took to fill in and the amount of work it required.

After the completion of the third Standard in 2009, the Forum decided to completely redesign it, taking members' feedback into consideration.[81] The new assessment tool was launched in September 2011; members were given more flexibility in terms of deciding which months they would participate the amount of time they had to fill it in. The new design aims to "make it shorter, simpler, easier to fill in with easier advice of what we were looking for in terms of evidence," says Joy Dearden, another BDF staff member working on its implementation for fall 2011.[82] The Standard now has 10 questions instead of 100 that focus on 10 areas of business, so different people from various departments can fill in their respective sections.

6.1.3 Financial Matters

The BDF has more or less maintained the same funding model throughout its many years of experience, which has granted it a great deal of flexibility and freedom. However, this model, which makes the organization's functioning dependent on membership fees and membership renewal, will not necessarily deliver sufficient funds to undertake new activities and projects. For example, remarks Scott-Parker, "there's no extra money for research and innovation."[83]

The BDF must work to retain its members to sustain itself financially. Part of the function of the Member Services team is to make sure that BDF members feel that they are getting value for money out of their membership through good relationship management, so that they renew their subscription annually. The BDF must also show employers that it remains on the cutting edge, constantly producing innovative products and services to offer, especially as increasing numbers of newly created organizations begin to encroach on their niche area of operation, disability and business. The BDF's Head of Business Development, Ian Hastie, explains that because of the difficult economic climate, some members are leaving.[84]

A point of note, however, is that the Forum's funding model had proved to be successful throughout its 20 years of operation. "I think that it's an excellent business model and I don't think it should change," Board member Stephen Duckworth says, although, he does agree that some of the finer details could use some tweaking.[85] The overall retention rates of 80%, which includes Gold and Standard members and both public and private sectors, and 94% for the more expensive Gold membership, reflect the fact that even in

difficult financial times, employers continue to value the services and expertise they are receiving from the organization.[86]

6.1.4 Breadth of Mission

Another important challenge that the BDF faces is balancing its opportunity to expand its global reach with maintaining its focus on and directing
its resources into the UK business community. The BDF has helped set up
an organization operating with a similar model in Australia, the Australian
Network on Disability,[87] and, during the summer of 2011, was working with
businesses in Madrid to help create an employers' network there. Board member and Disabled Associate Stephen Duckworth raises this issue: "I think that
the challenge for me is the balance between the internationalization and
maintaining and growing the UK base. . . . I am concerned about the stretch
that it places on the organization to deliver those two components."[88]

6.1.5 Future of Dynamic Leadership

The BDF is arguably a self-sustaining organization; however, it has been led
by a sole individual since the organization was founded. Many of the staff and
members attribute the organization's success to the thought leadership, ambition, commitment, and gregarious nature of Chief Executive Scott-Parker. One
Board member comments, "I think that it's got fantastic leadership, which is a
strength and a weakness."[89] It is unknown whether the organization's dependency on its founder will prove to be precipitous in the future: "[T]here is no
one out there being primed. . . . If Susan disappears, an awful lot of the relationships and the engine will splutter. It's too dependent on one person," elu-
cidates another member of the BDF Board.[90]

6.1.6 Expanding the Business Disability Forum's Role

Several interview participants expressed the desire for the Forum to expand its
thought leadership function. Implicit in this would be taking on a more vigorous
public affairs role and focusing more attention on prospective policy work with
the aim of triggering social change. Acting Director of Policy and Campaigns
of the disability charity Scope explains the advantages of prospective policy
work: "[As] a body that represents a good amount of high profile employers and
links to the disability sector, [the BDF] could be in there at quite a senior level
in strategy within government."[91] On the topic of what the BDF could do differently, Helen Chipchase, Disability and Care Lead of British Telecom, remarks,

"I think it may be extending their impact beyond the people who already agree with them and trying to find a way to reach people within an organization that are professionals in other areas."[92] Taking on additional roles, however, would require at the very least more staff, and thus, additional financial means.

6.2 External Challenges

6.2.1 The Move from Disability toward Diversity

With the passage of the Equality Act, several diversity strands or protected characteristics were brought under one antidiscrimination law. Although people with disabilities still remain protected under the law, there no longer exists legislation that exclusively concerns disability. Many businesses have established Equality and Diversity roles that address all of the diversity strands, and not specifically disability. As Tim Taylor comments, "There are so many messages out there and so many people competing for air time, that the message doesn't always get through about disability."[93] One challenge for the Forum is persuading members to continue their memberships by emphasizing the importance of belonging to an organization that offers a wealth of expert advice and knowledge on disability and employment, as opposed to diversity more generally.

The Forum is also working to spread its influence beyond human resources and diversity departments. In general, businesses delegate disability issues, especially if they are related to employment, to these departments. This is a potential issue of concern for the BDF, as the organization wants its message to cut across all departments and areas of business.[94]

6.2.2 Impact of Intermediary Disability Organizations

When looking for work, a disabled individual will likely encounter any number of intermediary organizations before even speaking with an employer. Although the BDF tries to influence disability organizations, recruitment agencies, and service providers through its work with government and employers, it is first and foremost an employers' organization and therefore cannot always directly influence intermediaries when issues concerning employment support and the pathways to work arise.

6.3 Maximizing Impact

The Forum's members employ 20% of the UK workforce;[95] however, there still remains the other 80%. Over the past few years, its membership base has hovered between 350 and 400 employers. Its success begs the question: How can the Forum maximize its impact and reach more employers through-out the United Kingdom? This is a difficult task, explains Chief Executive Scott-Parker: "We'll never have 50,000 members because we're in a leadership role, and we tend to attract the more enlightened organizations, attract companies that have individuals working for them that can see that investing in building their own capability in this space delivers mutual benefit."[96]

Top-performing members and high-profile executives in the President's Group may prove to be beneficial in the BDF's efforts to increase the participation of lower-performing members and recruit potential members. These companies act as role models for other businesses, providing examples of best practice on disability and sharing novel strategies on serving disabled customers and clients with other members at BDF events,; they may incite other businesses to improve simply because of the competitive nature of business.

7. RECENT AND FORTHCOMING ENDEAVORS

Although the BDF is currently facing a range of challenges, it is persistently working to overcome them. Some of its current endeavors include utilizing the influence of the Business Taskforce on Accessible Technology to make organizations IT-accessible, developing a procurement charter to which employers will formally commit, and expanding its model internationally.

7.1 The Business Task Force on Accessible Technology

In the United Kingdom, the law requires business to take steps to ensure that their technologies do not disadvantage people with disabilities, but not all businesses fulfill their legal obligation. The Business Task Force on Accessible Technology (BTAT) is a BDF member initiative to galvanize businesses to adopt accessible and usable technology, such as Web sites, office systems, application software, and Web-based services, in alignment with the BDF's mission to make it easier to employ and do business with people with disabilities. In addition to people with disabilities, accessible technologies will also benefit other demographics, such as older people, individuals with lower levels of literacy, and speakers of different languages. The BTAT currently has 33 members and developed a charter detailing ten points of best practice on accessible technology, which members elect to sign to pledge their commitment. The creation of the BTAT also facilitates the extension of the BDF's influence to new areas of business. Lloyds Banking Group's Senior Manager in IT Accessibility explains, "So the challenge that the BDF has got is that their prime contacts are generally in the diversity-[human resources] space, which means they'll have a more limited reach within the organizations. So I think the work of things like BTAT to actually get IT directors brought in is really important."[97]

7.2 Procurement

Procurement is another area on which the Forum has been focusing its efforts. Businesses should consider disability equality when establishing relationships with suppliers and partners to ensure that all aspects of business are accessible to disabled employees as well as customers. Matthew Thomas of Ernst and Young provides an example of his firm's progress in this area, "We did a lot last year speaking to our suppliers, saying these are our demands of you, if you're going to win a contract with Ernst & Young, we want you to display that you're disability-friendly, that you're members of the BDF and those requirements around that."[98]

7.3 Disability Means Business as Usual

Several members expressed the hope of reaching a point where disability becomes integrated into all areas of business and business practices, no longer being understood as supplemental or an add-on to daily duties that is insisted upon by the company's Human Resources or Equality and Diversity departments. "It's less about saying that disability is another thing that you have to remember, it's more about going through the day-to-day things that that an individual does," explains Helen Chipchase of BT.[99]

Other members contemplated the more distant future, imagining a day when the BDF—and their individual contributions—will no longer be needed. Graeme Whippy confidently asserts:

> Over the next two years I hope not to have a job, basically. One of my criteria is that I'm not needed anymore ... we've got to the point where disability is integral to the way we do business; we have defined policies and processes and practices that are self-sustaining.[100]

Although Whippy's comment may appear quixotic on the surface, it is an important goal to set and strive toward, and Lloyds Banking Group is certainly heading in the right direction. When Lloyds TSB merged with HBOS their disability performance dropped, largely due to the logistics of the merger. However, in only a few years, there exists substantial evidence of the bank's improvement, now under the name Lloyds Banking Group.

However, the experiences of members vary depending on size of the organization, which industry or sector they belong to, and their level of experience. NHS Blood and Transplant, for example, a newer member, is still in the early stages of this journey: "Practically, from a disability point of view, we've really needed the support of the Business Forum because we really didn't have a clue. And where we have...well-written documents and policies, it's the implementation where people don't understand about disabilities."[101]

7.4 Global Presence as Disability and Employer Organization

As mentioned, the Forum has already helped establish a similar organization in Australia. It has also worked to develop employers' networks in Argentina, Australia, Brazil, Canada, Germany, Russia, Spain, Sri Lanka, and Vietnam.[102]

It also appears that the BDF's terminology of "disability confidence" has expanded across the globe—at least in the disability sector. For example, a community business organization created a resource guide for employers in Hong Kong and Singapore that repeatedly references the BDF and its material and is titled *Towards Disability Confidence*.[103] Scott-Parker believes that this is one example that represents a "fundamental shift" toward recognizing the importance of disability equality by businesses occurring in many parts of the world.[104] Furthermore, the World Health Organization's (WHO) *World Report on Disability* features the Business Disability Forum in a substantial chapter on employment and describes it as an organization that "has developed innovative approaches for changing perceptions about disability."[105]

7.5 Replicability

The success of the BDF raises questions and points about its replicability. As discussed, the Forum has been involved in the successful establishment of similar networks elsewhere, mostly notably in Australia. As Paul Day explains, "Clearly, we are far more knowledgeable about UK law than Canadian law or South African law, but our best practice advice is still similar."[106] Yet, countries still have different cultural conceptions of disability and how employment inequalities should be addressed, and therefore, not all businesses and governments may be as receptive to the Forum's ideas.

The topic of BDF extending its global presence will be a predominant point of discussion at future board meetings. One board member argued that it would be strategic for BDF to look to the BRICs and other emerging economies are places to develop similar models that would be part of an employers' network on disability.[107]

8. CONCLUSION

Over the course of its 20 years of work engaging employers in the process of identifying and removing barriers to work and accessing services and products, the Business Disability Forum has achieved many victories and provides some valuable lessons in effecting social change.

8.1 Overview of Main Findings

Significant improvements in members' performance on disability have been made since the introduction of the Standard evaluation tool in 2005 in areas including, but certainly not limited to: physical accessibility, removing discriminatory features of recruitment and selection processes, and garnering senior management commitment to disability-equality. Of note, however, is that the Standard results also reveal that very limited progress has been made in other areas, specifically career advancement and internal monitoring.

The Forum's ability to impact employers and deliver mutual benefit to business and people with disabilities is directly linked to its innovative and unique approach to disability and employment. This approach includes, first, its successful creation of a nonjudgmental space for employers to learn, develop, and be challenged; and second, its strategic focus on the domain of disability as it affects business. Also essential to the Forum's success is that it equips its members with comprehensive and practical guidance and tools to teach them how to improve. Member retention is also a critical piece of the Forum's achievements, and thus tailored services and personal relationship management are of great import.

The Business Forum's success, however, has not come without its challenges. The BDF must balance its work with members with external projects and policy work. It also must make critical decisions about extending its model internationally. Moreover, the organization, like many other not-for-profits and businesses operating in the current economic climate, must work to sustain itself financially.

In addition to the Forum's distinctive approach to disability and employment, this study has revealed two key features that are integral to the Forum's success.

8.1.1 Member Engagement

As this case study has made apparent, member engagement is requisite to the Forum's successful functioning. The Forum has had the greatest impact on its members that use the BDF's services and resources, complete the Standard assessment, and act on their results. Whereas the Forum offers very effective tools, training, and services, it is up to members to utilize their membership. High-performing engaged members not only meet legal requirements, they also set the standard for best practice on disability performance and act as thought leaders in the field of disability and employment as they influence government and other businesses in the hopes of engendering social change.

8.1.2 Strong Leadership Is a Must

Additionally, the leadership of Scott-Parker has been a key component of the Forum's success and global presence. She is an inspiring and influential voice within the disability and employment movement and her name has become known amongst UK disability organizations. Since she founded the Forum, Scott-Parker has been making lasting connections with many UK senior business figures, which have likely encouraged their engagement and eagerness to improve. Although the Forum's activities and success are certainly not dependent on the chief executive's role as a thought leader and public figure alone, findings from this case study illustrate the importance of her strong leadership since the Forum's establishment.

8.1.3 Support from Government and Rights Legislation

Finally, a critical underpinning of the Forum's achievements has been the passage of particular legislation in the United Kingdom, specifically the Disability Discrimination Act which was replaced by the Equality Act in 2010. Such legislation makes the BDF's offering desirable to businesses—because discriminating against people with disabilities equates to contravening the law. One caveat of BDF's intentions to replicate this model globally is that such supportive rights-based legislation is absent in many countries around the world. This begs the question of what the organization's approach and experience can contribute elsewhere. This area of inquiry has not, however, gone unattended by the BDF; the organization's emphasis on best practice provides a means to address this issue and experiment with promoting its strategies on disability and employment elsewhere.

ACKNOWLEDGMENTS

The author would like to thank the McGill Institute for Health and Social Policy, and especially supervisors Tinka Markham-Piper, Magda Barrera, and Jody Heymann for the mentorship, support, and practical advice they provided throughout the process of preparing for and carrying out this case study. The author would also like to thank everyone from the Business Disability Forum and many other organizations who took the time to participate in interviews. This case study would not be possible without their great generosity and warm reception to the project.

NOTES

1. In October 2012, the organization changed its name from the Employers' Forum on Disability to the Business Disability Forum. Hereinafter, the Business Disability Forum will also referred to as "the Forum" and "BDF."
2. Business Disability Forum (2013). About us. Retrieved October 3, 2013, from http://businessdisabilityforum.org.uk/about-us.
3. For the purposes of this report the terms "business," "company" and "organization" will be used interchangeably to describe the Forum's members and apply to both public and private sector bodies.
4. Department for Work and Pensions (n.d.). Disability Facts and Figures: An Overview of Official UK Disability Statistics from the Office for Disability Issues. Retrieved September 10, 2011, from http://odi.dwp.gov.uk/disability-statistics-and-research/disability-facts-and-figures.php#1.
5. Ibid.
6. Sayce, L. (2011). *Getting in, Staying in and Getting On: Disability Employment Support Fit for the Future.* London, United Kingdom: Department for Work and Pensions.
7. Author Unknown (n.d.). Employment Rights and the Equality Act 2010. Retrieved September 10, 2011, from http://www.direct.gov.uk/en/DisabledPeople/Employmentsupport/YourEmploymentRights/DG_4001071. The Equality Act states that employers must make reasonable changes for disabled applicants and employees. Adjustments should be made in all cases where a disabled person could be put at a disadvantage compared to a non-disabled person. This includes making changes to an employee's working arrangements or any physical aspects of the workplace. In addition, if it is reasonable, the employer needs to provide an extra aid, such as special or adapted equipment, to ensure that the disabled applicant or employee is not put at a disadvantage. In determining what is "reasonable" employers may take several factors into account including: how effective the change will be, cost, practicality, the size and resources of the organization, the availability of financial support. When disagreements arise, an employment tribunal will ultimately determine what is reasonable.
8. Equality and Human Rights Commission (n.d.). Making Reasonable Adjustments for Disabled Employees. Retrieved September 10, 2011, from http://www.equalityhumanrights.com/advice-and-guidance/before-the-equality-act/.
9. Ibid.
10. Shah, S., & Priestley, M. (2011). *Disability and Social Change: Private Lives and Public Policies.* Bristol, United Kingdom: The Policy Press.
11. Sayce (2011). *Getting in, Staying in and Getting On,* 58.
12. Shah & Priestley (2011). *Disability and Social Change.*
13. Ibid.

14. Sayce (2011). *Getting in, Staying in and Getting On,* 56.
15. Office for Disability Issues (2010). Equality Act 2010: Guidance. Retrieved September 10, 2011, from http://odi.dwp.gov.uk/equalityact
16. Sayce (2011). *Getting in, Staying in and Getting On,* Notes.
17. Glasgow Centre for Inclusive Living (2011). The Social Model of Disability and Its Implications for Language Use. Language—A guide. Retrieved September 10, 2011, from http://www.gcil.org.uk/resources.aspx
18. Susan Scott-Parker (Chief Executive, BDF). Interview, 2 June 2011.
19. Ibid.
20. Ibid.
21. Ibid.
22. Ibid.
23. Ibid.
24. Ibid.
25. Paul Day (Chief of Staff, BDF). Interview, 20 June 2011.
26. Ibid.
27. Susan Scott-Parker (Chief Executive, BDF). Interview, 8 July 2011.
28. Ibid.
29. Susan Scott-Parker (Chief Executive, BDF). Interview, 27 June 2011.
30. Kate Nash (Disabled Associate and Director, Kate Nash Associates). Interview, 27 June 2011.
31. David Goodchild (Director of Business Development, BDF). Interview, 22 June 2011.
32. Rick Williams (Disabled Associate and Managing Director, Freeney Williams Ltd.). Interview.
33. Graeme Whippy (Senior manager of the group disability program, Lloyds Banking Group). Interview, 15 June 2011.
34. Equality and Human Rights Commission (n.d.). Public Sector Equality Duty. Retrieved September 10, 2011, from http://www.equalityhumanrights.com/advice-and-guidance/public-sector-equality-duty/.
35. Helen Chipchase (Disability Care Lead, British Telecom). Interview, 15 July 2011.
36. Scott-Parker. Interview, 2 June 2011.
37. Scott-Parker. Interview, 27 June 2011.
38. Brendan Roach (Senior Disability Consultant). Interview, 10 June 2011.
39. Joy Dearden (Disability Consultant, BDF). Interview, 10 June 2011.
40. Scott-Parker. Interview, 8 July 2011.
41. Communication from Susan Scott-Parker, discussed during BDF staff meeting May 25, 2011.
42. Scott-Parker. Interview, 8 July 2011.
43. Employers' Forum on Disability (n.d.). Realising Potential. Retrieved September 10, 2011, from www.realising-potential.org.
44. Graeme Whippy (Senior manager of the group disability program, Lloyds Banking Group). Interview, 15 June 2011.
45. Samantha Goldberg (Training and Events Manager, BDF). Interview, 31 May 2011.
46. Scott-Parker. Interview, 2 June 2011.
47. Simon Devereaux (Learning and Talent Specialist, Channel 4). Interview, 5 July 2011.
48. Nigel Howard (Detective and Treasurer for the Disability Enabling Network, City of London Police). Interview, 11 July 2011.

49. Alison Walsh (Disability Executive, Channel 4). Interview, 14 July 2011.
50. Marcia Wolfe (Equality and Diversity Officer). Interview, 16 June 2011.
51. Walsh. Interview, 14 July 2011.
52. Wolfe. Interview, 16 June 2011.
53. Relationship managers are BDF Disability Consultants who manage the accounts of Gold members and account managers handle the accounts of Standard members.
54. Nick Bason (Policy and Public Affairs manager, BDF). Interview, 27 May 2011.
55. Chipchase. Interview, 15 July 2011.
56. Disability Standard Team (Ed.) (2009). *Disability Stardard: Benchmark Report.* London, United Kingdom: Business Disability Forum.
57. Matthew Thomas (Senior Manager of Employee Relations, Ernst & Young). Interview, 16 June 2011.
58. Tim Taylor (Diversity and Inclusion Manager, Lloyds Banking Group). Interview, 1 July 2011.
59. Scott-Parker. Interview, 27 June 2011.
60. Bason. Interview, 27 May 2011.
61. Stephen Duckworth (Disabled associate and Director Serco Institute, Serco plc.) Interview, 14 July 2011.
62. Williams. Interview, 9 June 2011.
63. Scott-Parker. Interview, 2 June 2011.
64. Joanna Wooten (Director of Member Services, BDF). Interview, 3 June 2011.
65. Emma Mamo (Policy and Campaigns Manager, Mind). Interview, 24 June 2011.
66. Disability Standard Team (Ed.) (2009). *Disability Stardard.*
67. Seven private sector businesses and 14 public sector organizations scored an average of 80% or more in 2009.
68. Wolfe. Interview, 16 June 2011.
69. Chipchase. Interview, 15 July 2011.
70. Miriam Futter (Employer Brand Manager, John Lewis Partnership). Interview, 7 July 2011.
71. Taylor. Interview, 1 July 2011.
72. Susan Scott-Parker (Chief Executive, BDF). Interview, 11 October 2011.
73. Ibid.
74. Bason. Interview, 27 May 2011.
75. Bela Gor (Legal Director, BDF). Interview, 22 June 2011.
76. See World Health Organization & World Bank (2011). *World Report on Disability.* Geneva, Switzerland: World Health Organization, Chapter 8.
77. Office for National Statistics. Social and Vital Statistics Division (2009). Quarterly Labour Force Survey, January—March, 2009. In Office for National Statistics (Ed.). Labour Force Survey Series. London, United Kingdom: Office for National Statistics.
78. Sayce (2011). *Getting in, Staying in and Getting On,* 13.
79. Whippy. Interview, 15 June 2011.
80. Chipchase. Interview, 15 July 2011.
81. Suzi Mackenzie (Senior Disability Consultant, BDF). Interview, 12 July 2011.
82. Dearden. Interview, 10 June 2011.
83. Scott-Parker. Interview, 2 June 2011.
84. Ian Hastie (Head of Business Development, BDF). Interview, 9 June 2011.
85. Duckworth. Interview, 14 July 2011.
86. Scott-Parker. Interview, 27 June 2011

87. See http://www.and.org.au/
88. Duckworth. Interview, 14 July 2011.
89. Ibid.
90. Graham Bann (Business In the Community). Interview, 11 July 2011.
91. Marc Bush (Acting Director of Policy and Campaigns, Scope). Interview, 30 June 2011.
92. Chipchase. Interview, 15 July 2011.
93. Taylor. Interview, 1 July 2011.
94. Scott-Parker. Interview, 8 July 2011.
95. This statistic is regularly calculated by the Forum using published statistics on each member's staffing.
96. Scott-Parker. Interview, 8 July 2011.
97. Whippy. Interview, 15 June 2011.
98. Thomas. Interview, 16 June 2011.
99. Chipchase. Interview, 15 July 2011.
100. Whippy. Interview, 15 June 2011.
101. Wolfe. Interview, 16 June 2011.
102. See World Health Organization & World Bank (2011). *World Report on Disability*, Chapter 8.
103. Community Business (2011). *Towards Disability Confidence: A Resource Guide for Employers in Hong Kong and Singapore*. Hong Kong, China: Community Business.
104. Scott-Parker. Interview, 27 June 2011.
105. World Health Organization & World Bank (2011). *World Report on Disability*, Chapter 8.
106. Day. Interview, 20 June 2011.
107. Bann. Interview, 11 July 2011.

CHAPTER 5

Employability and Inclusion in a For-Profit Company

Serasa Experian's Employability Program for Persons with Disabilities

KALI STULL

1. BACKGROUND

1.1 Disability and (un)Employment in Brazil and São Paulo

According to Brazilian law, disability is defined as "any loss or abnormality of a psychological, physiological or anatomic function or structure resulting in a lack of ability to perform an activity within the range considered normal for the human being."[1] The Brazilian census of 2000 reports that 24.56 million people, or 14.5% of the national population, have a disability.[2]

Reducing unemployment for people with disabilities is incredibly important to improve equality for reasons including and beyond economic inclusion. However, once employed, there are still significant inequalities. Thirty percent of persons with disabilities in Brazil receive less than the minimum wage.[3] The average income for people with disabilities is US $250 per month, compared with US $295 for those without disabilities.[4] The government does provide a stipend for people with disabilities who are unemployed, but it is too low to support oneself financially.

Since 1991, Brazilian law requires that people with disabilities account for between 2% and 5% of the workforce of a company that has more than 100 employees; 2% for companies with up to 200 employees, 3% for companies with between 201 and 500 employees, 4% for companies with 501 to 1000 employees and 5% for companies with more than 1,000 employees. The current reported employment rate of people with disabilities is an average of 2.7% for companies with up to 200 people, 2.9% for companies with 201 to 500 employees, 4% for companies with 501 to 1000 employees, and 3.6% for companies with more than 1,000 employees.[5] These statistics of reported employment rate, however, are highly contested and thought to be inflated.

The legislation has had an impact. In 2001, 1,000 people with disabilities were employed in Brazil. As of August 2011, about 300,000 people with disabilities were employed (800,000 people with disabilities would be employed if the quota were fulfilled). The composition of what type of disability is employed reveals a discrimination and preference for particular types of disability. Of the people with disabilities employed, 50% have a physical disability, 20% are deaf, 5% have a cognitive disability, and 5% have a visual disability.[6]

The minister of labor is responsible for defending and enforcing the law by following up with companies to ensure that they are making an effort to comply with the quota. If a company is identified as falling short on their legal obligations to employ people with disabilities, they are given 120 days to address that shortcoming. The goal is not to fine companies or to increase the sheer numbers of employees, but rather to improve the quality of employment for people with disabilities. Therefore the minister of labor and his team of labor inspectors use their discretion to evaluate specific scenarios and apply timelines to fit each case. If the company continues to make no effort, they are fined. Although the quota has existed for 20 years, the penalization has only become strict and the fines more regularly applied in the last five years. Currently, there is a deficit of about 2,000 auditors in Brazil, which makes enforcement difficult.

1.1.1 Quota Reception

The quota legislation is a contentious issue for businesses. Many companies complain that the responsibility to address inequalities for people with disabilities should not fall onto the private sector. However, the hefty fine for companies that neither comply nor demonstrate an effort to comply with the quota pressures companies to register people with disabilities as employees. Unfortunately, these employees are often paid minimally by the company to stay home, maintain peripheral work, or are segregated in a specific low-level department with minimal responsibility.

Companies may try to make a deal with the minister of labor to illegally bypass the quota system by donating money to philanthropic organizations working in the disability field. Companies often think that hiring someone with a disability is a cost rather than an investment and prefer to take action from a charitable model of disability. João Ribas, a leader in disabilities rights says, "If I give money to the NGO I don't have to have responsibility to employ these people because it's a much different thing to live with people with disabilities inside the company . . . inclusion means you put people to live together, this is important."[7]

1.2 Overview of Serasa Experian and the Employability Program for Persons with Disabilities

Serasa Experian is a for-profit credit information services company headquartered in São Paulo that provides data and analytical tools to help client businesses manage credit risk, prevent fraud, and automate decision-making processes. In Brazil's largest state, São Paulo, 5.8 million of the 37 million inhabitants have a disability.[8] The 2003 study conduced by Fundacão Getúlio Vargas e Fundacão Banco do Brasil found that 54% of the disabled population in Brazil is unemployed, as compared with 32% of the nondisabled population. These figures do not include persons with disabilities who can work but are outside of the labor force. In the state of São Paulo, the legislated employment target is 50% reached.

Within Serasa's Human Resources Department and the Corporate Citizenship Team, the Diversity and Inclusion area runs the Employment Program for Persons with Disabilities (EPPD). The EPPD is designed to increase the rates of employment and improve the conditions and inclusion of people with disabilities by training and employing people with disabilities at Serasa Experian and sharing knowledge about employment for people with disabilities with partner companies and the public.

The EPPD was founded at Serasa Experian in 2001 in response to increased pressure from the minister of labor to address the company's lack of employment of people with disabilities and a concerted effort by current Serasa Experian leadership to be more "socially responsible." The program was created and continues to be coordinated by João Ribas. Ribas is a wheelchair rider, anthropologist, and former professor focusing on disabilities studies and the labor market. He has worked as an advisor to the government and to private companies about employing people with disabilities.

Components of the EPPD include company, institutional and governmental partnerships; a four-month-long training program for people with disabilities; sensitization and awareness-raising efforts, provision of technology and accommodations; and a triennial forum on employment for persons with disabilities. Of the 2,600 Serasa Experian employees in Brazil, 83 have a disability.

2. CASE STUDY DESCRIPTION

The main objective of this case study is to investigate the EPPD's impact on the graduates of the training program, the employees at Serasa Experian, and Serasa Experian's partnerships. The case study researches how the EPPD impacts people with disabilities' professional lives and overall quality of life as well as the structures of equity in the workforce for persons with disabilities. It examines the EPPD program objectives as they relate to the lived experiences of program participants, companies, organizations, and the state. This case study aims to provide evidence of effective strategies and actions to improve professional and social inclusion and equality of employment for persons with disabilities. Serasa Experian's EPPD was chosen for its well-respected 10-year involvement in the effort to increase and improve the quality of employment for people with disabilities in São Paulo using an innovative methodology.

2.1 Research Methods

This case study was conducted using qualitative research methods to describe and analyze the EPPD's methodology, practice, and impact on the levels of employment and inclusion for people with disabilities. The study is based on 52 semi-structured interviews conducted in 2011 with employees with and without disabilities, leaders of the EPPD, employees and leaders of companies in São Paulo, training program participants and instructors, and government officials.

Other sources of data collection include direct and participant observation of meetings, sensitization trainings, and classes at the training program, as well as tours of nongovernmental organizations (NGOs) and partner companies, and primary and secondary source material about disability in Brazil and São Paulo. Any statistical information regarding the EPPD refers to July 2011 data.

The case study includes participants of varying levels and kinds of disability, employment experience, tenure at Serasa Experian, and level and area of employment. Beyond Serasa Experian, participants were selected to increase understanding of partnership efforts, the reputation of the EPPD, and Brazil's legislation. Quotations have been anonymized for participants who preferred that their identity remain private.

3. SERASA EXPERIAN'S EMPLOYABILITY PROGRAM FOR PERSONS WITH DISABILITIES

3.1 Program Strategies

3.1.1 "Two-Way Street" Framework

The founder and director of the Employability Program for Persons with Disabilities, Ribas, describes social and professional inclusion for people with disabilities as "a two-way street"; both the workplace environment and the individual with a disability must be adequately prepared for fulfilling inclusive employment. The employer must know effective methods to train and qualify people with disabilities, optimize their potential, and integrate them into the workplace. Simultaneously, people with disabilities must demonstrate their potential, pursue their own growth and professional development, and show autonomy and independence. Ribas says, "Like everyone else, people with disabilities will only be professionally competent if they are qualified and are provided with the equipment and resources necessary for their development."[9]

People with disabilities at Serasa Experian subscribe to the "two-way street" methodology as an effective means for inclusion. They expect to be treated with respect and for the workplace to be accessible, while taking responsibility as an employee with a disability to include themselves and prove their working potential. Lincoln, a blind employee in public relations for four years shares, "I think that the philosophy of the company is what allows me to have the software on my computer and be able to work in the same way as the people here work and be demanded in the same way. . . . Both parties have to try to understand each other. I have to show what I can do and you have to be interested in learning what I can do."[10] Julianna, a blind proofreader, affirms, "To keep your job here, it depends on the . . . . capacity of the professional and not the existence of the program [EPPD] by itself."[11]

Abrahan, a supervisor—also referred to as "leader" at Serasa Experian— of two employees with disabilities, says, "My biggest concern wasn't only to treat [people with disabilities] better or worse, it was to treat them the same. If I treat worse, they would feel rejected, and if I treat better, they wouldn't grow or learn."[12] Luiza, a coworker then supervisor of two blind employees for nine years in public relations shares what she's learned, "Don't be paternalist, don't underestimate them. Demand goals or demand work, this is really important."[13] Simultaneously, Luiza and her coworkers make the environment welcome for their coworker with a disability to work by changing the format of texts and training the blind employees thoroughly for the public relations department. Once the area was prepared, employees with disabilities could stop performing menial, repetitive jobs and begin to have the same requirements and expectations and have the opportunity to be included.

3.1.2 Quality over Quantity

In order to put the "two-way street" methodology into practice, the EPPD has a "quality over quantity" approach; they employ only as many people with disabilities as they can fully support through preparing the individual and the environment. Ribas says, "That's a specific kind of methodology that's very important. I don't want to train a lot of people with disabilities. I don't want quantity, I want quality. . . . I think this program is a personal program. . . .

it's important that I accompany these people for their growing here in the company."[14]

3.1.3 Investment Rather Than Cost

The EPPD's methodology pivots around the idea that hiring people with disabilities is an investment, not a cost. Training people with disabilities for employment and making physical, structural, technological, and attitudinal adjustments improve the quality of work and inclusion for people with disabilities. The EPPD holds that these expenses should not be seen as "costs," but rather as "investments," both in the person with a disability and in the company.

3.2 The Training Program

3.2.1 Education for People with Disabilities: Background

According to the 2003 study conduced by Fundacão Getúlio Vargas and Fundacão Banco do Brasil, 27% of people with disabilities in Brazil have never been to school and 72% of people with disabilities in Brazil over the age of 15 are illiterate.[15] (The national rate of illiteracy in 2009 was 25%.)[16] Until 10 years ago, people with disabilities were not integrated into public schools. According to a national census in 2000, people with disabilities comprised 0.12% of the university student population.

Although federal legislation requires that all Brazilians attend school until they are 14 years old, 78.7% of the people with disabilities in Brazil report having seven years or less of schooling in 2006.[17] In 2003, 27.61% of people with disabilities in Brazil did not have the opportunity to study.[18] Amongst those making it through high school, fewer people with disabilities receive advance training.

3.2.2 The Employment Program for Persons with Disabilities Training Program

These disparities in educational opportunities between people without and with disabilities motivated the EPPD to develop a training program that offers preparatory education to qualify people with disabilities to work at Serasa Experian and partner companies. The EPPD has run a four-month-long training program twice a year since 2001. From 2001 to 2007, 12 people attended the program every semester. In 2008, when the EPPD formed partnerships with other companies, the training program expanded, training 30 people with disabilities for Serasa Experian and its partner companies. Since 2001, more than 200 students have graduated from the training program.

3.2.3 Application and Selection Process

The program requires that participants of the training program have a high school education (with an exception for participants with cognitive disabilities) and a working knowledge of computers, which leaves out a significant portion of the disabled community who do not meet that requirement. Applicants continuously outnumber available positions largely because of Serasa's well-known reputation as a company that inclusively hires people with disabilities.

The class monitor of the EPPD training program, Angela, had concerns that the entering education requirements (high school education and some computer knowledge) were too demanding and exclusive. Angela says, "The selection is outside of the Brazilian reality. It's too hard, too tough…they don't have many opportunities to qualify themselves. And these people that have disabilities, they have even less qualifications, even less opportunities or even more difficulties. So I think the selection should be more broad."[19] Yet she also negotiated that the training program might be too demanding for people that came with less education.

The EPPD favors enrollment for people who demonstrate independence, self-motivation and self-esteem. Finally, participants are selected based on the needs and available positions of Serasa Experian and their partner companies, so participants enter the training program knowing what position in which company they may secure upon graduation. Every training session, around five graduates work at Serasa Experian, in the entry-level position of auxiliary.

The training program enrolls participants with diverse types of disabilities. The EPPD's ideal balance is one third of students with a visual impairment, one third with a physical disability, one third with a hearing impairment, and one person with a cognitive disability. This is done in part as an effort to manage the imbalance of companies who request deaf employees more frequently than people with other disabilities.

3.2.4 Program Curriculum

The training program curriculum consists of 42 hours of professional behavior and administrative routine, 36 hours of financial math, 90 hours of computer (Word, Excel, PowerPoint), and 90 hours of Portuguese, divided into deaf and hearing-able sections.

The professional training portion of the program focuses on appropriate professional behavior and business dynamics. Milena, a deaf student, explained that the professional training portion set the Serasa Experian training program apart from others: "It's because here at Serasa Experian they have one focus . . . they teach us how to be really a professional inside a company and I was really happy about that."[20]

The professional behavior unit includes self-esteem. Alberto, a physically disabled participant in the training program, shared, "Yes you have a disability but you don't have to be closed in a cocoon and you can grow because of that, in spite of that. So I think it was really important in the beginning when we worked with the self-esteem."[21]

3.2.5 Logistical and Methodological Framework for the Program

The EPPD training program provides financial and professional support. The companies pay for their future employees to be trained. The participants are awarded a stipend primarily, and a salary later in the program. The class monitor, Angela, attends every class to ensure participants are receiving all the support they need. For instance, a participant with a cognitive disability in sessions observed, Felipe, had an additional monitor, a trained psychologist who is with him twice a week, on test days, and at his future workplace. Maria, a blind employee in the Diversity and Inclusion area at Serasa, serves as a link between companies and training participants. She addresses any concerns the students have at the training program or at their future workplace.

3.2.6 Fitting Employment Positions

Some training program participants were overqualified in previous jobs and entered the training program to secure more fitting and fulfilling positions. Making a good employment fit is possible by matching participants to positions in partner companies that interest them. Alex, a participant in a wheelchair, graduated with a BA in Sociology and was working as a telemarketer. Through the training program, he was able to find a position in what he was interested in, sustainability at the company Fluery. He says, "It's really good because the first impression is that they're going to treat me as a professional, beyond the chair."[22]

Karla, a partner of the EPPD and leader in deaf rights in São Paulo says, "The first concern is if what she's going to do in the company is going to be satisfactory to her professionally. If the person for instance works in IT, she won't adapt to an administrative area."[23] Lincoln, a blind journalist in public relations shared, "I think this is the difference of this program, that they have the sensibility to have people work with what they studied and this is not something that happens in all companies."[24]

3.3 Addressing Accessibility of the Workplace Environment

A physically accessible workspace has a significant impact on including employees with disabilities professionally and otherwise. As extrapolated in the social model of disability, disability is not inherently part of an individual; rather, it is created out of inaccessible institutional structures and physical barriers.[25] Likewise, structural accommodations, such as addressing communication barriers and negotiating working conditions, are necessary for full professional participation.

Consistent with the "two-way street" concept, the EPPD addresses issues of physical and structural accessibility and is able to ask the same results from people with disabilities as those without. Ribas argues that accessibility needs must be seen as an investment in standard work equipment like computers or telephones. He says, "I think technology is determinant for social inclusion."[26] It cannot be seen as a cost, and certainly not as a favor. Tech-support and tutorials are also available for disability-related technology.

3.3.1 Physical Accessibility

In 2003, the headquarter building of Serasa Experian, where 60 of the 83 employees with disabilities work, was the first Brazilian company to receive the certification as a building accessible to people with disabilities in compliance with the NBR 9050 accessibility standard. The certificate defines accessibility as, "possibility and condition of reach for utilization, with security and autonomy."[27] The standard recognizes that Serasa's building complies with the precepts of Universal Design; the building's environment, products, and objects may be accessed by wide-ranging categories of users, accommodating the functional needs of everyone. Examples of measures of physical accessibility at Serasa include ramps, adapted bathrooms, elevators with voice synthesizers, signs in Braille, parking spaces reserved for people with disabilities, software such as voice synthesizers like "Virtual Vision" (computer screen readers for blind employees), Braille printers, and high relief loupe electronics.

The three Serasa Experian satellite offices have varying degrees of physical accessibility, but none meet the NBR 9050 standard. The certified accessible main office building was not significantly more expensive than the other offices to build. However, remodeling a satellite office to meet accessibility standards would be far more expensive. In comparing Serasa Experian to other companies in terms of accessibility, Fernando, a sales employee in a wheelchair in the main Serasa Experian office shared, "There were much more difficulties to enter the other companies than Serasa Experian. They weren't adapted…and all the difficulties possible were there."[28]

Employees with disabilities can ask for accessibility improvements through the EPPD, either by talking directly to Ribas or going through their supervisor. For any oversights, Ribas welcomes people with disabilities to share their individual accommodation needs. For example, one deaf employee asked to be moved from a corner position as she needed to better communicate with her coworkers.

3.4 Structural Accessibility

In addition to preparing the physical and technological aspects of the office, the EPPD attends to structural adjustments that prepare Serasa Experian for the reception and inclusion of people with disabilities. For example, an interpreter of Libras (Brazilian sign language) and Portuguese is available for every meeting or event that a deaf employee attends. Kim, one of the owners of the EPPD's consultant group for deaf needs, K&K Libras, with Karla, remarked at how diligent the EPPD is with providing translation, "Serasa Experian is another world. It's the ideal world for people with disabilities. There isn't another company that offers as many resources as Serasa Experian offers...Serasa Experian is as concerned with a meeting of five minutes as a meeting of eight hours."[29]

Other examples of structural adjustments that occur include adjusting tasks throughout the team to fit with the abilities and limits of a person with disabilities; for example, not having a blind employee responsible for graphs or a deaf employee communicate over the phone. Julianna, a blind proofreader, provides an example: "The majority of things that had to be adapted was the type of work. For instance, I can't do the review of the printed material and in this my team works well, everyone knows that."[30] Isabel, the manager of a satellite office, says, "It's not difficult to work to make an environment that is adapted to the person, to recognize where she can't really help me and not give a task to her...because she has the capacity to do other tasks."[31]

Carolina, a senior analyst, provides examples of space considerations that improve work for two employees with disabilities in her area: "The person in a wheelchair, I try to put him in a place with lots of space so he can move and get things with less difficulty. I always try to put the deaf person sitting next to me so he can read my lips."[32]

In addition to providing translators, the EPPD once offered a three-month Libras course for employees at Serasa Experian at two office locations at the request of coworkers and supervisors who want to communicate better with deaf employees. It has not been offered since, most likely because the requests subsided. Occasionally, Serasa Experian employees independently organize taking Libras courses outside of the office to improve communication at work.

Bianca, an employee in Serasa's knowledge center, explains the structural adjustments made for Laura, her coworker with Down's syndrome: "When [Laura] first came, we didn't know anything about Down syndrome so they hired a psychologist to explain about Down syndrome."[33] Laura's workdays are four hours and her roles and responsibilities adjust according to her abilities. Bianca sees these "adjustments" as a process for every new employee. Abrahan, a manager at a satellite office, shares Bianca's perspective: "People think differently, they act differently, they have different needs and we, as leaders, need to think that they are not machines, they have to work, [we need to] conform to everyone's abilities."[34]

3.5 Knowledge Sharing with External Groups

3.5.1 Institutional Partnerships with the Government and Nongovernmental Organizations

As a prominent figure in the disabilities world in São Paulo and as a "benchmark company" for employing people with disabilities, Serasa Experian partners with other local efforts to share knowledge and reduce the inequalities for people with disabilities. According to Ribas, one of the EPPD's missions is to take their example to other groups and show what is possible. Serasa makes these partnerships to network and maximize the unique skills and resources that nonprofits, companies, and governmental groups have.

The EPPD gives, on average, one presentation a year to the Brazilian congress to share their successes and methodology with the government. Serasa also participates in a group hosted by the minister of labor, the Camera Paulista. This group is comprised of companies, NGOs, and people with disabilities who are working to change legislation and public policy for people with disabilities in Brazil.

The position of the EPPD as a benchmark program is influenced by the positive relationships that it has developed and maintained in the past 10 years with government at the municipal and state level. Although the EPPD has no formal influence on governmental policies or procedures, Ribas has communicated its strategy with the Ministry of Labor and collaborates with other government officials on committees and groups. The Minister of Labor, when approaching companies who are not making an effort to comply with the quota, often references Serasa Experian to prove that it is possible to employ people with disabilities. He says, "For us, it's very important to have good examples to show."[35] He recommends to companies that show apprehension about meeting the quota that they partner with the EPPD training program.

The EPPD links with NGOs to find participants for the training program and share strategies for employing people with disabilities. They partner with organizations such as ADIDI and Congruencia to train people with Down's syndrome and other cognitive disabilities to provide support throughout employment, and with K&K Libras to find people with hearing impairments to train and employ, for interpretation support, and to run the Portuguese for deaf students portion of the training program.

An ongoing project that links government, NGOs, and the EPPD is Multa Moral (Moral Fine), a campaign to promote awareness about and secure the rights of people with physical disabilities to have parking spaces designated with a disabilities sign respected by the public. Serasa Experian funds the project, hosts meetings, and has their logo printed on the promotional material.

3.6 Partnerships with Companies

In 2008, seven years after the EPPD's inception, the EPPD decided to invite private companies to partner with them. Companies that partner with the EPPD receive graduates from the training program to work in their company, trainings on how to employ and work with people with disabilities, information about the methodology of the EPPD, and continued support through ongoing correspondence with Ribas and the EPPD. Serasa Experian actively solicits partnerships by reaching out to companies. Since 2008, the EPPD has partnered with 40 companies in São Paulo and currently has 12 partner companies, including well-known multinational corporations such as Deloitte and Terra.

3.6.1 Motivators and Deterrents for Partner Companies

Serasa Experian provides support and knowledge about structural, technological, and physical accommodations for their partner companies. Three of the primary obstacles that companies in São Paulo face for fulfilling the quota of employees with disabilities are prejudice, lack of information, and nonqualified staff.[36] Because inclusively employing people with disabilities is relatively new for most companies, they often do not feel confident embarking on the process without outside knowledge and guidance. The EPPD attempts to address and alleviate these obstacles by providing support and knowledge about structural, technological, and physical accommodations.

The EPPD offers a streamlined way to employ qualified people with disabilities through the training program and can include partners in a network of people committed to the inclusive employment of people with disabilities. Ribas says, "This kind of work, social inclusion, professional inclusion...you can only do if you have a network."[37] The EPPD shares the overall perspective steering the program and shows partner companies that it is beneficial to hire people with disabilities and make investments in their accommodations.

The most common reason why companies would choose not to form a partnership with Serasa is the cost. The partner companies pay more than US $2,500 for each individual to participate in the training program. Those companies that choose to pay do so because they believe it will supply them with some of the best qualified people with disabilities in the market, and they value the expertise, support, and networking that the EPPD can provide.

3.6.2 Sensitization Training

The EPPD invites employees at partner companies and Serasa to partake in a half-day sensitization training twice a year to improve relationships and communication with people with disabilities. The objective of the training is to destigmatize disabilities and show that people with more severe disabilities can be desirable employees. It does this by educating their coworkers about the daily life, abilities, and needs of people with disabilities as well as how to work with people with disabilities of varying types.

At the sensitization trainings, participants rotate through four mini-workshops: one addressing motor disabilities, one addressing visual disabilities, one addressing hearing disabilities, and one addressing cognitive disabilities. The objective is that, by discussing details such as about how a person in a wheelchair gets in and out of the wheelchair, how a blind person uses a computer and rides buses, and how a deaf person wakes up with an alarm clock and communicates with non-deaf people, coworkers will become more familiar and thus more comfortable with disabilities. The sensitization also ideally eradicates prejudices that companies have against blind people, people with cognitive disabilities, and wheelchair users and shifts the preferences that companies have for deaf people to being open to employees of all kinds of disabilities.

Alice, a deaf employee at a satellite office in São Paulo who has worked at Serasa Experian for nine years explains, "It's important for the companies to be open to have seminars on how to live with people with disabilities without prejudice, without fear. There are many places that don't have this knowledge that they have in Serasa Experian. Serasa is disseminating the knowledge to the other companies."[38]

3.6.3 General Knowledge Sharing

Since 2003, Serasa Experian has hosted the Forum for Persons with Disabilities three times a year for people in the disabilities field and the public to attend free of charge. The goal of this forum is to exchange information so that employment for people with disabilities grows and social inclusion for people with disabilities improves in Brazil by "re-including society in the discussion."[39] Once a year, Serasa Experian invites an international leader in disabilities rights. The forum has drawn up to 200 people physically attending and 2,000 people tuning in to the real-time broadcast over the Internet.

Serasa Experian has a knowledge center in the headquarter office that serves as a resource center with publications, computers, and reports available to anyone to browse through and check out. The knowledge center has several theses and dissertations about people with disability in Brazil and many pamphlets about how to include people with disabilities in the workplace, several written or co-written by the EPPD.

4. IMPACT OF THE EMPLOYMENT PROGRAM FOR PERSONS WITH DISABILITIES

4.1 Impact on Employees with Disabilities

4.1.1 Numbers and Retention

From June 2009 to September 2011 the number of employees with disabilities employed at Serasa Experian fluctuated from 80 to 93. In September 2011, 83 people with disabilities were employed; 41 employees with a physical disability, 23 with an auditory disability, 19 with a visual disability, and one with a cognitive disability. Of the people with disabilities employed, 38 were men and 45 were women. These numbers indicate that Serasa Experian is not fulfilling the quota, because only 3.2% of the workforce has a disability. (The law requires 5% for companies of more than 1,000 employees, and Serasa Experian has 2,600 employees.)

Ribas explains: "Why are we not complying [with] the law? It's because we don't want to employ 2,000 people at the same time. If I employ five people with disabilities per semester I can give attention for these people.... We don't have a program just to tell the government."[40] Ribas adds, "I doubt you will find a company that will have the entire quota."[41] Serasa Experian has not been fined since the inception of the EPPD. The program is recognized and respected for its efforts and is therefore not penalized for its shortcomings in terms of numbers.

Numbers of retention of people with disabilities at Serasa Experian and partner companies are not officially maintained. However, Ribas estimates that graduates of the training program typically remain at their placement company for at least two or three years, and 80% remain for more than three years. Of the remaining 20%, half choose to leave and half are dismissed. The 83 employees with disabilities working at Serasa in 2012 began working in the following years: two since 1988, one since 1993, one since 2000, one since 2001, three since 2002, eight since 2003, four since 2004, thirteen since 2005, eleven since 2006, eleven since 2007, three since 2008, ten since 2009, five since 2010, and ten since 2011.

Although retention numbers are valuable as a way of displaying the general satisfaction of employees with disabilities at Serasa Experian, the EPPD does not see these numbers as a clear measurement of success. Their goal in the training program is to qualify people with disabilities for work in general, at Serasa and beyond. If a person with a disability leaves Serasa Experian for another employment opportunity, the employability program has achieved its goal.

The average salary of employees with disabilities working at Serasa Experian is US $1,175 per month. The average salary at Serasa Experian, US $1,920 per month and the minimum wage in Brazil, US $398 per month.[42] There are three people with disabilities holding leadership positions and higher salaries, or 3.6% of the 83 employees with disabilities. The disparity in average wages between people with and without disabilities exists because of the unequal distribution of people with disabilities in leadership positions.

In addition to a salary, all Serasa Experian employees receive benefits that include health and dental insurance, a US $256 per month meal card, tax cuts with a bank account, life insurance, and money for retirement. When salaries of people with disabilities at Serasa are compared with those of people without disabilities in the same position, there is no salary distinction. This is noteworthy because, throughout Brazil, people with disabilities earn on average US $64 a month less than coworkers in the same position.[43]

4.1.2 Inclusion

In addition to gaining work experience and professional inclusion, the impact on employees with disabilities extends to their inclusion as members of a community and participation in society. Many employees with disabilities report increased feelings of inclusion and respect since their employment at Serasa. A blind proofreader, Julianna, commented that socially, her life has been positively impacted through being in contact with more people daily.

Employees expressed that the ability to participate as a consumer felt like a form of inclusion. A blind employee, Lincoln, shared, "It's really important, I think that having a job and being inserted in the job market is what gives you the biggest equality in a social world, so it's been really important. The professional insertion creates a big cycle of things because when you get money, you spend money. You start traveling, you start going places, so the conquer of a job allows you to have other achievements."[44]

4.1.3 Self-Esteem

The training program addresses self-esteem because people with disabilities are disenfranchised and this discrimination can negatively affect their self-esteem. Professional success and recognition are powerful sources to improve self-esteem. Andrea, a physically disabled employee of one year says, "To have a job is important because people with disabilities usually are more retracted and so it's important for them, not only professionally but also personally to have something. That will work with your self-esteem, making you feel better with yourself."[45]

4.1.4 Independence

One of the intentions of the EPPD program, as Ribas explains, is "to make people with disabilities grow up."[46] By this, he is referring to dismantling the patronizing attitude that many people and the government hold toward people with disabilities that creates forms of dependency, particularly financial (whether through the state or family). Gustavo, a blind employee, explains, "I'm more independent. I can help my family or help myself. I felt myself responsible for things in my house. My father used to be the only money and now it's not the case anymore. So, I can feel responsible, I could decide things in my life."[47]

Beyond finances, gaining familial independence is an empowering experience. Luiza commented on her blind coworker's employment playing a role in his family relations and independence. She says, "He proved himself professional, the family started to see him as someone capable of doing something."[48] Lincoln says, "The fact that I got a job allowed me to discover the world, the fact that I leave my house, I go to work, I leave early, I walk at night, I have to walk on the streets to get a bus, a subway, these things let me know the world, let me know people."[49]

Two of the current participants were previously employed by their families and they found that the insular environment was not a fulfilling or particularly interesting source of work for them. Teresa, a leader in cognitive disability rights in Brazil, reports that working for one's family can result in stress for the family and the individual, who cannot feel independent in many ways.

4.1.5 Fulfilling Work

It has been a unique experience in the context of the Brazilian environment that many of Serasa Experian's employees with disabilities have their interests and abilities line up with their area of work. It is common practice for companies hiring people with disabilities to place all employees with disabilities in the same area without regard to employees' personal interests and abilities, allowing the presence of a disability to determine the type of work. Gabriela, a deaf employee, describes her relationship with coworkers at Serasa as more personable and inclusive than her former work experience. "Here it's different. There it was production and they could talk a little but with lips and it was boring. They didn't want to learn Libras and also they didn't want to talk with me that much."[50]

Bruno, a logistical coordinator at Serasa Experian, comments on a similar observation with his former company. "[Deaf people] used to do repetitive jobs and tasks and it's something that people do a lot with deaf people and in my opinion it's terrible because it's underutilization of the person, underestimation."[51] About Serasa Experian Bruno shares, "People are utilized, they are optimized in all the potential."[52]

The EPPD does not make limiting assumptions that allow the type of disability to determine the area of work. For instance, Serasa Experian has a blind proofreader and a traveling salesman in a wheelchair. Lincoln, a blind employee in public relations, says, "I'm a journalist and I have never found out about another place that I could work even though I have a deficiency."[53] An employee with a physical disability commented, "[The EPPD] has the sensibility to have people work with what they studied and this is not something that happens in all companies. Usually the work for people with disabilities is patronized, so I think this is a really, this is a course that has a high quality and a high sensibility for people."[54]

4.2 Impact on the Company

4.2.1 Coworkers' Perception of People with Disabilities

The EPPD has an effect on the employees without disabilities as their prejudices and preconceptions about people with disabilities are challenged. In addition to the intentional practices of the EPPD to educate employees without disabilities about people with disabilities, most coworkers highlight the power of coexistence with coworkers with disabilities to dispel prejudices.

Many spaces remain largely segregated between populations with and without disabilities in São Paulo. Teresa says, "I think this is the thing like in Brazil, we don't live with people with disabilities and this is really hard...to break this segregation in Brazil that people with disabilities don't like have a regular life and go to regular school, to have the regular job."[55]

Segregation results in an inequality of education and employment for people with disabilities and a lack of opportunity for people without disabilities to live with and understand the abilities and realities of people with disabilities. Public awareness campaigns and education about people with disabilities are only recent endeavors by the government. At Serasa Experian, the shared space and daily interaction with employees with disabilities has thus been unique and illuminating for people without disabilities. As the EPPD has existed for 10 years, people with disabilities have a strong presence in the company. Ribas says, "You see people with disabilities always; in the corridors, in the work stations, in the elevator, in all places here at Serasa Experian."[56]

Many coworkers and supervisors of people with disabilities have recognized prejudices they unknowingly held when they began to work alongside an employee with a disability. Luiza, an employee without a disability says, "I didn't have an inclusive education...I didn't really know how to talk, how to act, and then you find all the prejudice in you."[57] She goes on to say, "The possibility of living with people...it opens the head to realize that many barriers are in our heads."[58]

Bianca explains the "ripple effect" of challenging prejudices through her working closely with Laura. She says, "I think that when you put someone with a disability working in a regular environment you change the people that work in this environment and these people will go out and change the world. They will change their families and the education of their kids. I have two kids and they know Laura, so they deal with disability in a much better way."[59]

Isabel, the agency manager at a satellite office, says, "I've grown a lot as a person. It was kind of funny how the team got involved [because] we were scared how we would be able to communicate when Gabriela came because she was deaf. And so, we found out that living together, every day, seeing each other, it changes everything."[60] Isabel goes on to say, "Seeing the work that Serasa Experian does and having people on my team with a disability and knowing their potential, they have a lot of quality to add to the team. So it is with our vision we look at them like this, not as a number to just...fulfill the quota."[61]

4.2.2 Diversity and Reputation

The president and upper management view the EPPD as part of Serasa's efforts to be socially responsible. Serasa Experian is a for-profit company, so although their being socially responsible may have real positive benefits for individuals and the community, the company has one overall objective, to make money. Upper management wants to increase diversity through employing more people with disabilities to improve overall functioning of employees and problem-solving abilities. As the president of Serasa Experian shares, "I think [diversity] a good element in terms of getting different perspectives from life. I think it's very important for new insights that can provoke innovation."[62] Serasa also wants to create a company reputation as an ethical and socially responsible company as a strategy to increase profits by influencing consumers through its positive role in the community and also by avoiding fines from the government.

There are varying opinions about whether increased profit through an improvement in Serasa's reputation is an impact of the program. Antonio, the manager of Corporate Citizenship, does not think that the EPPD is a money-maker for Serasa Experian: "I don't believe this program makes us better business…but, it helps us to build stronger relationships."[63]

The EPPD is a well-known and respected program in the disability world throughout São Paulo. The EPPD was selected by the International Labor Organization as a Best Practice in a report about employability and disability. A combination of the longevity of the program and the government's respect for its results contribute to the position of Serasa as a benchmark company.

4.3 Impact on Partner Companies

The impact of the EPPD on the partner companies has been on the quality of employees with disabilities and the "severity" of the employee's disability. For the majority of the partner companies, the number of people with disabilities employed has increased since partnering with Serasa Experian, but not dramatically. The partner companies have used other methods to recruit people with disabilities to work in addition to the EPPD.

All of the partner companies interviewed report that graduates from Serasa's training program are better qualified and more professional than past employees with disabilities, though the extent of that difference varies. Marcelo from the partner company Deloitte shares, "There were 65 people with disabilities working, and now there are 70, so the numbers haven't gone up but the quality of the work that the people with disabilities have delivered has gone up."[64]

The partner companies value having access to the expertise of the EPPD and Ribas. Since Deloitte became partners with the EPPD, they have learned the methodology and constructed a training program and online sensitization program, largely inspired by what they learned with the EPPD. Tozzini Freire, partners with the EPPD since 2008, have also created a sensitization course similar to that of Serasa Experian's. A coordinator at Tozzini Freire, Fabia, says, "Serasa Experian is a good company because usually after [people with disabilities] are hired they need following. So [the EPPD] can talk about physical adaptation, accessibility, relations, and they give us this support."[65]

The support and knowledge that the EPPD offers also makes companies more confident to hire people with more "severe" disabilities. Fabia says, "Serasa Experian introduced people with more severe disability and this is a tendency in the whole market, to hire people with light disabilities…this is important because bringing these professionals that need the job, they also need the training and the environment where they are going to work needs to be prepared. Serasa Experian can give you this support."[66] Marcelo, from Deloitte, says, "The training program of Serasa Experian made it possible for us to bring people with bigger disabilities. Like our first completely blind and completely deaf [employee], came through Serasa Experian and made us open the doors."[67]

By partnering with the EPPD, companies could become part of a community of leaders in the disability field in São Paulo. Fabia elaborates about the positive experience of networking, "Serasa Experian today in Brazil is the reference in inclusion, so to work with Serasa Experian is an opportunity to get to know other partners... We exchange experiences and João Ribas is a great guy who gives a lot of ideas and change[s] our concepts with some things. It's no doubt that it's a good partnership."[68]

Networking with Serasa Experian is beneficial to secure positive relations with the government and the minister of labor as well. Marcelo shared, "When Deloitte talked to Serasa about training, we were being heavily fined by the public minister and we needed to show that we were changing our actions. So the Serasa participation is a little bit political... It is something that the public ministry and the... regional legacy of work, they will see as something positive."[69]

5. CHALLENGES, LIMITATIONS, AND DISCUSSION

Although the overall successes of the EPPD outweigh its shortcomings, the program does face difficulties.

5.1 Challenges and Limitations

5.1.1 Promotions, Positions of Leadership, and Securing Fulfilling Work

Employees with disabilities at Serasa Experian expressed a shared concern and frustration with the difficulty of securing a promotion. According to the September 2011 data, 63 of the 83 employees with disabilities (or 76%) were at entry-level positions (auxiliary or assistant), 17 (or 20.5%) had mid-level positions, and three (or 3.5%) had leadership positions. Renan, a blind employee who has worked at Serasa for 22 years has been promoted twice. He thinks it is because he was unable to complete a college degree and Serasa Experian requires a college education for higher positions.

Mateus, a blind lawyer, particularly frustrated with the difficulty of being promoted, shares, "I have colleagues that are here for four years and haven't had a promotion yet. And the company hasn't resolved this problem yet. It's general, but I think it's harder for people with disabilities."[70] Antonio, a manager in the Corporate Citizenship area says, "You can see that part of them are moving, but I believe it's less than 10% you know, so it's something we have to deal with and this is one of the reasons sometimes that we lose some of them."[71]

Factors that increase one's enjoyment of work include diversity in what you're doing, opportunities for advancement, and autonomy.[72] Mateus, a blind employee who was promoted once after four years of working, says, "We don't just want a job and that's it, we want to have the opportunity to grow.... I really enjoy my job and I think the more responsibilities you have, the more motivated you feel and I think the more motivated you feel, the better job you do."[73]

Lack of promotional opportunities made employees less invested in staying at Serasa Experian long term. Every employee with a disability that I talked to reported that they felt included, both professionally and socially, at Serasa. However, only about half of the participants responded that they felt fulfilled professionally, that they were being fully utilized and challenged. Employees desire professional growth and promotions not only for an increased salary, as Mateus, a blind lawyer explains, "The big problem is not just the amount of money I make. The big problem is the lack of challenge. You arrive here everyday and do always the same thing and you think, 'no, it's not challenging, it's not fair.'"[74]

The majority of the employees with disabilities at Serasa Experian have completed the training program, which makes them more qualified than the average person with a disability in São Paulo and thus more likely to be able to find better positions in other companies. Ribas understands restricted vertical mobility is a limitation at Serasa Experian. He says, "If two, three years after he starts his job here, he wants to start his own company, it's okay because I know in the other company maybe he can grow much more than here."[75]

The problem of promotion, however, is a citywide and nationwide challenge. Companies may be particularly wary of promoting because Brazilian workers are highly protected by collective bargaining, so it is difficult to reverse a wage increase or a promotion unless a worker agrees to it. The Minister of Labor recognizes this shortcoming of the employment of people with disabilities in leadership positions. He says, "We have observed that the possibility of getting higher places is difficult and something that we are trying to check in to stimulate."[76] In addition, at Serasa Experian, in order to move to receive a promotion one must remain in a position for one-year minimum and it is difficult if not impossible to skip positions as one makes their way up in the ranks.

Renata, a blind woman in the training program, worked at a large computer company for four years without a promotion. When asked if she thought promotion for people with disabilities was a problem specifically at her former company she says, "I don't believe it was the company, I think it's general. There were 85 people with disabilities, only one got a promotion."[77] She says that people without disabilities get promotions more frequently. "A little bit because people think that a person with disabilities doesn't have that much development to become a leader, to have leadership. A little bit because of the culture, it takes more time for a people with disabilities to have access and this makes it harder to have leadership."[78]

This issue of lack of promotion at Serasa Experian is currently being addressed by having ongoing education supported by Serasa Experian. Serasa Experian offers subsidies and flexibility for employees (with or without disabilities) who have worked at Serasa Experian for at least one year and who want to pursue another degree in school. Ribas has additional plans to address this issue further by offering leadership training specifically for people with disabilities.

There are benchmark cases that are used to prove that promotion and employment in a leadership position is possible at Serasa Experian. One such is Fernando, a manager of sales, who has been promoted four times in the eight years that he has worked at Serasa and currently holds a leadership position as manager of external sales. He has ranked in the top-selling 10% in the department for three years.

Fernando was a manager of sales previous to coming to Serasa, before he became a wheelchair rider. When he entered, Fernando was placed in a much lower position that paid 90% less than his previous experience. He began at the low-level position of call center employee because the EPPD had that specific opening available. Even though Fernando did not enter through the training program, he was hired through the EPPD. The EPPD rarely has openings at a high level because it is rare for a person with a disability to be qualified for a high level position upon entering. Fernando chose to come to Serasa because he "believed in the program."[79] About being recognized for his abilities and being promoted, Fernando says, "[People with disabilities'] capacity has to be much bigger than our normal…people don't believe that we are capable."[80]

Victor, Fernando's supervisor, says Fernando's case is proof that hiring people with disabilities is not an act of charity, but, as with all employees, a benefit for Serasa Experian. Victor says, "Like Fernando, we get a lot from being open to these people because he's one of the top performers, I don't care if he can walk like I do. He is a top performer on my team, so I think it's more an example for other companies."[81]

5.1.2 Individual Prejudice and Lack of Leadership Support

The level of inclusion and opportunities for growth for an employee with disabilities at Serasa Experian is greatly influenced by their direct supervisor, a position referred to by Serasa Experian employees as "leader" interchangeably. An accommodating and respectful supervisor, or leader, can create a cohesive team that takes time to teach a new employee with disabilities how to fulfill tasks and learn what that employee needs in order to achieve those tasks. Alternatively, a supervisor who holds negative perceptions about people with disabilities in the workplace and acts discriminatingly and impatiently can repress the professional growth of employees with disabilities on their team. Although the EPPD makes efforts to eliminate prejudice and discrimination toward people with disabilities, anecdotal evidence shows that certain supervisors have maintained an attitude that creates challenges for the professional and social inclusion of employees with disabilities.

Many of the employees with disabilities expressed that, at first, they had one or a few coworkers who were prejudiced. With time, the coworkers' attitudes changed and prejudices subsided by seeing first-hand the capable work done by a person with a disability. Victor, a director of sales and supervisor of Fernando, the benchmark example of success, speaks highly of the program but also honestly shares what may be a common concern, "If you ask me, 'well, would you give an opportunity for a person with disabilities?' I have to be sincere…maybe in Brazil, this is a sales person, you have to go to the clients and we don't have a good infrastructure for people with disabilities in Brazil. Would I have concerns? Yes, I probably would because it's more difficult for them."[82]

Ribas admits that it is sometimes difficult to convince supervisors to take the time to train new employees with disabilities. He says, "You have to have the knowledge to help him in the first three months, because of course he needs special attention."[83] Luiza, a coordinator in public relations, has witnessed first-hand the problems that arise with a prejudiced supervisor. A blind coworker of hers, Paulo, was nearly released because his supervisor was impatient and unmotivated to search for the ways to create an environment in which he could work and succeed (e.g., by adjusting the format of certain texts). Luiza speculates that these actions stemmed from biased notions of what a blind person's limits were. Luiza says, "Our leader kind of gave up on him."[84] Paulo and his coworker made adjustments independent from the supervisor and proved his competence. Because of this support, Paulo was able to keep his position. Luiza suggests that the EPPD "invest more in the capacitation of the leadership."[85]

Efforts to address these issues at Serasa are ongoing. Julianna, a blind employee who experienced resistance from her supervisor even after sensitization training says,

> "Many leaders never had contact with a professional with a disability so they don't know how the work is done and how to interact with these people. So, at

the same time the leader has to be open to the professional, the professional has to be patient to show to the leader their capacities and limitations too . . . Maybe a training is not enough to take all the barriers that exist in the mind of a person. So, sometimes a prejudice is not broken like that, like from one minute to the other. So that's why I say that the two parts involved have to be patient, the leader and the professional."[86]

5.2 Discussion: Lessons Learned and Potential Replicability

5.2.1 Supportive Upper Management and Leadership

Although individual prejudice and lack of mid-level leadership support negatively affect employee work and inclusion, the existence and much of the success of the EPPD is reliant upon upper management's support. Initially, the president supported the idea of the program because Serasa Experian was being threatened with a fine for not making efforts to comply with the quota. Since then, two subsequent presidents have continued to support the EPPD. Their motivation for supporting the EPPD may be both to improve Serasa's reputation and to increase profit. However, they fully support Ribas and grant him autonomy to run the program without the upper management micromanaging or steering its direction.

At a lower level, a supportive team and leader are necessary for the inclusion, acceptance, and ultimate fulfillment of the employee with a disability. Gustavo, a blind employee, comments positively on the leadership support since entering Serasa Experian two years ago: "I think it's the boss, the manager that really wanted to be patient about teaching me new things, and believing that I would be able to [handle] that situation. And I would think [it was] nothing special that Serasa did, just believed it was possible."[87]

Abrahan, a leader at the Antonio Carlos branch of Serasa Experian, explains his mentality as a leader of people with disabilities, "This is my concern as a leader; the communication has to reach everyone. And so I will look at the disabilities that I have in my group and I'll try to find solutions to each disability."[88] He recognizes the need for employees in leadership positions to take responsibility: "The leader, he needs to have a really active analysis . . . so if someone is doing something wrong, he's not doing something wrong because he has a disability, but maybe because he didn't have the proper training or no one kept up with what he was doing and teaching him."[89]

5.2.2 Budget

The complete support and trust that the EPPD has secured from upper management and the economic success of Serasa Experian have provided the program with an ample and flexible budget. Ribas reports that he has more than he needs in terms of financial support. Upper management trusts Ribas to define what costs are necessary for the EPPD. Ribas provides an example, "When we are preparing the new budgets, if I ask Serasa Experian to change a Braille printer, they won't ask me if it's important, they trust me."[90] As the company's profits and budget increases, so does the budget for the EPPD.

Currently, the EPPD has a rough budget of US $2,000 for sign language interpretation a month, US $3,500 per month for equipment, US $1,100 for Bianca's support with Laura, and US $1,200 for a screen reader software. The forum they hold is another significant expense.

Although the salary of the person with disabilities is most often paid by the department where he or she is placed, occasionally the EPPD pays. This is used as an incentive for managers to hire a person with a disability to his or her team to save money on salary costs. Unfortunately, Ribas reports that occasionally this system prevents employees with disabilities paid by the EPPD account from getting promoted because the EPPD can only pay the starting salary from its budget.

5.2.3 Positive Work Environment

The EPPD is situated in a "people-oriented" company. Serasa Experian sees employees as indivisible—unable to be separated into a professional and a personal self. This approach encompasses the EPPD and its attention to the employee as an individual with both professional and personal needs and providing support for its employees and their community. The workplace atmosphere is generally described as positive, friendly, and calm.

Bianca, an employee at Serasa Experian's knowledge center, comments on the unique humanity of Serasa Experian, "I feel that Serasa Experian is a company that is really concerned with people. I see this difference between here and my previous jobs."[91] Gustavo, a blind coworker, agrees: "[My coworkers] are all my friends, I consider them more than family."[92] Serasa has been recognized as the best company to work for in Brazil and as the tenth best company to work for in Latin America, appearing on this list every year consecutively since 2004.

6. CONCLUSION

6.1 Overview of Main Findings

The Serasa Experian Employability Program for Persons with Disabilities' main goal is to increase professional and social inclusion, decrease inequalities in employment for people disabilities, fulfill the company's social obligation, and comply with the quota legislation. To reach these goals, the EPPD uses a diverse set of strategies, including creating a workplace that is physically and structurally accessible, providing training for incoming employees with disabilities and nondisabled coworkers, and partnering with companies, NGOs, and governmental bodies. The EPPD's methodology of "two-way street," quality over quantity, and investment rather than cost frames informs all of its strategies, helping make the program a benchmark example of inclusion in São Paulo.

The EPPD, with a unique methodology and level of expertise and experience, networks to share their knowledge. The EPPD partners with companies to provide trained employees with disabilities and support through knowledge and networking and hosting an open-to-the-public forum on employment and persons with disabilities.

The strategies employed by the EPPD have been successful overall, as measured by the positive impact on the lives of those in the training program, employees with disabilities at Serasa Experian and the partner companies. They have expressed feeling respect at work and independence and autonomy as they move through society.

There are difficulties, both internal and external to the company, which prevent the EPPD from reaching its goals completely. Greatly affected by the societal and educational context that puts people with disabilities at an inherent disadvantage upon entering the training program or the workplace. Moreover, there is a disproportionately low percentage of employees with disabilities in leadership positions. Despite the internal knowledge-sharing efforts and support offered to all employees in leadership positions by the EPPD about people with disabilities, some individuals remain prejudiced and continue to behave impatiently, unaccommodatingly, or discriminatorily toward people with disabilities, negatively affecting the fulfillment and growth potential of an employee with disabilities.

The EPPD's methodologies and strategies are potentially replicable by other for-profit companies to increase their inclusion of people with disabilities. However, the EPPD, as it exists at Serasa Experian, has specific elements that are fundamental to its success, namely, the support it receives from upper management.

When people with disabilities at Serasa Experian were asked what effect employability has had on their lives, two responses represent commonly expressed ideas. One employee shared, "It's really important, I think that having a job and being inserted in the job market is what gives you the biggest equality in a social world."[93] Another employee responded, "In everything…this changed life completely; you start to see society in a different way."[94] The success of the program reinforces the importance of employability as a means for equality and inclusion of people with disabilities both professionally and socially, as members of society.

ACKNOWLEDGMENTS

This case study would not have been possible without the incredible cooperation and participation of Serasa Experian; all of the employees, trainees, Ribas, and Pricilla. Thanks to Serasa's partner companies, NGOs, and individuals. Thank you Tinka, Leo, Magda, Gonzalo, and Jody from the IHSP. Finally, thank you Fernanda for translating.

NOTES

1. Presidência da República (1999). Decreto Nº 3.298 de 20 de Dezembro. Retrieved February 19, 2013, from http://www.planalto.gov.br/ccivil_03/decreto/d3298.htm
2. Instituto Brasileiro de Geografía e Estatística (n.d.). Demographic Census 2000: Population and Household Characteristics—Universe Results. Retrieved February 19, 2013, from http://www.ibge.gov.br/english/estatistica/populacao/censo2000.
3. International Disability Rights Monitor (2004). Brazil. 2004 IDRM Country Report. Retrieved on February 19, 2013, from http://www.ideanet.org/idrm_reports.cfm.
4. Neri, M., Pinto, A., Soares, W., & Costilla, H. (2003). *Retratos da Deficiência no Brasil*. Rio de Janeiro, Brazil: FGV/IBRE.
5. Ibid.
6. Araújo, J.P., & Schmidt, A. (2006). A inclusão de pessoas com necessidades especiais no trabalho: a visão de empresas e de instituições educacionais especiais na cidade de Curitiba. *Revista Brasileira de Educação Especial* 12(2), 241–54.
7. João Ribas (Coordinator of Diversity and Inclusion at Serasa Experian, São Paulo). Interview, June 13, 2011.
8. Instituto Brasileiro de Geografía e Estatística (n.d.). Demographic Census 2000.
9. Ribas, Interview, July 4, 2011.
10. Lincoln (Assistant in Public Relations, Serasa Experian, São Paulo). Interview, June 15, 2011.
11. Julianna (Auxiliary of Communication, Serasa Experian, São Paulo) Interview, August 5, 2011.
12. Abrahan (Manager of Operations of Agencies, Serasa Experian, São Paulo). Interview, July 18, 2011.
13. Luiza (Public Relations Coordinator, Serasa Experian, São Paulo). Interview, June 29, 2011.
14. Ribas, Interview, July 4, 2011.
15. Neri, Pinto, Soares, & Costilla (2003). *Retratos da Deficiência no Brasil*.
16. Instituto Brasileiro de Geografía e Estatística (2010). Síntese de Indicadores Sociais: Uma Análise das Condições de Vida Da População Brasileria. Retrieved February 19, 2013, from http://www.ibge.gov.br/home/estatistica/populacao/condicaodevida/indicadoresminimos/sinteseindicsociais2010/default.shtm
17. UN Enable (2007). Disabilities and Employment. Fact Sheet 1. United Nations Department of Public Information. Retrieved on February 19, 2013, from http://www.un.org/disabilities/documents/toolaction/employmentfs.pdf

18. Neri, Pinto, Soares, & Costilla (2003). *Retratos da Deficiência no Brasil.*
19. Angela (Monitor of Serasa Experian Training Program, São Paulo). Interview, July 19, 2011.
20. Milena (Serasa Experian Training Program Participant, São Paulo). Interview, July 12, 2011.
21. Alberto (Serasa Experian Training Program Participant, São Paulo). Interview, June 16, 2011.
22. Alex (Serasa Experian Training Program Participant, São Paulo). Interview, July 19, 2011.
23. Karla (Libras Translator, Serasa Experian Consultant, São Paulo). Interview. August 9, 2011.
24. Lincoln, Interview, June 15, 2011.
25. Shakespeare, T. (2010). The Social Model of Disability. In L.J. Davis (Ed.). *The Disability Studies Reader Third Edition* (New York: Routledge), 266.
26. Ribas, Interview, June 13, 2011.
27. Author Unkown (1994). Section 3.1 of NBR 9050, ASSOCIAÇÃO BRASILEIRA DE NORMAS TÉCNICAS. Acessibilidade de Pessoas Portadoras de Deficiências a Edificações, Espaço, Mobiliário e Equipamento Urbanos. NBR 9050. Rio de Janeiro, Brazil: ABNT.
28. Fernando (Manager of External Sales, Serasa Experian, São Paulo) Interview, August 5, 2011.
29. Kim (Libras Translator, Serasa Experian Consultant, São Paulo). Interview, August 9, 2011.
30. Julianna, Interview, August 5, 2011.
31. Isabel (Manager of Serasa Experian Santo Andre Office, São Paulo). Interview, July 27, 2011.
32. Carolina (Senior Analyst at Serasa Experian, São Paulo). Interview, July 12, 2011.
33. Bianca (Knowledge Center Assistant, Serasa Experian, São Paulo). Interview, June 22, 2011.
34. Abrahan, Interview, July 18, 2011.
35. Dr. Carlos de Carmo, (Labor Inspector for the São Paulo Ministry of Labor and Employment, São Paulo). Interview, July 14, 2011.
36. Rocha Olivier, J., and de Camargo, M.R. (2006). A Empregabilidade para Pessoas Surdas: Inclusão e Exclusão Social. São Paulo, Brazil: UniFMU.
37. Ribas, Interview, July 4, 2011.
38. Alice (Analyst for Tech Suport, Serasa Experian, São Paulo). Interview, June 30, 2011.
39. Ribas, Interview, June 13, 2011.
40. Ribas, Interview, August 1, 2011.
41. Ibid.
42. Martelo, A. (2011). Mantega anuncia que salário mínimo será de R$ 545 a partir de fevereiro. *O Globo*, January 14. Retrieved February 19, 2013, from http://g1.globo.com/economia/noticia/2011/01/mantega-anuncia-que-salario-minimo-sera-de-r-545-partir-de-fevereiro.html
43. Neri, Pinto, Soares, and Costilla (2003). *Retratos da Deficiência no Brasil.*
44. Lincoln, Interview, June 15, 2011.
45. Andrea (Assistant in Payroll, Serasa Experian, São Paulo). Interview, June 22, 2011.
46. Ribas, Interview, June 13, 2011.

47. Gustavo (Administrative Assistant, Serasa Experian, São Paulo). Interview, June 13, 2011.
48. Luiza, Interview, June 29, 2011.
49. Lincoln, Interview, June 15, 2011.
50. Gabriela (Auxiliary at Serasa Experian, São Paulo). Interview, July 27, 2011.
51. Bruno (Logistical Coordinator, Serasa Experian, São Paulo). Interview, July 1, 2011.
52. Ibid.
53. Lincoln, Interview, June 15, 2011.
54. Andrea, Interview, June 22, 2011.
55. Teresa (Consultant of Serasa Experian and Psychologist at ADIDI and Congruencia, São Paulo). Interview, June 29, 2011.
56. Ribas, Interview, June 13, 2011.
57. Luiza, Interview, June 29, 2011.
58. Ibid.
59. Bianca, Interview, June 22, 2011.
60. Isabel, Interview, July 27, 2011.
61. Ibid.
62. Ricardo Loureiro (President of Serasa Experian, São Paulo). Interview, July 27, 2011.
63. Antonio (Manager Corporate Citizenship, Serasa Experian, São Paulo). Interview, August 1, 2011.
64. Marcelo (Human Resources Consultant, Deloitte, São Paulo). Interview, July 11, 2011.
65. Fabia (Coordinator Human Relations, Tozzini Freire, São Paulo). Interview, July 29, 2011.
66. Ibid.
67. Marcelo, Interview, July 11, 2011.
68. Fabia, Interview, July 29, 2011.
69. Marcelo, Interview, July 11, 2011.
70. Mateus (Junior Lawyer, Serasa Experian, São Paulo). Interview, July 1, 2011.
71. Antonio, Interview, August 1, 2011.
72. Walton, R.E. (1973). Quality of Working Life: What is it? Sloan Management Review 15(1), 11–21.
73. Mateus, Interview, July 1, 2011.
74. Ibid.
75. Ribas, Interview, July 4, 2011.
76. Dr. de Carmo, Interview, July 14, 2011.
77. Renata (Serasa Experian Training Program Participant, São Paulo). Interview, July 7, 2011.
78. Ibid.
79. Fernando, Interview, August 5, 2011.
80. Ibid.
81. Victor (Director of Sales, Serasa Experian, São Paulo). Interview, July 6, 2011.
82. Ibid.
83. Ribas, Interview, June 13, 2011.
84. Luiza, Interview, June 29, 2011.
85. Ibid.
86. Julianna, Interview, July 5, 2011.
87. Gustavo, Interview, June 13, 2011.

88. Abrahan, Interview, July 18, 2011.
89. Ibid.
90. Ribas, Interview July 4, 2011.
91. Bianca, Interview, June 22, 2011.
92. Gustavo, Interview, June 13, 2011.
93. Lincoln, Interview, June 15, 2011.
94. Gustavo, Interview, June 13, 2011.

CHAPTER 6

Assistive Technology and Employment in Low-Resource Environments

JOYOJEET PAL

1. INTRODUCTION

Since the opening of the United Nations Convention on the Rights of Persons with Disabilities (CRPD) in 2007, there has been a renewed energy in global concerns over the availability of low-cost access to assistive technology (AT). With 154 signatories, 126 ratifications, and 76 ratifications of the optional protocol,[1] the CRPD is one of the most widely embraced pieces of international legislation in history.

For people with disabilities in a number of nations, the convention has been the first instance of legal provision of rights and accessibility. The rights-based view of disability that the CRPD brings to the table has much potential to bring greater attention to economic and social inclusion.

And yet, people with disabilities in low-income nations often face additional challenges in ensuring economic rights embodied in the CRPD because of limited state capacity, public funding, and implementation. Although there has been a significant amount of research on disability in low-income regions, a majority has been on one of two general areas of work—the first has been research on disease burden,[2] focusing on the enumeration and prevention of physical impairments, or examining the economic impacts of disability through one specific variable of analysis. The second area has been anthropological and philosophical work on disability, approaching it from cultural frames of social or rights-based models.[3]

The early years of implementation of the CRPD have led to an increase in scholarly research relating to disability rights and accessibility in low- and middle-income countries,[4] including on the need for and scope of assistive technology for increasing social and economic inclusion.[5] This chapter offers an overview of assistive technology and accessibility for people with disabilities, focusing on workers with visual disabilities, and discusses some of the key issues ahead in bridging the cost and context divide between these technologies to better fit the needs of people in low- and middle-income countries.

2. INTERNATIONAL LAW AND THE IMPORTANCE OF ASSISTIVE TECHNOLOGY

The CRPD comes at the end of three decades of international legal discussions around the issue of disability. The UN General Assembly adopted the World Program of Action concerning disabled persons over three decades ago, which promoted the full participation of persons with disabilities in social life. The idea of "promotion" implied nothing legally binding, but the specific inclusion of "all countries regardless of their level of development" into the World Program of Action meant that there was already recognition that, irrespective of the state of economic development, disability rights needed prioritization. The decade immediately following—from 1983 to 1992—was declared the UN Decade of Disabled Persons. At the end of this, in 1993, the General Assembly adopted the Standard Rules on the Equalization of Opportunity for Persons with Disabilities, which required states to remove obstacles to equal participation. A Special Rapporteur was appointed as a monitor for the implementation at national levels, but the Rapporteur's recommendations were again not legally binding.

An argument against a specific convention on the rights of persons with disabilities was that the existence of a Universal Declaration of Human Rights ought to extend to all people. However, the movement for a separate classification was supported by a number of factors. First, a number of states legislated these disability rights, in spite of having general citizen rights constituted, thus highlighting the recognition for a separate discussion on disability. Second, the Decade of Disabled Persons had not led to much quantifiable progress. Finally, the UN's recognition of a distinction beyond the general "human rights" definition in its creation of a Convention on the Rights of the Child (which also explicitly mentioned disability) strengthened the case for a separate convention. The ad-hoc committee meetings for the convention began in 2002, and culminated in a General Assembly adoption of the final convention in 2006, which was opened to signing by nation-states on March 30, 2007.

The potential role of international law in the development of legal protections at the national level is an interesting question. In general, international conventions have limited real enforceability against nation-states because of state sovereignty and a broad cultural resistance to global governance of any form.[6] The ability of nation-states to interpret international law has typically meant that the implementation of several such conventions is largely dependent on the appropriation of the nation-state in question, as has been seen in the cases of human rights,[7] women's rights,[8] and torture.[9] From an international law perspective, greater specificity has the benefit of highlighting the importance of one set of rights, but also offers the risk of the blatant non-fulfillment of those mentioned provisions. The mention of AT in articles of the CRPD thus brings attention to it worldwide, but the specific citing of a class of technology that at present-day prices is outside of most low-income regions' ability to provide to its citizens introduces a strange conundrum. Is the mention of AT then purely lip service, and if so, does it reduce the credibility of nation-states' commitment to the convention altogether?

Yet, for many groups of people with disabilities, such as those with vision impairments, creating an inclusive society requires investment in assistive technologies. From basic spatial navigation to communications and computing, just about every means of social participation for people with vision impairments can be significantly enhanced by assistive technologies on mobile or computing devices. Unfortunately, the lack of serious action on the part of signatory states to bring down the cost of AT and make it available outside of what has been a fairly lukewarm market-driven increase in access to AT calls to question the seriousness with which several states (including many who have signed on to the optional protocol) have considered implementation specifics. Although there has been some work on the scope of the convention[10] and on the education of children with disabilities in relation to the convention,[11] there has been little detailed research on what it really means in practice to contextualize AT to the needs of populations in low- and middle-income countries.

There are both explicit and implicit roles for assistive tools in implementing the convention to its intended spirit. By explicit we mean those places where AT and accessibility are specifically noted; and by implicit we mean those parts of the CRPD that could not be implemented without the use of AT. As an example, in several countries where governance and the economy are increasingly technology heavy, the right to work or the right to political and public life—both defined in the Convention—may not be actionable without adequate access to computing resources. In addition, there is much evidence that assistive technology significantly improves educational and workplace opportunities for people with disabilities.[12]

The following articles in the Convention specifically refer to AT or accessibility in some form:

- Article 4 (General Obligations), Sections 1(g) and (h): Section 1(g) refers to states' commitment to undertake or promote research and development of new technology and give priority to technologies at affordable costs. Section 1(h) commits states to providing accessible information about assistive technologies.

The specific note of promoting research at affordable costs is important because most research on AT is currently done in the industrialized world, and consequently at the costs reasonable for markets in those countries.

- Article 9 (Accessibility), Section 2(g) and (h) commit states to promoting the design, development, production, and distribution of accessible ICTs at an early stage, such that these technologies become accessible at a minimal cost. The mention of "early stage" here is likewise important because it implies that nation states need to work accessibility into the production of new technologies, to ensure that the legacy problem of inaccessible products and devices is minimized for the future. Legacy problems stretch from architectural accessibility issues with built environments, which can be difficult to retroactively make accessible, to issues with technologies on the hardware and software sides that did not deal with accessibility prior to widespread adoption.

There are several examples of such technologies—such as the Flash multimedia platform (formerly Macromedia, now Adobe), which had a number of accessibility problems. The quick widespread adoption of Flash by Web designers exacerbated the difficulty of the Web-browsing experience for many people with vision impairments. Another important challenge on software accessibility is that of forms. Complex forms with multiple layers of authentication have historically been challenging for people who use screen readers; as more countries start implementing e-governance or e-commerce platforms, this may significantly increase challenges over time.

- Article 20 (Personal Mobility), Section (b) commits states to facilitating access to quality mobility aids and assistive technologies for persons with disability. Section (c) commits states to encouraging entities that provide assistive technologies to conduct needs assessments of people with disabilities. Reference to personal mobility is of immediate relevance to people with a range of disabilities that can impact physical access or wayfinding. In the case of people with vision impairments, this could have important implications to the availability of cellular devices with wayfinding capabilities. Further, the specific mention of needs assessment can help support designers of locally appropriate assistive technology.
- Article 21 (Freedom of expression and opinion, and access to information), Section (b) commits states to facilitate augmentative and

alternative communication (AAC). Section (c) commits states to urging private entities with an Internet presence to providing information in accessible and usable formats. Section (d) commits states to urge the same to mass media. From the perspective of people with vision impairments, Sections (c) and (d) of Article 21 will require states to pay attention to ensuring both that future online information is made more accessible for screen readers, and also that other emerging forms of content such as narrative captioning of films and other content are as well.

- Article 26 (Habilitation and rehabilitation), Section 3 requires that states promote assistive technologies for rehabilitation. Article 29 (Participation in political and public life), Section (iii) requires that states facilitate assistive technologies for the voting process. Articles 26 and 29 are worded in terms of "promotion" and refer to the availability of assistive technologies, potentially provided by the state. The explicit note of the voting process would imply the need for accessible secret ballot devices.

- Article 27 (Work and employment), Section 1(d) commits states to enabling persons with disabilities to have effective access to technical and vocational guidance. Most significantly, Section 1(i) commits states to ensuring reasonable accommodation is provided to persons with disabilities in the workplace. Technology is central to this particular item, especially in the case of vision-impaired persons in the labor market who require accessible computing tools. This is one of the really important articles because it underlines the need for reasonable accommodation in the workplace, which for people with vision impairments would imply at the very least the provision of screen reading technology at the employer's expense.

In summary, the articles clearly note the importance of AT, and are thorough in noting various aspects of the production chain—including research, early-stage development, production, and dissemination. Importantly, the expansion of AT into various low-income regions could significantly impact the larger state of research and development because the need for technology at lower prices would require new innovations in design. Likewise, low-income regions will necessitate new languages, infrastructures, and interfaces. To consider these in detail, we examine the specific technologies within a subset of AT—those technologies developed for people with vision impairments. We discuss the major technologies in this space, as well as their applicability to the needs of new populations in parts of the world that have not had adequate access to AT, and finally how some of these new directions may impact the availability and use of AT around the world.

3. TYPES OF ASSISTIVE TECHNOLOGY FOR PEOPLE WITH VISION IMPAIRMENTS

For people with vision impairments, the importance of assistive technologies in economic and social participation has been fairly well documented in the last decade, especially as computing has become ubiquitous in the workplace.[13] The discussion on Web accessibility and assistive technologies such as screen reading and mobile applications in low- and middle-income countries is still young, but growing.[14] It is useful here to examine briefly the kinds of assistive technology that exist for people with vision impairments and to what extent they are at a point of "market readiness" for use in low- and middle-income countries.

There are various ways of classifying the types of AT, but we explore them here from two categories—framework technologies, and output/hardware technologies. Framework technologies are defined here as those technologies that do the fundamental computing tasks but typically operate at the back end. Framework technologies can be thought of as comparable to an operating system—thus the technology that serves as the scaffolding for applications to be mounted on. The second category is that of output and hardware technologies: the audio, tactile, or magnified output, or the hardware device used by the end user fall under this category. There is another category one can conceptualize coming from this frame: the application level. This refers to those technologies layered over existing hardware but operating at the software level.

3.1 Framework Technologies

Framework technologies are primarily those applications that allow for the translation of computing applications and data to an output format that is appropriate for a person with a disability. Very broadly this includes three main technology groups—optical character recognition (OCR) tools, Braille translators, and screen readers. OCR tools have wide-ranging applications in document management, and consequently represent a much larger research and product agenda than the framework technologies specifically used only by people with vision impairments. While specific Braille translator and screen reader products are used primarily by people with vision impairments, they each have individual components that apply across various technologies.

3.1.1 *Optical Character Recognition Tools*

Optical Character Recognition is a mechanical or electronic translation of scanned text into machine-encoded text through calibration to certain fonts.

It is used mainly to convert written text to electronic form, and also to synthetic speech. Optical Character Recognition has been fundamental to the AT space since the Kurzweil Reading Machine was released in 1975, and there has been significant progress since then on converting printed material to digital text. OCR technologies are reasonably mature in terms of typed print material, and with the growth of mainstream applications in document processing, including a number of massive digital library projects, there is much enthusiasm for the increase in available digital material that can be accessed by people with vision impairments.

In the past, individuals may have needed standalone OCR applications alongside scanners, but this has increasingly moved to the cloud: a number of companies have started offering OCR services online through remotely located servers that process a range of documents in several languages to digital text. Much of the research and new product development in the OCR space has moved to new domains including OCR on photographic and moving images such as security applications, handwritten documents, or improved OCR algorithms. Exact estimations of the global size of the OCR industry are hard to come by because of the level of integration of OCR into various tools, but by one estimate in May 2012, the market for OCR software is in the range of US $347 million, with about 23 major companies operating in this space.[15]

For many of the low- and middle-income nations, the major challenge with OCR is support for native scripts. For example, OCR for Roman/Cyrillic scripts is far more advanced than for other languages, although there are tools that are effective for some forms of printed material in a number of Asian and Middle Eastern written scripts. For people with vision impairments who need to access printed or written material in less represented languages in digital formats, this continues to be a major challenge and is likely to be an important area of technology research in the near future. Countries like India had already started moving towards better OCR for larger languages like Hindi, Bangla, Telugu, and Tamil,[16] whereas smaller languages such as Oriya,[17] Kannada,[18] and Malayalam[19] have also seen important progress in recent years. Likewise, there has been progress with other less dominant scripts, such as Amharic,[20] Tibetan,[21] and Sinhala.[22] A region of the world that needs more progress on this front is Southeast Asia/Indochina, where alphabets like Khmer, Burmese, and Lao still do not have a significant presence in digital document processing research.

Given that OCR has several mainstream uses for the sighted community, applications as diverse as character recognition on postal services[23] have contributed to the increase in research in this space, but the leap from OCR in situations such as numerical or typeset recognition to functional use with a vast range of texts in written forms of very high variance represents a very significant challenge. It may indeed be several years before the vast majority of written materials in the native languages of people with vision impairments in low- and middle-income countries can be easily accessed in digital formats, but the overlap of heritage preservation with this need, as elicited in Article 21 of the CRPD, bodes well.

3.1.2 Speech Recognition

Speech recognition (SR) tools have significant interest within the developers of computing applications because of their widespread application for both disabled and nondisabled populations. These users include people with vision impairments, people who have difficulties reading, and also others with repetitive stress injuries or motor impairments that make them unable to utilize market-standard keyboards, as well as those who simply prefer to use speech. Although some speech recognition applications in the English language are fairly well developed (specifically the product Dragon Speaking Naturally) and use approaches such as training the engine to the voice and intonation of a specific user, the process of speech recognition is itself extremely complex.

A number of factors, including the size of the vocabulary (i.e., open speech versus limited vocabulary), the variability in the speech, background noise conditions, and tonality of the language offer a range of significant challenges to building speech recognition engines. There are a few projects that are looking at speech recognition in languages with a smaller digital footprint, including Arabic,[24] Hindi,[25] and even tonal languages such as Vietnamese,[26] Mandarin,[27] and Thai.[28] But much of this work is at a very experimental level, unlike work in the English language, which is well-established in the product space. Interestingly, some of the developments in SR tools have come from technologies that serve the needs of another socially excluded population: illiterate people.[29] Research into speech recognition is of much greater immediate concern among populations with neuromuscular conditions or an inability to use touch interfaces than to people with vision impairments, because of the relative ubiquity of QWERTY and Braille keyboards, and more recently of cellular interfaces.

3.1.3 Braille

A Braille translator is a back end tool that forms the connecting link between the operating system and a Braille output device. The Braille file created by the translator is sent to a Braille printer or read on a Braille display or smaller personal device. There are a range of products, including Duxbury Megadots and Viewplus Tiger Software, which can be combined with Braille embossers (printers) to print Braille characters alongside a written alphabet. While different languages frequently have different Braille characters, the challenge in supporting these is minimal. One of the major challenges faced by

Braille-based technology has been the physical cost of production of Braille materials—either in the paper format (special paper) or in the electronic format (cost of Braille displays). However, because tactile material is particularly useful in certain specialized domains, Braille translators will continue to play a role for an important niche market.

Braille keyboards are used to type in Braille alphabet using eight keys, six for each Braille dot, one for spaces, and one more for special characters and capitalization. To type one letter, all of the keys that correspond to the dots in that letter are pressed at the same time. Mechanical Braille keyboards have historically enjoyed a relatively small market share, but this is in part due to their historically high cost (roughly in the range of US $500), as a result of which most low-income people with vision impairments in many parts of low- and middle-income countries mainly relied on styluses for writing. Electronic Braille keyboards come in different shapes and formats, from those that can be directly plugged into a computer's USB port to those that come with their own screen readers, inbuilt memory and stand-alone operation capability. A typical keyboard is priced anywhere between US $70 and US $300, which can be fairly steep in low-income nations, but the keyboards with integrated braille displays can cost several thousand dollars. A reason why the size of the Braille keyboard market has been difficult to estimate in recent years is the lately popular approach of Braille overlays, which can be as cheap as US $10 over a conventional QWERTY keyboard. For many low- and middle-income countries, one challenge may be transitioning mechanical keyboard users to QWERTY keyboards if individuals prefer to stay with a Braille input interface, because typing new languages on QWERTY keyboards is fairly straightforward. Approaches such as screen overlays for conventional keyboards are also relatively straightforward to implement in new languages for which the keyboard combinations are fairly standardized.

3.1.4 Screen Readers

Screen readers are perhaps the most important domain of AT for people with vision impairments, as it is a fundamental prerequisite for a nonvisual computing interface. Screen readers are software programs that channel output through a speech synthesizer or Braille translator and allow a user to interact with material on a computer screen. A screen reader is the necessary interface between the computer's operating system, its applications, and a vision-impaired user. The most widely used screen readers are Freedom Scientific's JAWS, which has historically had a very large market share worldwide, and the free and open source NVDA (NonVisual Desktop Access).[30]

JAWS (Job Access With Speech) and Window-Eyes are the screen readers that rank highest in functionality and support the range number of applications, and both cost roughly $1,000. In general, JAWS and Window Eyes control something of a monopoly comparable to the Windows leadership of the operating system market, and wherever possible, users tend to prefer trial or pirated versions of these rather than the available open source alternatives. Even the major agencies working with people with vision impairments tend to donate copies of these rather than promote free or open source technologies. As a result, even though open source tools exist, the more expensive proprietary tools are an overwhelming majority. However, the growth of NVDA is remarkable, up from only 2.9% market share in 2009 (though the users surveyed are mostly from Europe and North America) to being the second most used screen reader in 2012.[31]

However, more importantly, most "power users" of screen readers tend to prefer one of the popular proprietary screen readers due to application support. This is a key technological issue going ahead, especially given the large number of legacy and custom-made applications that screen readers need to support in individual work places. In many low- and middle-income countries, although the proliferation of JAWS has happened due to weak international intellectual property protection, this is unsustainable and poses the risk of regular JAWS users losing the ability to continue using it. Although this will most likely not come to pass for home and public computers, there is a very serious risk that employers will be unwilling to pay high license fees for expensive software. Indeed, the same study showed that vision-impaired job seekers were training themselves in free screen-reading programs as a means of making themselves more "marketable" to companies, and major companies have started investing in application support on NVDA as a means of avoiding buying copies of proprietary software.

Significant challenges to the adoption of open source tools like NVDA still exist. A recent study of screen readers in India showed that factors such as the quality of voice output are extremely important for users at early stages of selecting screen reading technologies, but that these in turn become less important as one becomes an advanced user. However, by the time one does get hooked on to a certain technology, switching costs become very high.[32] In effect, people mentally bundle together the screen reader with the output, and in turn end up comfortable with one overall interface that then becomes difficult to quit.

Language support is also likely to be an important issue given that a large proportion of vision-impaired populations are not speakers of the languages dominant on the Internet. Unlike some of the Braille-based technologies, which are largely restricted to those among the visually-impaired population that are relatively better off because they had access to education, audio-based output technologies have the potential for broad-based reach. Both JAWS and NVDA already support a number of languages, but this will probably need to increase in the coming years. As we see in Table 6.1, there is a significant discrepancy between languages commonly spoken and used by people and the representation of those languages on the Internet. The skew toward a small

Table 6.1 LANGUAGE USE WORLDWIDE AND GROWTH OF LANGUAGE CONTENT ONLINE

Language	Speakers[33] (million)	Language-speakers	Internet users in primary language (million)	Language	Webpages (Million) (2000)[34]	Webpages (Billion) (2010)[35]	Language-speakers	Wikipedia pages ('000) (2011)[36]
Mandarin	845 (1025)	English	536.5	English	214 (68.4)	4.42	English	3669
Spanish	329 (390)	Mandarin	444.9	Japanese	18.3 (5.9)	0.87	German	1252
English	328 (1800)	Spanish	153.3	German	18.1 (5.8)	0.56	French	1119
Arabic	221 (452)	Japanese	99.1	Chinese	12.1 (3.9)	17.17	Italian	815
Hindi-Urdu	182 (490)	Portuguese	82.5	French	9.3 (3.0)	0.35	Polish	811
Bengali	181 (250)	German	75.1	Spanish	7.6 (2.4)	0.40	Spanish	780
Portuguese	178 (193)	Arabic	65.3	Russian	5.9 (1.9)	0.59	Japanese	756
Russian	144 (250)	French	59.8	Italian	4.9 (1.6)	n/a	Russian	728
Japanese	122 (123)	Russian	59.7	Portuguese	4.3 (1.4)	0.20	Dutch	711

few Western languages is probably of most concern in those countries where one of the colonial languages is used commonly, as in most of South Asia, Sub-Saharan Africa, or where indigenous languages do not exist widely in a written form. For users of these languages, the amount of digital information available in their native language is fairly limited. Consequently, the relatively small market creates limited incentives among private firms to build high quality AT tools.

New language support for screen readers will require building an infrastructure of developers interested in creating language add-ons and improving content extraction, on users adding to the corpus of translated and transliterated data, and on machine-learning technologists refining the tools that translate. One of the exciting possibilities for the future may be the ability to crowdsource some of the language content and application support for screen readers. There is scope for a hybrid approach in which governments work on the framework side of the basic screen reading technology, and some form of crowdsourcing can be used to refine the tools in the event that there is no group of dedicated professionals to hone the quality of these tools. However the larger issue of lacking content online is still one that needs addressing.

The last and most important issue on screen reading is going to be the portability of screen readers to mobile devices. This is discussed in greater detail under the subsection on Mobiles.

3.2 Output and Hardware Technologies

As with input devices, output for people with vision impairments depends on their level of functional vision and hearing, which will determine whether a tactile, visual, or audio output system is appropriate. Visual output devices are typically magnifiers that can be either handheld or integrated into the computing environment. Audio output would include products such as screen readers or mobile-based systems. Tactile output devices allow users to perceive through touch—broadly through either a range of Braille-related products, or increasingly, advanced haptic devices that not only allow access to textual material but also to feedback on shapes, texture, vibrations, and motion. Although we recognize the importance of some of these advanced technologies, as well as several innovations in technology-aided wayfinding such as electronic white canes, in the context of this chapter we are discussing only mature technologies of immediate relevance to people with vision impairments in low- and middle-income countries. Importantly, the hardware for people with vision impairments is more than just output devices, as it contains functional elements as well. This is especially important as mobile devices expand in capabilities.

3.2.1 Speech Synthesizers

Speech synthesizers are the primary audio output technology for screen readers. The speech synthesizer is a computer system used for artificially producing human speech and can be implemented in software or hardware. The text to speech (TTS) conversion is implemented in the speech synthesizer. Speech synthesis systems use two basic approaches. The first, text-to-phoneme conversion, involves a large dictionary containing all the words of a language and their correct pronunciations being stored by the program and matched to the spelling. In the other approach, rule-based conversion, pronunciation rules are applied to words to determine pronunciation based on their spelling. Speech synthesizers can thus generate sound based on stored human voice samples or through electronically generated artificial machine approximations of sounds. For the listener the technological approach used could give the impression of output being either "natural sounding" or "mechanical sounding."

As mentioned when discussing language support in the section on screen readers, the text-to-speech synthesis process is technically complex and involves a fair amount of engineering and machine learning, and is consequently fairly expensive to develop. A TTS is typically a separate product from the screen reader itself, and can be either sold separately or bundled with proprietary screen readers; Eloquence and ViaVoice are popular examples of the latter, and they offer a very high quality human-sounding voice in their output in the English language. Even though these products are not technically incompatible with free and open source screen reading products, the companies that own them impose licensing restrictions that do not allow them to be integrated with other screen readers. Thus, users of free screen readers such as NVDA typically need to use open source speech synthesizers such as eSpeak, which is free but offers a somewhat less human sounding output.

In low- and middle-income countries, speech synthesis offers a second challenge: the problem of regional localization. Right now, speech synthesis works very well for languages like English, French, and Japanese, but not for some of the smaller languages in the world. From the perspective of building low-cost technologies for developing regions, a text-to-phoneme approach is quick but fails if it is given a word not contained in its dictionary. As a result, a challenge for new languages involves getting a large enough corpus of words in place. The text-to-phoneme conversion method is more convenient for phonetic scripts like Indic languages than for writing systems that use morphosyllabic characters (as are common in East Asia). For example, Mandarin Chinese is difficult to synthesize due to the range of characters, which have different pronunciations depending on the context, and wherein the intonation is critical in conveying the appropriate meaning. Furthermore, dialectical differences make it difficult to obtain agreement from native speakers on what constitutes an accurate pronunciation of certain phonemes. In short, building high quality screen readers is likely to be very expensive, and companies that have built these are likely to want to capitalize on their efforts.

Text to speech development efforts have nonetheless been underway in a number of countries around the world, building tools for local languages ranging from Romani languages[37] to Kiswahili[38] and Xhosa.[39] Such initiatives, while still often funded in part or whole by university and international academic initiatives, may soon move to state-funded research (as it already has in some countries like India), aligned with the spirit of Articles 4 and 9 of the CRPD. Historically, the work on building TTS has had a fairly large component of university research, and this is likely to be true for the perceivable future of speech synthesis for new languages. The challenge for many of these efforts is moving from lab experiments to full-fledged products. However, as in the case of speech-recognition technology, speech synthesis also benefits from the existence of mainstream applications and there is good reason to hope that the near future will have many high-performing products in this space.

The importance of high-quality local language speech synthesis cannot be understated. While spoken language acquisition for persons with vision impairments follows much the same patterns as that of sighted persons, the case for second language acquisition can be complicated, especially in cultures wherein much language learning depends on visual reinforcement.[40] Findings among neuropsychologists that people with vision-impairments process auditory language stimuli faster than sighted people further underlines the importance of screen readers in facilitating learning.[41] In short, not only is it imperative that there be high quality tools in local languages, there is also an argument for these to be introduced at early ages for children with vision impairments.

3.2.2 Braille Embossers

Braille embossers are printers that provide Braille output. They are impact printers that render Braille on special paper or, nowadays, even on normal paper. These embossers are either mechanical or use special ink. The mechanical ones involve piercing pins into the paper; the thermal method uses special inks that swell up on heating, producing Braille output. There are also traditional Braille typewriters such as the Perkins or Mountbatten Braillers or the larger scale mechanical Braille printing that uses metal plates on which the text is etched and then the plate is impressed upon special swell paper that produces the Braille output. Thermoelectric and impact-based processes have replaced Perkins quite significantly in recent years, similar perhaps to the way typewriters were replaced by word processors.

Modern Braille embossers range from small portable devices that can print out small signs to commercial-grade printers. Commercial grade-printers are comparable in output potential to a multifunction printer for sighted users. Whereas the latter category of printers may cost no more than a few thousand dollars and are easily accessed by the general population either at print shops or in the workspace or educational institutions in the industrialized world, commercial-grade Braille printers can cost upwards of US $80,000 for double-sided printing and are therefore rarely available for people with vision impairments who need material printed except at select academic institutions or public libraries; Indeed, access to Braille printed material continues to be a huge challenge in the industrialized world as well.

In a recent visit to Sierra Leone, we found that there was only one functioning Braille embosser in the entire country (to the knowledge of our affiliates) and that was a fairly basic machine. One can imagine that, for a number of low- and middle-income countries, the problems of the printing, maintenance, durability of output on pin-type Braille, and special paper are all very significant challenges. A few promising directions are emerging—researchers at Northeastern University have experimented with a US $200 embosser that replaces ink cartridges with motor-operated embossing wheels.[42] Although this works very slowly at present (1 character per second), there is scope for such technologies to do better in the near future. Given that Braille embossers have no perceivable use for the mainstream population, this may be one of the areas of research that need significant state-funded research to create less expensive options.

3.2.3 Braille Displays

Braille displays offer tactile output by electronically raising and lowering different combinations of nylon, metal, or plastic pins in Braille cells. These may be used in addition to audio output, depending on individual preferences, though where the user is deaf-blind, these are the primary means of communication. Most Braille displays available in the market are in flat panel formats, with 40 or 80 cells per panel in a straight line. The cells refresh as the user moves a finger along the material. Such panel-based Braille display devices rely on piezoelectric materials for pin actuation; each cell (of 8 dots) has specific dots raised or lowered depending on the character displayed. Because of the complexity of producing a reliable display that will cope with daily wear and tear, these displays are expensive and out of reach for many potential consumers. For Braille displays language is not an issue, because Braille translators take care of that problem.

The larger issue is how to build low-cost Braille displays, which currently cost anywhere between US $2,000 and US $15,000; given the nature of the engineering involved and the relatively small size of the market at that price, this cost may not fall significantly in the near future. One of the interesting innovations in this space has been a rotating-wheel Braille display, in which the Braille dots are placed on the edge of a spinning wheel. This allows the user to read text continuously using a stationary finger as the wheel spins around at a selected speed. Because the Braille dots are set in a simple scanning style and the Braille characters are set by an actuator, the cost and complexity of manufacturing a unit is reduced greatly compared with traditional displays. This is therefore unlike the panel format display, in which each cell has a cost associated with the fabrication of every individual pin and of the rotating wheel. As an area of research, Braille displays offer an interesting spectrum because work in this space involves elements of materials science and electrical and mechanical engineering. For instance, dielectric elastomers (DE) are a new direction in the development of tactile surfaces that may significantly reduce the cost of Braille displays. These electroactive polymers are smart material systems that basically transform electric energy directly into mechanical work.[43] DE have high elastic energy density but are also lightweight and can be used as electric actuators for refreshable Braille displays such as PolyBraille[44] and sheet-type display panels.[45]

3.2.4 Screen Magnifiers

Screen magnifiers are used by people with functional vision, and can either be bundled into computing devices as software, or be sold as standalone hardware that uses a lens to magnify a stationary object and thereafter project to a surface. Computer-based magnification technology is an area in which the basic technology issues have been more or less solved but improvements continue to be made, and new application support (for cellular interfaces, for instance) is the main area of new work. On the other hand AT for the magnification of print materials is constantly improving, and with the market for senior citizens growing throughout most of the industrialized world, there is a healthy research agenda and continuous investment in new product development. There is a range of products from portable or handheld LCD scanners that start at roughly US $200 to stationary high-resolution magnifiers with large monitors that can be combined with computing devices and can cost in the range of US $2,000 to US $4,000.

Despite the value of high quality print and computing-based magnification technologies, for the low-income populations with low-vision all around the world most digital magnification technologies can be prohibitively expensive. As a result, reliance on mechanical tools for print magnification and the basic magnification tools that come built into operating systems are most commonly used. One of the areas of possible future development is cellular-based magnification apps. With smartphones rapidly decreasing in price toward the $50 price point for low-end devices, there has been a very significant increase in smartphones in the past five years to over 500 million units annually.[46] Although these do not perform currently at very high resolution, the technology is rapidly catching up to where cellphones will provide the functionality of handheld LCD magnifiers at a significantly lower price. The apple iPhone magnifier app, for instance, retails at $0.99. Devices that can combine various functions—such as the KNFB reader (which works on Symbian-based phones) can be used as an OCR mobile reader and processor of digital material.

3.2.5 Mobile Phones

Finally, mobile phones have played an increasingly large role as AT devices for people with vision impairments. Although we list mobiles here as an output technology, the increase of smartphones and the breadth of mobile applications (typically abbreviated as apps) have made smartphones an essential part of the AT discussion for people with vision impairments. Applications range from basic accessibility tools such as speech synthesis to complex apps that combine various features of the mobile device (camera, calculator, and speakers) and the range of infrastructure it can exploit (Web, GPS, crowdsourcing). For most parts of the world, a basic screen reader (such as Nuance Talks on Symbian platform phones) can cost between US $150 and US $200 as an add-on, but higher-end mobile phones can have their own inbuilt or supported screen readers—such as VoiceOver on Apple's iPhones, the open source TalkBack on Google's Android platform phones, Oratio on Blackberry, and MobileSpeak on WindowsMobile phones.

For many low- and middle-income nations, appropriate language support on mobile platforms is possibly even more essential than it is in the personal computing space because of the fairly widespread proliferation of mobile devices among people with vision impairments, including the phenomenal increase in access to smartphones. Both general apps and apps specifically designed for people with vision impairments are an important part of the AT environment because there is increasingly a movement to make apps accessible. Several tools and guidelines exist to test the accessibility of mainstream apps as well as to help app developers plan for better accessibility right from the early design stages. The range of specific apps available for smartphones is a good indicator of how AT options are dramatically evolving in the last few years. From recognizing currency notes to finding restaurants or social connections, office applications and wayfinding, apps are rapidly becoming central to the daily social and economic realm of people with vision impairments who use smartphones.

However, the two basic technologies that remain starter apps for people with vision impairments are magnifiers and screen readers. Nuance Talks, which runs on Symbian phones, is an extremely popular mobile screen reader throughout low- and middle-income regions. In these areas of the world the low-cost Symbian-based Nokia phones are extremely popular, though Nuance Talks is also compatible with other operating systems, which is important as Symbian phases out and Android emerges as the fastest growing platform for smartphones globally. Android, Windows Phone, Apple, and Samsung each have their own screen reading options. However, users with vision impairments may become locked into a certain device type based on the screen reader interface they are used to, or worse, that they have a renewable license for. As cellular phones reduce in shelf life, changing phones can become problematic for users who rely on specific applications.

For researchers in low- and middle income countries, building on the basic capabilities of screen reading on cellular phones is likely to be an important area of the near future. As with desktop screen readers, open source alternatives such as Android TalkBack offer an interesting range of possibilities, and language support and speech synthesis capabilities are critical. In addition, given the widespread use of mobile telephones and text messaging by people in their native language but using Roman script, there is also the possibility of using this corpus to hone existing speech synthesis tools. Advancements in natural language processing have made translation and transliteration from various languages fairly accurate, especially for limited vocabulary scenarios, and these can be overlaid on cellular screen reading technologies. Although much research and product development needs to be done to bring such technologies to the point of being market-ready, the ubiquity of cellular phones and the spectacular growth of smartphone users carries great promise.

4. ASSISTIVE TECHNOLOGY AND EMPLOYABILITY IN LOW- AND MIDDLE-INCOME COUNTRIES

Alongside social exclusion, employment continues to be among the major challenges for people with disabilities. Studies show that people with vision impairments are frequently faced with gentle nudges toward certain professions, such as massage therapy in parts of Europe, the Middle East, and East Asia[47] and petty vending or lottery sales in Europe, Thailand, and Latin America.[48] The importance of "channeling" in the economic lives of people with vision impairments is underlined by the fact that even academics use the term "professional blind" to refer to the use of blindness as a means of economic sustenance.[49] Much work has discussed the economic segregation of people with vision impairments from the mainstream population[50] and the lack of opportunities to grow fruitfully within organizations.[51] People with vision impairments face both architectural/structural barriers that prevent their physical access to workspaces[52] and social barriers such as a lack of social support systems in the job market.[53]

The important questions are whether or not this is changing, and also whether the advent of and increasing access to assistive technologies has made the ability of people with vision impairments to participate intellectually, economically, and socially with the mainstream significantly easier. But few studies tell us about how this plays out on the ground because of the relative newness of AT in many countries, which in turn has meant that widespread traditional attitudes toward the workplace ability of people with vision impairments continue to prevail. The key findings of empirical work from three recent studies that have looked at AT and vision impairment are summarized here to discuss some of the challenges ahead.

The three studies were a 2008 qualitative study of assistive technology centers for people with disabilities in four countries of Latin America (Guatemala, Ecuador, Mexico, and Venezuela),[54] a study of assistive technology preferences of people with vision impairments in India,[55] and a narrative exploration of people with vision impairments talking about their experiences with employability in Peru and India.[56] The three studies collectively represent the voices of about 250 people with vision impairments, and highlight several of the key issues that people with disabilities in low- and middle-income countries face when they join a workforce that lacks the infrastructure and social supports to include them.

The three studies of AT all find that the CRPD comes at a time when there has been a fairly significant increase in technology access for people with vision impairments, even though the overall population of people with disabilities who actually have access to AT remains relatively negligible. The studies find that all six countries have fairly well-developed core groups of advanced AT users who are both pushing the boundaries of technology and creating a vanguard of persons with disabilities in the workplace.

4.1 Attitudes Toward Hiring People with Disabilities

An important starting point in understanding challenges on the hiring of people with disabilities is that constraints faced by people with disabilities in employment around the world have been found to be relatively comparable on a number of aspects. Studies have consistently found socioeconomic factors and perceptions of vision impairment as impacting employability.[57] A study specifically looking at global comparisons found that the top five factors cited include poverty (and the structural factors that come with it), discrimination, lack of education, employers' lack of knowledge on disabled peoples' abilities, and finally, lack of access to technologies.[58]

The last two points are of particular importance to us here—the discussion of assistive technology is inherently tied to employers' opinions. Employers' lack of knowledge refers to a larger point about a lack of cultural appreciation of issues around disability.

The cross-cultural study of disability has typically focused on issues around the perception of disability in various regions around the world. Thus, disability is typically defined in cultures worldwide in three important ways: by its cause, by its effect, and by the status of the disabled.[59] Research exists on workplace culture and disability,[60] but little such work has focused on low- and middle-income countries, or, more importantly, on the impact of assistive technology on workplace culture. The path ahead for policymakers and society as a whole involves significant efforts to create laws that ensure equity of access, but also to make fundamental social investment to educate people on disability and employment.

4.2 The State and Accessibility Champions

One of the key impacts of the CRPD has been to increase the discussions in countries over legal mechanisms to increase the employment of people with disabilities. Beyond legal policymaking, the existence of a serious champion in the government was an important part of the push for greater recognition of disability rights. A great example came from Ecuador, where vice president Lenin Moreno is himself disabled.

Now with the disabled Vice President, it has helped a lot, because before, years ago, it wasn't like it is now. They didn't take us into account they didn't help us. We didn't have job opportunities, not in every company like now with the Vice President's help. They respect us and everything, not like before.[61]

IS, 23, Quito, Ecuador

Indeed some of the other major politicians who have campaigned for greater rights for people with disabilities include Cambodian Prime Minister Hun Sen, who lost an eye during the Cambodian Civil War and frequently speaks at disability-related events. The role of a publicly prominent champion is not by any means unique to low- and middle-income countries—in the United States, there have been important champions like Ed Roberts,[62] but such champions have typically been more activists than politicians. The obvious concern for something like this is the complexity of creating champions. While the value of champions as change advocates as well as icons has worked in some contexts such as product development,[63] there is an inherent risk in relying on individuals rather than on a collective disability movement.

Although there is a gradual increase in the number of jobs available, an issue consistently noted by all three papers is the lack of faith among employers in the abilities of the users.

I have trained hundreds of candidates (in screen reader use). I come to know from them that most of them do not get a job for which they study or get trained. Some of them are technically well trained but are offered a telephone operator's job…. I am totally convinced, that whatever be the capabilities of the blind, the society never once accepts them as equal to normal…. If they raise their voice, they fear that they may even be removed from the job itself.[64]

LA, 55, Bangalore

The quote above from an assistive technology trainer is fairly telling of the risks of underemployment that candidates face. An advanced screen reader user can have computing skills comparable to a non-disabled person, but the problem of underemployment persists and is potentially exacerbated by placement through quotas that candidates and employers treat as allotments rather than merit-based jobs. In Guatemala, a training center that offered screen reader access to people with vision impairments took to making first-hand demonstrations to potential employers of its students:

When we go to a company, we do a presentation…we explain to the company about our programs, we actually show them how they work because that's quite an important part because they always wonder how a blind person is actually able to use a computer. [O]nce we have designed a simulation we invite them here, to sit down with our students and watch how they are able to manage and use the program….. Then we go to the company, we install the program, we fit the program to work as best as we can with the company, then we stay a few days with them too, watching how they work as well as explaining to them how it works. If they have any doubts we are there to explain it to them and look for a response. The longest we have had to stay is just a few days so that they can adapt to working and using the program.[65]

GU, Guatemala City

Both that such a service exists and that people with disabilities may be expected to accept this—the need to have a physical person to reassure an employer that one is able to do the work one is technically already certified to do—is a stark reminder of how distant the job market is from mainstreaming people with disabilities in the workplace.

4.3 Familiarity with Accessibility Issues and Knowledge of AT

The Guatemalan case described above is an extreme though important indicator of just how significant the barriers to employment even for the best trained AT users can be. The guarded attitude that employers took towards job candidates in Guatemala was mirrored in India and Peru, and research showed that part of the problem was very limited knowledge of assistive technology, not just broadly in society, but even specifically among people with disabilities and professionals who worked on disability issues.

No educational institutions in the countries where the studies took place required courses on assistive technology or disability studies as part of the general higher education curriculum. Even specialized institutions for people with disabilities often lacked state-of-the-art AT for vision impairments, which resulted in most people accessing AT only as adults. In India, in particular, the lack of adequate knowledge about disability issues frequently led to situations in which a person with a vision impairment lived without any knowledge of AT for several years before finding out about AT options.

At a hospital, they told me about it (the computer training course). Till then, I had not known that even blind can study computer. I was doing my first year degree when I got to know about it.[66]

SN, Ananthapur, India

Throughout most low- and middle-income countries, there is both a lack of adequate resource centers for people with disabilities as well as integrated educational facilities for children with disabilities. Often parents are unaware of assistive technologies, especially in rural areas, and this in turn leads to children being segregated to home environments. This further impacts the willingness and ability of parents to invest in career choices for children with disabilities.

When my parents (who are illiterate) came to visit me when I was in my 5th grade, I took them to the computer room and typed their name and the computer spoke it out. My parents were amazed and realized that I could learn computer on my own. From that day onwards they have been supporting me in all my endeavors and encouraging me to become independent. I would have been languishing in a room corner in a village if there was not a chance to show my parents that I can operate computers with the help of AT.[67]

VA, HR executive, Bangalore

The case of VA cited above is a particularly troubling situation. On the one hand it depicts the apparently victorious story of a young girl who managed to get access to assistive technology, but, on the other, it shows that children from rural areas are often moved to urban areas, and sometimes separated from their families, to be able to access assistive technology. This could change significantly in the future; although some forms of training, such as Braille literacy, may require specialized attention, many of the audio-based interfaces can be taught by teachers in remote villages.

4.4 Career Recalibration and Employment Engineering

Both the studies on India and Peru found multiple cases of people recalibrating their medium- or long-term career goals based on information available at various stages of their lives. In part, this was due to the frequent reinforcement of lack of opportunities in the economic sphere, but also to prevalent trends on what were perceived as "appropriate jobs" for people with disabilities. To a significant extent, this also depended on the ignorance of teachers or people working at institutions offering services to people with disabilities.

I was interested in accountancy. I got into one of the colleges; again the teachers had apprehensions as to how I will manage with accounts with numbers in columns and rows. Again in 12th grade, I stood first in commerce stream for the handicapped category (competing with students without vision impairments).[68]

KA (female), office administrator

Although a good number of the respondents cited did end up rejecting channeling toward certain careers or educational choices, for most, the primary point of career calibration happened at the entry point to higher education. This was typically the first point at which a vocational choice had to be made, and individuals often felt a sense of dependency on advice from immediate circles for their perception of what was feasible.

Some of the research subjects in India noted that they frequently calibrated their educational and career goals around the early college stage, influenced by their own assumptions and also by recommendations from people or institutions. Access to assistive technology created a greater sense of agency in one's own ability to evaluate possibilities. People report that their career aspirations changed either due to a new awareness of possibilities, or due to an extension of networks related to assistive technology training or through online social networks.

An interesting corollary to the career recalibration is that of "employment engineering," which refers to the channeling of people with disabilities to certain occupations. The new wave of employment engineering can be seen as a more modern avatar of the older crude diversions of people with vision impairments toward massage or lottery sales. It is instead a more complex condition wherein assistive technology training centers nudge people with vision impairments toward certain jobs. There were a few manifestations of this. Telemarketing and phone-based jobs are two specific vocations that have grown significantly in the last few years in several of the countries where the studies were conducted, especially in Mexico and India.

Taking the course [in computer use with JAWS] is fundamental for finding a job.... More than anything at banks, in the famous telemarketing. There are specific areas where one can develop customer service, which is mainly where people who have learned JAWS work.[69]

AL, Mexico City

In many cases, such training for jobs was extremely limited to one specific task that it was perceived the future employee needed to carry out in day-to-day work. Rather than broad training in assistive technology use, which would allow the individual to think of what careers he or she may be interested in, the focus was on acquisition of a single skill, which in turn creates the risk of making the individual highly suitable for one job but inadequate for many others.

We did a little HTML, but other than that nothing. We actually asked our lecturers to teach us some applications, but they told us that the job opportunities in that field are less. We were asked to concentrate on medical transcription. But now the opportunities in this field (MT) also have reduced. Since we are already into this field, it is very difficult for us to move to another field.[70]

KU (male), medical transcriptionist, Bangalore

The paternalism inherent in past waves of employment engineering is surprisingly evident in the three studies even in an era of much improved access to technology as well as increased public consciousness of disability issues from a rights-based perspective. The channeling of people toward transcription jobs in particular exposed them to the risks of employment volatility in a particularly competitive field of work, telemarketing, which is known both for the high degree of employee turnover, and the unpredictable nature of work, given its reliance on international contracts. Arguably, the late introduction of assistive technologies into the lives of people with vision impairments in parts of low- and middle-income countries is also important in these forms of employment engineering; candidates frequently do not have access to AT at younger ages either due to cost or to the lack of AT in schools, and thus enter the AT training centers at a point where they are already thinking in terms of work options.

4.5 Social Networks and Workplace Options

An unusual trend noted in the AT study in India was the understanding of specific firms as being "accessible" and having reputations for employing AT users. This turned out to be a very important finding for AT-using people with vision impairments and their employment prospects, because of their relatively short history of employment in white collar sectors in India and arguably in other countries. The study found that companies that offered jobs to people with vision impairments quickly developed reputations as desirable employers within the community of AT users, so much so that interviewed individuals who were asked what they perceived as career goals would mention working in those companies as specific long-term aspirations. This on the one hand is somewhat at odds with how people in general perceive aspiration or career goals (such as "I would like to be a chef, business owner, etc." as opposed to "I would like to work at Company X") but it does relate well to existing literature on the ways in which other economically excluded groups have perceived workplace aspiration. Studies on employability preferences around race/ethnicity[71] and gender[72] have likewise shown that the recognition of a certain firm or line of work as being friendly to a particular group can influence employment.

The most common manifestation of this came from individuals at AT training classes, who interacted with senior colleagues who had graduated and found work at certain companies in jobs they enjoyed. This in turn frequently built the impression of those companies as favorable workplaces.

More broadly, seniors at AT training classes or companions on social networking sites served in a range of advisory or exemplary functions for other persons with visual impairments, given that they were perceived as having a shared experience of vision impairment and an understanding of employability issues. AT training cohorts and peer groups can thus become much more than just a job-training cohort and can offer advice on issues relevant to a range of career and life decisions.

While undergoing (screen reading) training at this NGO, I met many VI (people with Vision Impairments) who were already working in MNCs (Multinational Companies) and in IT (Information Technology) companies. I used to enquire with them as to how they got the job, how they prepared for the same.... From all these discussions, I got the confidence that I can also get a job and the motivation was there when I came across all these people who are suffering like me, but have overcome their difficulties and are being independent, working in reputed companies. Then my goal was to get a job. Once I got a hold on the screen reader technology, my confidence improved.... Many companies are hesitant to take VI people. If they employ 1 or 2 VI, they will come to know about the abilities of VI.[73]

TE (female), Clerical administrator, Bangalore

The studies suggest that the importance of peer groups and social networks, especially in low- and middle-income countries where such groups have themselves been rare because of the lack of institutional development to support the needs of people with vision impairments, needs much examination.

4.6 Access to AT in the Workplace

For people with vision impairments, firms that already had some history of having employees that needed assistive technology were reported to offer a greater comfort with working conditions, especially in the service sector. However, the relative complexity of some assistive technology could be a significant challenge, in part because of the lack of experience. In particular, this represented a problem for small call centers or medical transcription firms because these were highly cost-sensitive and unwilling to spend on software needs for employees with disabilities. Even among large firms, one should not make the assumption that an employee with disabilities could easily access the necessary technology.

There are two fundamental problems—the first, as we note, is the actual cost of most screen-reading technology. The second, and the one that is actually much more challenging, is compatibility of firm-specific software and legacy systems. Many of these systems were not written to work with screen reading software, and likewise many existing screen readers do not work very well outside of some of the fairly standardized consumer software.

They inserted me in this [call center job], but it is turning out to be very difficult for me because . . . JAWS doesn't enter the Orion program that this company uses. It enters Excel but it doesn't read Orion. . . . [It] depends on my boss to tell me if I can stay with Excel. The engineer from [the job-placement NGO] went to install JAWS at the company, but that did not work. The company said that it was going to contact [the job-placement NGO] to try to help me, but until now I don't know what has happened, they haven't told me anything.[74]

CL, Quito, Ecuador

For some companies that are relatively more invested in ensuring accessibility for employees with vision impairments, this could mean investing either in upgrading their own software or in making existing screen readers work better with their in-house tools. This approach has already attracted some investment to developer groups working on NVDA in India[75] and may in fact be one of the key ways in which open source tools like NVDA can pose a serious challenge to the more established products like JAWS and WindowEyes, which currently have better application support. Although the cost of JAWS was found in all three studies to be relatively less challenging for individuals because of the widespread availability of pirated versions of JAWS both online and at small software shops, the challenge was the use of pirated software at workplace computers.

Major nonprofits working with people with vision impairments were fairly clear in their policies about putting their stakeholders above the structural complexities of providing "legitimate" copies of the screen reading software—in short, facilitating where needed, pirated copies of JAWS. The distributor of JAWS (Freedom Scientific) was aware of this piracy but they were generally more focused on the market of corporate buyers and individuals who preferred to pay for a full-feature stable version on their laptops. In fact, piracy probably helped create a legion of very loyal JAWS users, because a lot of AT users make decisions based on word-of-mouth. In general it is much easier to get tech support from within the community for JAWS-related issues. Activists for open source assistive technology rue the dependencies this created, especially given that almost all the training centers for people with vision impairments started their students off on JAWS.

However, although some offices may encourage people to bring in their own machines with installed versions of screen readers, others not only prohibited this for company policy reasons but also were not enthusiastic about buying full versions for their in-house machines.

The informatics guy came here and deleted all my screen readers because they said that as we don't have licenses, they didn't want me to have it, so they deleted it. So I said "how am I going to work," "that's not my problem" he said.... So I ask "why don't you buy it?," (they say) "oh, because it's not considered in the budget"[76]

AN, Lima

In short, for someone with vision impairment, finding a company willing to adequately support AT needs can be a challenge. Frequently it is left to the employee to figure out his or her requirements. This means both that the employee would have to be able to afford his or her computer, and also that the systems at the workplace are such that personal machines are allowed to operate on the network. For employees without either choice, the only option could be the demo version of JAWS, working with which could be practically impossible.

JAWS costs around 15000 pesos [US $1000] on average.... There is a free version in Spanish; we can download it on the website of ONCE. It is a demo version that works for 34 minutes [thereafter you need to restart the machine to make it work again].[77]

AL, Mexico City

One common factor that stood out in all three studies was the ubiquity of donated materials as part of the infrastructure of technology for people with vision impairments. Donations of screen reading software was extremely common—with certain international disability rights agencies such as ONCE donating copies of JAWS in several technology centers throughout Latin America. As a result, the choice of technologies could also depend not on individual preferences or experience, but on what donors were willing to provide, and can lead to needing to learn and adapt to new complex approaches that may or may not be the best fit.

For the past two years we had been working with Magnus, which is a very, very good magnifying program, but we recently had to switch to Zoom Text because it is compatible with Windows Vista. Programs like these ... there aren't many on the market. There are very few companies that develop software such as these that work with the idea of disabilities. And JAWS is one that is very complex. We receive this software as a donation, a donation managed by Microsoft and the OAS [Organization of American States].[78]

GU, Guatemala City

4.7 Barriers to Switching Assistive Technologies

The final, but perhaps particularly important finding related to AT use in low- and middle-income countries is a sort of culmination of the distribution issues related to AT and the specifics on how the technology is learned and used. McCarthy's research on screen reader use suggests that people with vision impairments show a lesser tendency for switching technology, potentially because of the perceived productivity loss. The screen reader, for many users, was perceived as an information lifeline, especially when people came into assistive technologies as adults and had a certain perception of their own productivity pre– and post–screen reader access.

I tried [NVDA] once very briefly, but the problem for me is if I have to switch to another screen reader, effectively I need at least one week or ten days to familiarize myself with it, and for that period of time I'm not able to work productively because I'm still discovering these things.[79]

NM, JAWS user, Bangalore

McCarthy's second important finding was that of the trade-off between quality of voice output and application support for screen reader users. Interestingly, screen reader users valued the quality of voice output very significantly when they were novice users—thus, the more human sounding the voice, the more the users were likely to prefer it. However, as users became advanced users, they valued voice a lot less compared with application support.

Thus, novice users strongly preferred the "natural sounding voice" of JAWS, which uses the eloquence TTS, over the formant-based, more mechanical-sounding eSpeak TTS. Ironically, as the same users became more advanced, they would typically speed up their audio output—to a level almost unintelligible to the untrained ear, that ended up sounding very mechanical. By this point, however, the individual was probably already a fairly well-established JAWS user and unwilling to switch interfaces.

Ensuring people with vision impairments can use AT they have been trained on and not repeatedly need to switch is more in the realm of recommendations for accommodation than requirements because it implies a cost to companies for which it may be difficult to enforce compliance. In McCarthy's study of AT use in India, the cost of JAWS was cited as one of the primary reasons for companies investing in alternatives to proprietary screen reading software

Middle-level and startup companies... cannot afford to spend about 1000 dollars (per license of JAWS).... If people start using open source screen readers like NVDA, it's easy to convince an employer to give an employment opportunity to these candidates, and it's easy for them to get in onto the payrolls.... I recommend our trainees to learn using NVDA because it's easy for us to generate employment for them... (but) since it's existed for quite some time, people are actually addicted with the Eloquence synthesizer (on JAWS), because the quality of the speech is pretty good.[80]

SC, Accessibility Consultant, Bangalore

Moving to open source products was probably one of the biggest dilemmas faced by users and companies alike in all the countries studied. On the one hand there was a clear preference among users for JAWS, but on the other hand there is a push toward free technologies that companies were more willing to invest in. A few major companies in India have already started investing in developers to build tools for custom applications on NVDA. This interesting trend in open source software development makes a lot of sense for low- and middle-income countries, where investment into free tools that can be adapted to use for local needs is crucial to ensure that more people can appropriately access assistive technologies. Language accessibility is also a challenge:

"So, in the first act, people are forced to use screen reader English, for English screen reader. And when it comes to a specific reading purpose, there is where they want it in Indian language . . . there's a demand. Growing demand, really really growing demand for this [Indian language screen readers]."[81]

SN, screen reader trainer, Bangalore

In India, as in several other parts of low- and middle-income countries, a huge challenge in getting quality assistive technologies in local languages has been that those individuals with vision impairments that get to the point of being able to use assistive technologies are already drawn from slightly higher economic strata. For these people, using a screen reader in English, French, or whatever international language is locally prevalent has not been a problem. This in turn opens up a much broader set of questions around the dominance of a few large languages in the international business domain and the impact they have on the market for language support for screen readers. This is perhaps one of the strongest arguments for greater state support of research and development into assistive technologies, as noted in Articles 4 and 9 of the CRPD.

5. CONCLUSION

There is much scope for optimism that access to assistive technologies will grow dramatically for people with vision impairments in low- and middle-income countries due to the timing of the CRPD around a period of much technological advancement in assistive technologies. This chapter has both outlined the key technologies that require attention and discussed employment from the perspective of assistive technology use.

Examining the state and use of assistive technologies for visually-impaired populations helps us understand key technology gaps and how these gaps manifest in real workplace scenarios. Looking at the sheer pace at which mobile technologies (in particular accessible apps on smartphones) are changing the way AT is used and incorporated into peoples' lives, it is entirely possible that a survey in the future would look much harder at mobile devices as being the primary device to improve the employment of people with vision impairments. Between the writing of this piece and its publishing, the number of new mobile apps for various functions will have grown dramatically, and such developments will require that researchers in this field perpetually update their assertions and, in some cases, research directions entirely. Nonetheless, the issues with desktop environments such as software compatibility, low-cost desktop screen reading, language extension, and Braille support are not going away in the short term, and are going to need urgent attention on various fronts to ensure the inclusion of all people with vision impairments.

In the spirit of the CRPD, the overwhelming majority of the research points to technology as playing a key role in surmounting the structural inequities that have impacted the working lives of people with disabilities. Yet a crucial finding, and one that applies as well to populations with other disabilities, remains that many of the needed improvements to assistive technology may not find takers in the private sector, which highlights the importance of a public role.

Although AT is likely to play a critical role, any argument for change that relies too heavily on technology should be approached with caution. As has been seen with the Information and Communications Technology and Development field in the last few years, technology is only one part of the issue, possibly even the smallest. As highlighted here, there are a range of social issues around employment for assistive technology users, and, although the promises of technology are many, a larger transformation of social attitude towards the inclusion of people with disabilities in the public sphere needs to come first. For social scientists working on themes related to disability, such as employment, there is an important case here for collaboration with engineers and technologists working on improving and innovating existing AT. Even today, there is not much available research; although a few venues have started taking issues of accessibility seriously, practitioners and users of AT need to be included in the research.

The best technology at the lowest prices still counts for little if the professional environment is stacked with negative attitudes towards hiring people with disabilities. Technologists will not solve these problems in isolation, nor will social scientists, governments, civil society, industry bodies, or indeed the most critical players—activists and technology users themselves. A multistakeholder approach is not just a desirable ideal, it is an absolute must.

NOTES

1. The Optional Protocol delineates a process whereby a central Committee may receive communications and conduct investigative proceedings regarding potential violations of the Convention by signatory parties to the Protocol.
2. Simeonsson, R. (1991). Early prevention of childhood disability in developing countries. *International journal of rehabilitation research* 14(1): 1–12; Murray, C. & Lopez, A. (1997). Global mortality, disability, and the contribution of risk factors: Global Burden of Disease Study. *The Lancet 349*(9063), 1436–1442; Snow, R.W., Craig, M., Deichmann, U., & Marsh, K. (1999). Estimating mortality, morbidity and disability due to malaria among Africa's non-pregnant population. *Bulletin of the World Health Organization* 77(8), 624–640; Maulik, P. & Darmstadt G. (2007). Childhood disability in low-and middle-income countries: overview of screening, prevention, services, legislation, and epidemiology. *Pediatrics 120*(Supplement), S1–S55.
3. Jackson, H. & Mupedziswa, R. (1988). Disability and rehabilitation: beliefs and attitudes among rural disabled people in a community based rehabilitation scheme in Zimbabwe. *Journal of social development in Africa 3*(1):, 21–30; Devlieger, P. (1995). Why disabled? The cultural understanding of physical disability in an African society. In B. Ingstad & S. Reynolds White, *Disability and culture* (Berkeley and Los Angeles, CA: University of California Press), 94–106; Stone, E. & Priestley, M. (1996). Parasites, pawns and partners: disability research and the role of non-disabled researchers. *British Journal of Sociology* 47(4), 699–716; Rösing, I. (1999). Stigma or sacredness. Notes on dealing with disability in an Andean culture. In B. Holzer, A. Vreede, & G. Weight, *Disability in different cultures: Reflections on local concepts.* New Brunswick, NJ: Transcript, 27–43.
4. Hernandez, V. (2008). Making Good on the Promise of International Law: The Convention on the Rights of Persons with Disabilities and Inclusive Education in China and India. *Pacific Rim Law & Policy Journal 17*(2), 497–527; Kett, M., Lang, R. & Trani, J.-F. (2009). Disability, development and the dawning of a new convention: A cause for optimism?, *Journal of International Development 21*(5), 649–661; Szymanski, C. F. (2009). The Globalization of Disability Rights Law-From The Americans with Disabilities Act to the UN Convention on The Rights of Persons with Disabilities. *Baltic Journal of Law & Politics 2*(1), 18–34; Ahmad, M. & Ahmad, M.M. (2010). *Who should pay the price: state or disabled rural individuals?: a low-income countries' perspective.* Singapore: Singapore Therapeutic, Assistive & Rehabilitative Technologies Centre; Aldersey, H. M. & Turnbull H.R. (2011). The United Republic of Tanzania's National Policy on Disability: A Policy Analysis. *Journal of Disability Policy Studies 22*(3), 160–169; Meekosha, H. & Soldatic, K. (2011). Human Rights and the Global South: the case of disability. *Third World Quarterly 32*(8), 1383–1397.
5. Dias, M. B. & Brewer, E. (2009). How computer science serves the developing world. *Communications of the ACM 52*(6), 74–80; Eide, A. H., & Oderud, T. (2009). Assistive technology in low-income countries. In M. MacLachlan & L. Swartz (Eds.). *Disability & international development: Towards inclusive global health.* New York: Springer, 149–160; Pearlman, J., Cooper, R., Chhabra, H.S., & Jefferds, A. (2009). Design, development and testing of a low-cost electric powered wheelchair for India. *Disability & Rehabilitation: Assistive Technology* 4(1), 42–57; Simpson, J. (2009). Inclusive information and communication

technologies for people with disabilities. *Disability Studies Quarterly 29*(1), 1–13; Kelly, B., Lewthwaite, S. & Sloan, D. (2010). Developing countries; developing experiences: approaches to accessibility for the real world. *Proceedings of the 2010 International Cross Disciplinary Conference on Web Accessibility*, Article 3; Borg, J., Lindström,A., & Larsson, S. (2011). Assistive technology in developing countries: a review from the perspective of the Convention on the Rights of Persons with Disabilities. *Prosthetics and Orthotics International 35*(1): 20–29.

6. Paul, J. (2000). Cultural Resistance to Global Governance. *Michigan Journal of International Law 22*, 1–84.
7. Hathaway, O. (2001). Do human rights treaties make a difference? *Yale Law Journal 111*, 1935–2042.
8. Cook, R. (1989). Reservations to the Convention on the Elimination of All Forms of Discrimination against Women. *Virginia Journal of International Law 30*, 643–709; Venkatraman, B. (1994). Islamic States and the United Nations Convention on the Elimination of All Forms of Discrimination against Women: Are the Shari'a and the Convention Compatible. *American University Law Review 44*, 1949–2027.
9. Miller, D. (2002). Holding States to Their Convention Obligations: The United Nations Convention Against Torture and the Need for a Broad Interpretation of State Action. *Georgetown Immigration Law Journal 17*, 299–324.
10. Kanter, A. (2006). The Promise and Challenge of the United Nations Convention on the rights of Persons with Disabilities. *Syracuse Journal of International Law and Commerce 34*, 287–322.
11. Hernandez (2008). Making Good on the Promise.
12. Beijen, J., Mylanus, E.A.M., & Snik, A.F.M. (2007). Education qualification levels and school careers of unilateral versus bilateral hearing aid users. *Clinical Otolarynology 32*(2), 86–92; Parette, H. & Petersen-Karlan, G. (2007). Facilitating student achievement with assistive technology. *Education and Training in Developmental Disabilities 42*(4), 387–397.
13. Mackelprang, R. W. & Clute, M.A. (2009). Access for all: Universal design and the employment of people with disabilities. *Journal of Social Work in Disability & Rehabilitation 8*(3-4), 205–221; Fok, D., Polgar, J.M., Shaw, L., & Jutai, J.W. (2011). Low vision assistive technology device usage and importance in daily occupations. *Work: A Journal of Prevention, Assessment and Rehabilitation 39*(1), 37–48.
14. Chandrashekar, S. (2010). *Is Hearing Believing? Perception of Online Information Credibility by Screen Reader Users who are Blind or Visually Impaired.* PhD thesis. University of Toronto: Canada; Pal, J., Pradhan, M., Shah, M., & Babu. R. (2011). Assistive technology for vision-impairments: an agenda for the ICTD community. *Proceedings of the 20th international conference companion on World wide web pages*, 513–522.
15. IBISWorld (nd) Optical Character-Recognition Software Developers in the US: Market Research Report. *IBISWorld*. Retrieved on February 15, 2013, from: http://www.ibisworld.com/industry/optical-character-recognition-software-developers.html
16. Pal, U. & Chaudhuri, B. (2004). Indian script character recognition: a survey. *Pattern Recognition 37*(9), 1887–1899.
17. Mohanty, S., Dasbebartta, H. N., & Behera, T.K. (2009). An Efficient Bilingual Optical Character Recognition (English-Oriya) System for Printed Documents. *Proceedings of the 2009 Seventh International Conference on Advances in Pattern Recognition*, 398–401.

18. Kunte, R.S. & Samuel, R.D.S (2007). An OCR System for Printed Kannada Text Using Two-Stage Multi-Network Classification Approach Employing Wavelet features. *Proceedings of the International Conference on Computational Intelligence and Multimedia Applications*, 349–353.

19. Rahiman, M. A. & Rajasree, M. (2009). Printed Malayalam Character Recognition Using Back-propagation Neural Networks. *Proceedings of the Advance Computing Conference*, 197–201.

20. Meshesha, M. & Jawahar, C. (2007). Optical Character Recognition of Amharic Documents. *African Journal of Information & Communication Technology* 3(2): 1–14.

21. Ding, X. & Wang, H. (2007). Multi-Font Printed Tibetan OCR. In B.B. Chaudhuri (Ed.).*Digital Document Processing* (London, United Kingdon: Springer-Verlag), 73–98.

22. Chanda, S., Pal, S., & Pal, U. (2008). Word-wise Sinhala Tamil and English script identification using Gaussian kernel SVM. *Proceedings of the 19th International Conference on Pattern Recognition*, 1–4.

23. Pal, U., Roy, R.K., Roy, K., & Kimura, F. (2009). Indian Multi-Script Full Pin-Code String Recognition for Postal Automation. *Proceedings of the 10th International Conference on Document Analysis and Recognition*, 456–460.

24. Vergyri, D., Kirchhoff, K., Duh, K. & Stolcke, A. (2004). Morphology-based language modeling for Arabic speech recognition. *Computer Speech and Language* 20(4), 589–608.

25. Kumar, M., Rajput, N., & Verma, A. (2004). A large-vocabulary continuous speech recognition system for Hindi. *IBM journal of research and development* 48(5.6), 703–715.

26. Vu, N. T. & Schultz, T. (2009). Vietnamese large vocabulary continuous speech recognition. Presented at the IEEE Workshop on Automatic Speech Recognition and Understanding, Merano, Italy, 13–17 Dec.

27. Lei, X., Siu, M., Hwang, M.-Y., Ostendorf, M., & Lee, T. (2006). Improved tone modeling for Mandarin broadcast news speech recognition. *Proceedings of Interspeech*, 16–19.

28. Kasuriya, S., Sornlertlamvanich, V., Cotsomrong, P., Kanokphara, S., & Thatphithakkul, N. (2003). Thai speech corpus for Thai speech recognition. *Proceedings of the International Conference on Speech Databases and Assessments*, 54–61.

29. Plauche, M., Nallasamy, U., Pal, J., Wooters, C., & Ramachandran, D. (2006). Speech recognition for illiterate access to information and technology. *Proceedings of the International Conference on Information and Communication Technologies and Development*, 83–92.

30. WebAIM (2010). Screen Reader User Survey #3 Results. *WebAIM*. Retrieved on February 15, 2013, from: http://webaim.org/projects/screenreadersurvey3/; WebAIM (2012). Screen Reader User Survey #4 Results. WebAIM. Retrieved on February 15, 2013, from: http://webaim.org/projects/screenreadersurvey4/

31. WebAIM (2009). Screen Reader User Survey #2 Results. *WebAIM*. Retrieved on February 15, 2013, from: http://webaim.org/projects/screenreadersurvey2/

32. McCarthy, E., Pal, J., Cutrell, E, & Marballi, T. (2012). An Analysis of Screen Reader Use in India. *Proceedings of the International Conference on Information and Communication Technologies and Development*, 149–158.

33. First number refers to primary speakers, the second number refers to the number of people who can speak the language, including as a second or third language.

34. There are vastly varying calculations of this, although there has been much progress. A study by Inktomi as far back as in 2000 found that English language held 86.5% of all material on the Internet. See Pimienta D., Prado, D., & Blanco, A. (2009). *Twelve years of measuring linguistic diversity in the Internet: balance and perspectives*. Paris, France: UNESCO.

35. Data from Zuckerman, Ethan (2009). What percentage of the Internet is in English? In Chinese? *My Heart's in Accra*. Retrieved on February 15, 2013, from: http://www.ethanzuckerman.com/blog/2009/06/01/what-percentage-of-the-internet-is-in-english-in-chinese/

36. Data as on June 30, 2011.

37. Rusko, M., Darjaa, S., Trnka, M, Zeman, V., & Glovna, J. (2008). Making Speech Technologies Available in (Serviko) Romani Language. *Text, Speech and Dialogue* 5246, 501–508.

38. Ngugi, K., Okelo-Odongo, W., & Wagacha, P.W. (2010). Swahili text-to-speech system. *African Journal of Science and Technology 6*(1), 80–89.

39. Roux, J. C. & Visagie, A.S. (2007). Data-driven approach to rapid prototyping Xhosa speech synthesis. *Proceedings of the 6th ISCA Workshop on Speech Synthesis*, 143–147.

40. Couper, H. (1996). Teaching Modern Languages to Visually Impaired Children. *Language Learning Journal 13*(1), 6–9.

41. Röder, B., Rösler, F., & Neville, H.J. (2000). Event-related potentials during auditory language processing in congenitally blind and sighted people. *Neuropsychologia 38*(11), 1482–1502.

42. Kornwitz, J. (2010). Engineering students win innovation prize. *news@ Northeastern*. Retrieved on February 14, 2013, from http://www.northeastern.edu/news/stories/2010/10/brailleembosser.html

43. Carpi, F., De Rossi, D., Kornbluh, R., Pelrine, R., & Sommer-Larsen, P. (Eds.) (2008). *Dielectric Elastomers as Electromechanical Transducers: Fundamentals, Materials, Devices, Models and Applications of an Emerging Electroactive Polymer Technology* (Amsterdam, Netherlands: Elsevier).

44. Carpi, F., Frediani, F., Sommovigo, A., & De Rossi, D. (2011). Refreshable Braille Display Based on Dielectric Elastomer Actuators. Poster presentation, First International Conference on Electromechanically Active Polymer Transducer and Artificial Muscles. Pisa, Italy, June 8-9.

45. Kato, Y., et al. (2007). Sheet-type Braille displays by integrating organic field-effect transistors and polymeric actuators. *IEEE Transactions on Electron Devices 54*(2), 202–209.

46. MobiThinking (2012). Global mobile statistics 2012 Part A: Mobile subscribers; handset market share; mobile operators. *MobiThinking*. Retrieved on February 15, 2013, from: http://mobithinking.com/mobile-marketing-tools/latest-mobile-stats/a#smartphone-shipments

47. French, S. (1993). The origins of physiotherapy as a career for blind and visually impaired people in Great Britain. *Physiotherapy 79*(11), 779–780; Gleitman, I., Kurssiya, Y., Miterani, R., & Marom, O. (2004). *Medical Massage–A Profession for Blind and Visually Impaired People in Israel*. Jerusalem, Israel: Ministry of Welfare.

48. Garvia, R. (1996). The professional blind in Spain. *Work, Employment & Society 10*(3): 491–508; Love, C. Y. (2001). Asian Americans and Pacific Islanders with Visual Impairments. In M. Milian & J.N. Erin (Eds.), *Diversity and Visual Impairments: The Influence of Race, Gender, Religions, and Ethnicity on the Individual*. New York: AFB press, 79–107; Pal, J., Freistadt, J., Frix, M., & Neff,

P. (2009). *Technology for employability in Latin America: Research with at-risk youth and people with disabilities*. Seattle, WA: TASCHA.

49. Garvia (1996). The professional blind; Scott, R. A. (1969). *The Making of Blind Men: A Study of Adult Socialization*. New York: Russell Sage.

50. de Jong, H. (2005). Employment strategies for the blind in Eastern Europe. *International Congress Series 1282*, 1134–1138.

51. Kaye, H. S. (2009). Stuck at the bottom rung: occupational characteristics of workers with disabilities. *Journal of occupational rehabilitation 19*(2), 115–128.

52. Crudden, A. & L. W. McBroom (1999). Barriers to employment: A survey of employed persons who are visually impaired. *Journal of Visual Impairment and Blindness 93*, 341–350; McCarty, C. A., Burgess, M, & Keefe, J.E. (1999). Unemployment and under-employment in adults with vision impairment: The RVIB Employment Survey. *Australian and New Zealand Journal of Ophthalmology 27*(3-4), 190–193; Shaw, A., Gold, D., & Wolffe, K. (2007). Employment-related Experiences of Youths Who Are Visually Impaired: How Are These Youths Faring? *Journal of Visual impairment and Blindness 101*(1), 7–21.

53. Cimarolli, V. & Wang, S. (2006). Differences in social support among employed and unemployed adults who are visually impaired. *Journal of Visual Impairment & Blindness 100*(9), 545–556; Gold, D., Shaw, A., & Wolffe, K. (2010). The social lives of Canadian youths with visual impairments. *Journal of Visual Impairment & Blindness 104*(7), 431–443.

54. Pal, Freistadt, Frix, & Neff (2009). *Technology for employability in Latin America*.

55. McCarthy, Pal, Cutrell, & Marballi (2012). An Analysis of Screen Reader Use in India. *Proceedings of the Fifth International Conference on Information and Communication Technologies and Development*, 149–158.

56. Pal, J., & Lakshmanan, M. (2012). Assistive Technology and Employability for people with vision impairments: Narratives from Lima and Bangalore. Draft.

57. Clements, B., Douglas, G., & Pavey, S. (2011). Which factors affect the chances of paid employment for individuals with visual impairment in Britain? *Work: A Journal of Prevention, Assessment and Rehabilitation 39*(1), 21–30.

58. Wolffe, K. E. & Spungin, S.J. (2002). A glance at worldwide employment of people with visual impairments. *Journal of visual impairment & blindness 96*(4), 245–253.

59. Groce, N. E. (1999). Disability in cross-cultural perspective. *The Lancet 354*(9180), 756–757.

60. Hall, E. (1999). Workspaces: refiguring the disability–employment debate. I R. Butler & H. Parr (Eds.), *Mind and Body Spaces. Geographies of Illness, Impairment and Disability*. London, United Kingdom: Routledge, 138–153; Schur, L., Kruse, D., Blasi, J., & Blanck, P. (2009). *Is disability disabling in all workplaces? Workplace disparities and corporate culture. Industrial Relations: A Journal of Economy and Society 48*(3), 381–410.

61. Pal, Freistadt, Frix, & Neff, (2009). *Technology for employability in Latin America*, 11.

62. McCarthy, H. (2003). The Disability Rights Movement. *Rehabilitation Counseling Bulletin 46*(4), 209–223.

63. Chakrabarti, A. K. (1974). The role of champion in product innovation. *California Management Review 17*(2), 58–62; Howell, J. M. & Higgins, C.A. (1990). Champions of change: Identifying, understanding, and supporting champions of technological innovations. *Organizational Dynamics 19*(1), 40–55.

64. Pal & Lakshmanan (2012). Assistive Technology and Employability, 7.

65. Pal, Freistadt, Frix, & Neff (2009). *Technology for employability in Latin America*, 27

66. Pal & Lakshmanan (2012). Assistive Technology and Employability, 7.

67. Ibid.

68. McCarthy, Pal, Cutrell, & Marballi (2012). An Analysis of Screen Reader Use in India.

69. Pal, Freistadt, Frix, & Neff (2009). *Technology for employability in Latin America*, 27.

70. Pal & Lakshmanan (2012). Assistive Technology and Employability.

71. Fouad, N.A. & Byars-Winston, A.M. (2005). Cultural context of career choice: Meta-analysis of race/ethnicity differences. *Career Development Quarterly* 53(3), 223–233.

72. Lightbody, P. & Durndell, A. (1996). Gendered Career Choice: is sex stereotyping the cause or the consequence? *Educational Studies* 22(2), 133–146.

73. Pal & Lakshmanan (2012). Assistive Technology and Employability.

74. Pal, Freistadt, Frix, & Neff (2009). *Technology for employability in Latin America*, 82.

75. McCarthy, Pal, Cutrell, & Marballi (2012). An Analysis of Screen Reader Use in India.

76. Pal & Lakshmanan (2012). Assistive Technology and Employability.

77. Pal, Freistadt, Frix, & Neff (2009). *Technology for employability in Latin America*, 80.

78. Ibid., 82.

79. McCarthy, Pal, Cutrell, & Marballi (2012). An Analysis of Screen Reader Use in India, 154.

80. Ibid., 153.

81. McCarthy, Pal, Cutrell, and Marballi (2012). An Analysis of Screen Reader Use in India, 156.

CHAPTER 7

Microfinance and Disability

Recommendations for Policymakers and Practitioners

LEIF ATLE BEISLAND AND ROY MERSLAND

1. INTRODUCTION

The provision of financial services to poor persons—microfinance—has been praised for its development effect. It has been an implicit assumption that access to microfinance services may improve the standard of living of poor people, particularly in low- and middle-income countries. Nonetheless, it is often contended that especially vulnerable groups of people, for instance persons with disabilities, are barred from accessing microfinance services.[1] Historically, such claims have been based on expert opinions[2] because "the academic literature on microfinance and disability published in peer-reviewed journals is basically non-existent."[3] Nevertheless, the topic is important; because persons with disabilities living in low- and middle-income countries often struggle to obtain a job, most of them turn to self-employment, and access to capital is thus a necessary ingredient for success. Moreover, the United Nations Convention on the Rights of Persons with Disabilities promotes equalizing opportunities for persons with disabilities. The paucity of research on microfinance and disability is therefore worrying and problematic.

Recent research on the developmental impact of microfinance has shown controversial results. In experimental studies conducted at family and village levels, researchers struggle to identify a positive causal relationship between access to credit and the improved well-being of poor individuals.[4] At the same time, researchers find that an increased penetration of microfinance reduces poverty at the country level.[5] As strange as it might sound, no effect at the micro level and a positive effect at the macro level may actually both be true.

The reason is that impact studies at the micro level, particularly experimental studies, may not measure the secondary effect of microfinance. A secondary effect could, for example, be that microfinance customers use their money to buy groceries at a neighbor's store or building materials in a nearby town. Microfinance customers' money may thus have a positive impact on other persons' lives. Regardless, the microfinance impact literature is certainly still in its infancy, and it is important to turn to theory to understand why policymakers recommend the penetration of microfinance and in particular the inclusion of persons with disabilities in microfinance efforts.

The most cited theory to support the necessity of making credit available for poor persons is found in the entrepreneurship literature, highlighting that access to credit is a vital ingredient in enterprise development. For persons with disabilities, access to credit is of special importance because employers normally resist hiring disabled personnel. Thus, persons with disabilities need access to credit to develop their entrepreneurial activities. In general, this starting point is not disputed. However, financial capital alone does not secure success in the marketplace. Other resources, for instance, human capital (e.g., knowledge, skills, attitude) as well as social capital (e.g., networks) can be equally or even more important than access to financial capital in regard to succeeding in a business venture. It is the combination of the different types of capital together with access to customers that determines whether a person succeeds with a business activity. Therefore, when we lay out knowledge related to microfinance and disability in this chapter, we want to emphasize from the outset that ensuring access to financial capital by itself may not necessarily benefit persons with disabilities.

A second point we want to emphasize at this point is that there are several other theories supporting the promotion of microfinance; however, these theories often tend to favor savings (and insurance) over credit. The theory most relevant for persons with disabilities is the "consumption smoothing theory." A great deal of variation in incomes and expenses is part of the poverty trap. On a daily basis, poor people must come up against uneven incomes and expenses. One day these people might have to pay medical expenses worth 200 while at the same time only having an income of 20, whereas on another day, their expenses might be 10 only and their income may be 100. Collins and coworkers explain in detail how one primary problem of being poor is figuring out how to match the uneven income and expense streams and how poor people save, both in cash and in kind (e.g., animals), to evenly distribute their daily consumption.[6] Thus, when discussing microfinance and disability, we cannot emphasize enough that the focus should include savings and not credit only.

The purpose of this chapter is to focus on how the use of microfinance schemes by persons with disabilities relates to, and possibly improves, employment rates and economic activities. We seek to describe existing knowledge, lessons learned, limitations, challenges, and future potential. Unfortunately, these categories are not easily explained due to the current paucity of relevant literature. One reason that the literature on microfinance and disability is scarce is that it is difficult to obtain access to data that facilitate rigorous academic research. First, researchers are faced with the difficulty of defining disability. The "disabled proportion" of a population is very sensitive to the definition of "disability" being applied. For instance, our previous research shows that the percentages of persons with disabilities range from approximately 3% to 20% of a given population.[7] Second, even if everybody agreed on the "correct" definition of a disabled person, researchers are still left with the challenging issue of categorizing citizens according to this definition and then accessing the data of the persons who can be included as disabled. Finally, to ensure random inclusion of a sufficient number of the various types of disabilities, datasets of a given population need to be very large, which is costly.

Despite the challenges and data limitations, there has been an increased focus on disability and microfinance over the past few years, and some academic research is currently becoming available. Therefore, the first aim of this chapter is to review the existing research, and the second goal is to provide practical recommendations and policy guidelines based on this knowledge.

This chapter is organized as follows: Section 2 begins with a presentation of the theoretical framework that is often applied to analyze microfinance and disability. The second part of section 2 discusses the empirical research on access to microfinance for persons with disabilities. Section 3 applies survey evidence from two Ugandan studies and uses Uganda as a case for a more in-depth empirical analysis of access to microfinance. Section 4 is the forward-looking section of the chapter. It combines hard facts from the presented research with subjective judgment based on several years of experience from both academic microfinance research and practical microfinance work in the field to assert suggestions for future applications of microfinance and disability. Section 5 concludes the chapter.

2. PRIOR RESEARCH

2.1 Theoretical Framework

Persons with disabilities are a low priority and a disadvantaged group in regard to socioeconomic integration.[8] According to the United Nations, employers often resist hiring persons with disabilities.[9] Even if "disability does not necessarily mean inability,"[10] statistics indicate that the vast majority of persons with disabilities in low- and middle-income countries do not have formal jobs; thus, most persons with disabilities resort to self-employment.[11] Because lacking access to capital can be a major problem for this group, access to microfinance should be a priority in pro-disability policies.[12] Nevertheless, it is generally assumed that persons with disabilities have low access to microfinance services.[13] Simanowitz defines four exclusion mechanisms, or barriers, that lead to the exclusion of disabled and other vulnerable persons from microfinance services: exclusion by other credit group members, exclusion by staff, exclusion by service design, and exclusion by the disabled person himself.[14] Bwire and coworkers add a fifth barrier to this list, physical and informational exclusion stemming from the disability itself.[15]

The first of the listed exclusion mechanisms—exclusion by other microfinance costumers—may be a serious barrier to persons with disabilities. This barrier can be attributed to the group methodology often applied in microfinance. For instance, in solidarity groups or village banks, the members themselves decide whom to include in the group.[16] Martinelli and Mersland contend that a core element in group methodologies is that all members are jointly liable for each individual's loan and "the poorer and the more vulnerable community members therefore tend to be excluded from such groups by 'stronger' persons."[17]

Stigmatization, discrimination, and perceived risk are explanations for the exclusion caused by the staff of microfinance institutions (MFI) and especially by their credit officers.[18] Bwire and coworkers contend that credit officers are often not able to see past the disability and recognize the real working ability of a person with a disability;[19] thus, the staff fails to distinguish between real credit risk and perceived credit risk. It is also suggested that if group methodologies are practiced, prejudiced staff may cause increased levels of exclusion by other group members.[20]

Exclusion by service design, often referred to as "credit design," is also a potentially important barrier for persons with disabilities. Microfinance products are often designed for nondisabled clients and do not acknowledge that persons with disabilities may have particular needs. For instance, frequent installments on loans may all too often represent an insurmountable hurdle for persons with various physical handicaps and reduced mobility if they have to pay in person. In general, according to Mersland and Martinelli, the credit methodology is often too standardized and inflexible, thereby hindering persons with disabilities from participating.[21]

Irrespective of pure design issues, the disability itself can be a serious hindrance for persons with disabilities. This exclusion mechanism is caused by physical and informational barriers.[22] Microfinance institutions provide information in both verbal and written form, inaccessible to many with visual or hearing impairments. Moreover, MFIs are often located so that stairs have to be climbed or crowds have to be penetrated to reach their premises.

Finally, although at first glance, self-exclusion may appear as a peculiar barrier to the use of microfinance services, as explained by Bwire and coworkers,[23] persons with disabilities often experience rejection throughout life. Repeated exclusion produces low self-esteem, and low self-esteem often leads to self-exclusion from public and private services such as microfinance.[24] Self-exclusion may also be attributed to the fact that some persons with disabilities and their families may have the expectation to constantly receive grants,[25] and are thus unwilling to pay the interest rates demanded by sustainable microfinance institutions.

2.2 Empirical Evidence

One of the most comprehensive studies on microfinance and disability was conducted by Handicap International. The empirical part of the study covers survey evidence from South Asia, East Africa, and Central America and field visits in seven countries; Afghanistan, Bangladesh, Ethiopia, India, Kenya, Nicaragua, and Uganda. Generally, surveyed MFIs indicated that they did not discriminate against persons with disabilities, although this segment was not their target population. Yet, only 0% to 0.5% of the costumers of the surveyed MFIs had a disability. Even if this number is somewhat underestimated because many of the institutions do not track disability status, the percentage was as low as 0% to 2%, even for organizations that kept track or could identify their clients with disabilities.[26] A general finding is that microfinanciers with a higher outreach to persons with disabilities are usually those providers for which poverty alleviation is a main objective.

Another finding in the Handicap International study is that in addition to MFIs, many disabled persons' organizations (DPOs) operate credit schemes for their members. These schemes are generally very small (often serving only a few handfuls of people), often rural-based, and not financially sustainable. Approximately half of these schemes only target disabled women, whereas the rest also include men. Nineteen percent of the schemes actually provide grants and not loans, whereas 16% of those schemes offering loans charge no interest rates. The rest charge rates between 10% and 24% per year. In contrast, MFIs in the survey charge annual rates of 20% to 58% per year.[27]

The study of Handicap International also investigates possible barriers to microfinance that persons with disabilities face. The results are reported separately for DPOs with credit schemes and MFIs. Among the DPOs, 95% affirm that persons with disabilities face specific barriers accessing microfinance services, and lack of education, low income, stigmatization, and lack of access to information are listed as the main barriers. In contrast, only 47% of the MFIs state that persons with disabilities face specific microfinance barriers. Among MFIs, lack of self-esteem, guarantees, and access to information are viewed as the most important barriers.[28]

The more detailed field studies, which may also be referred to as in-depth case studies, of Handicap International also revealed interesting aspects of the microfinance market of persons with disabilities. For instance, in Kenya, many persons with disabilities expected grants instead of loans, and "[the] recipients of the loans were much more committed to working seriously to develop their businesses compared with the grant clients."[29] Moreover, whereas evidence from Colombia suggests that it is important to make some adjustments in microfinance services for persons with disabilities if these persons are very vulnerable, a lesson learned in Nicaragua was that the inclusion of persons with disabilities in mainstream MFIs boosts the economic and social inclusion as well as self-confidence of these persons.

Based on the Handicap International study, de Klerk concludes that there is no single best solution to the funding of self-employment activities for persons with disabilities. The inclusion of persons with disabilities in existing microfinance institutions may be the preferred strategy due to sustainability and access to funds for the target group; however, de Klerk contends that many persons with disabilities in reality will not have access to conventional institutions. For instance, many persons with disabilities are too vulnerable; MFIs typically only provide services to clients with existing business activities, and persons with disabilities often have no business experience. Moreover, he indicates that the stigmatization by staff and self-exclusion by the disabled themselves are two primary explanations for why persons with disabilities do not obtain access to mainstream microfinance services.[30]

In addition to the large Handicap International survey, several studies covering limited geographical areas have been conducted. In a study of projects promoting savings and credit groups in Bangladesh, Thomas supports the contention that persons with disabilities have low access to microfinance services. Even if eight out of 12 projects include persons with disabilities, only 0.3% to 5% of the savings and credit group members are persons with disabilities. Moreover, in her sample Thomas finds that, even in specific disability rehabilitation projects, only 18% to 23.5% of saving and credit group members are disabled. She maintains that community development and disability rehabilitation projects lack selection criteria for the inclusion of people with disabilities into savings and credit groups.[31]

Thomas lists several hindering mechanisms that may exclude persons with disabilities:

> The common difficulties faced in including people with disabilities in the savings and credit groups are that the non-disabled persons do not accept disabled persons easily, disabled people expect charity funds rather than operating a savings scheme, the [perceived] credit worthiness of disabled persons is low, their motivation is low, their source of earning is less than others, many of them are very poor and unable to save, their families are not very supportive, it takes longer to prepare disabled persons to include them in this programme, their mobility is restricted, their ability to market their products is limited, and their attendance in the group activity is lower than the others.[32]

The author also maintains that attitudinal changes among nondisabled people and the families of persons with disabilities may be major steps to overcome these difficulties.[33]

In Uganda, Bwire and coworkers report results from a pilot project in which the aim is to enable persons with disabilities to access mainstream microfinance services. In this project, staff in mainstream MFIs is trained to be more disability-sensitive. As a result of the project, a change in attitudes has been observed and all MFIs report an increase in the number of clients with disabilities (on average, participating MFIs doubled their number of clients with disabilities, from 0.5% to 1%). The study stresses that the disability community is an untapped market opportunity for MFIs and that the institutions need to realize the potential of this group of customers. Bwire and coworkers list exclusion by staff and self-exclusion due to low self-esteem as major hindering mechanisms for microfinanciers; additionally, the study indicates the importance of informational barriers. The authors maintain that misinformation about MFI terms and conditions may be a primary explanation for why persons with disabilities do not approach these institutions.[34]

Also using Ugandan data, Labie and coworkers provide an in-depth empirical and theoretical analysis of one of the exclusion barriers, namely, exclusion by staff. Their main finding is that credit officers are more biased against disabled customers than are other employees. Because credit officers are the individuals with daily contact with the customers and are those who hold a large influence on whether a particular costumer is granted a loan, this finding is particularly unfortunate. However, Labie and coworkers emphasize that credit officers are often motivated by a genuine desire to be useful and do good. The bias can often be attributed to an overestimation of risk or an underestimation of the abilities of persons with disabilities to run viable businesses.[35]

Lewis analyzes microfinance from the perspective of women with disabilities in Zambia and Zimbabwe. The research illustrates that MFI staff can be a major barrier to microfinance. In many cases, the 30 women from the study reported that the staff often appeared to assume that persons with disabilities lack the ability to run a successful business and would likely experience repayment challenges. Moreover, Lewis presents evidence that MFIs require collateral of disabled but not of nondisabled credit applicants. The study also indicates inaccessible infrastructure and lack of appropriate adaptive equipment and resources as serious barriers. Additionally, an informational barrier is highlighted by the study: Many women did not know that community microfinance programs existed or that they would be eligible to participate.[36]

In a case study from Bamako in Mali, Ormazabal focuses particularly on persons with disabilities' ability to contribute to the double bottom line of MFIs, that is, to both the financial and social objectives of the organizations. She concludes that persons with disabilities can be better clients for MFIs than nondisabled persons. Nevertheless, she finds that persons with disabilities remain a stigmatized segment of the population.[37] This view that persons with disabilities are stigmatized and considered unproductive and risky clients is also observed in Pakistan.[38]

Collectively, the reviewed research confirms that access to microfinance services is limited for persons with disabilities. The importance of the barriers outlined earlier is emphasized by several studies; however, the perceived importance of the various barriers differs among the studies. However, all studies appear to take for granted that access to credit would benefit persons with disabilities. No study actually investigates to what extent access to credit improves the outcome of self-employment activities among persons with disabilities or whether better access to credit increases the portion of persons with disabilities being self-employed. Another weakness of the surveyed literature is that it focuses nearly entirely on credit and does not include savings (and insurance) services.

3. THE UGANDAN CASE

Recently, using Ugandan survey data, we conducted several studies to better understand the concept of "microfinance and disability."[39] The data come from two different surveys from 2008, one conducted by the National Union of Disabled Persons of Uganda (NUDIPU) and the other collected by the Association of Microfinance Institutions of Uganda (AMFIU). The Norwegian Association of the Disabled supported the surveys. The data from NUDIPU were collected in trainings organized for *economically active* persons with disabilities. An economic activity was defined as anything from the smallest farm or the tiniest kiosk. The AMFIU data were collected from MFI staff participating in awareness-creation sessions in MFI branches. Both surveys were originally designed to improve the design of a project in which NUDIPU and AMFIU had joined forces to increase persons with disabilities' access to mainstream MFIs. The following presents the main findings of four empirical studies.

3.1 Access to Microfinance

Although the first study does not speak to the overall access of people with disabilities to microfinance, it does demonstrate that, applying a broad definition of microfinance, *economically active* persons with disabilities have better access to microfinance than previously assumed.[40] Out of the 841 respondents, 748 (89%) have used at least one type of microfinance service. The survey splits microfinance services into two broad categories: informal and formal services. Membership in rotating savings and credit associations (ROSCAs)[41] or any type of traditional saving activity is regarded as informal microfinance, whereas formal microfinance services include savings and loans from banks, MFIs, or formally registered member-based organizations such as savings and credit cooperatives (SACCOs). The survey data show that a total of 72% of the respondents save money regularly, out of which 70% save in a formal institution (i.e., 50% of the respondents have a formal savings account). Moreover, 39% of the respondents have borrowed money formally; however, only 15% of the respondents had a loan at the time the survey was conducted.[42] Thus, the majority of those accessing credit have not been able to maintain the borrower–bank relationship over time.

Figure 7.1 relates the use of microfinance services to types of disability. The figure illustrates that persons with vision and hearing impairments have less access to microfinance services than persons with other physical impairments. Our past research also indicates that women in general have better access than men, and that those who are married have better access than those who are not. Moreover, the study strongly suggests that the use of microfinance services increases with education level.[43]

Using the NUDIPU survey, the use of microfinance services may also be related to income source and income level. There is a positive association between the respondents' estimates of monthly income and their use of microfinance services. This pattern is particularly strong for the use of formal services. For example, whereas only 33% of the respondents with monthly incomes less than 100,000 Ugandan shillings (approximately US $50) stated that they have obtained a formal loan, the proportion increases to 59% for monthly income levels in between 400,000 and 700,000 Ugandan shillings. This relation between the use of microfinance and wealth is further confirmed

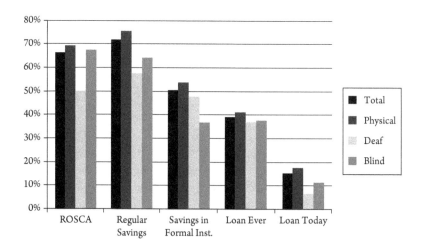

Figure 7.1
Disability Type and Access to Microfinance[44]

when the respondents' estimated business value replaces monthly income as the variable representing wealth.[45]

The NUDIPU survey also provides information on the relation between microfinance and primary source of income. Those persons whose primary source of income is farming or manufacturing generally use fewer microfinance services than those whose primary income source is from wholesale/retail or the service sector. This result is strongest for formal microfinance services. The survey also indicates, not surprisingly, that persons with farming as their primary source of income report the lowest income levels, whereas persons involved in wholesale or retail trading report the highest income levels. Thus, a major reason why most persons with disabilities in Uganda are poor is because more than 50% of them have farming as their primary source of income. Only 23% of the respondents have their primary incomes from wholesale or retail trading.[46] The dependency on farming is therefore a major constraint in regard to improving the outcome of business activities of persons with disabilities.

3.2 Barriers to Microfinance

The NUDIPU survey includes questions that can be related to the barriers to microfinance presented earlier. The main advantage of applying the NUDIPU survey to study barriers is that the study provides the persons with disabilities' *own view* on the importance of the barriers. Much of the previous research on the barriers to microfinance has not included empirical evidence from the clients themselves. Note that this part of the NUDIPU study has a microcredit focus because the questions focus on borrowing, not saving.

Based on the NUDIPU survey, our research shows that there is some fear among the respondents that they would be rejected by the staff of the institutions because of their disability. Specifically, 22% of the respondents express such a fear. However, more respondents (30%) fear that existing (nondisabled) credit group members would not accept them as members because of their disability. Another important barrier is the disability itself; 28% of the respondents state that their disability would make it difficult to access the banks' premises or to attend regular meetings. In contrast, self-exclusion appears to be less relevant than expected; only 12% of the respondents would feel shy or embarrassed if trying to apply for a loan.[47]

Exclusion by credit design emerged as the most important barrier in the study. Forty-six percent of the respondents of the study fear that the loan conditions may not suit their needs. However, a weakness in the survey is that the interest rate level is entangled with the question about the loan amount and period. Thus, we cannot know whether the barrier is actually the interest rate or whether it is related to other design issues. The relative importance of the barriers as measured by the NUDIPU survey is summarized in Figure 7.2.

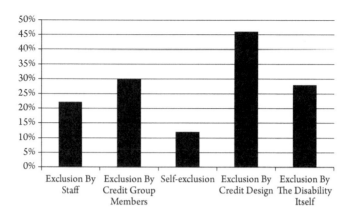

Figure 7.2
Barriers to Microfinance: The Customer's Perspective[48]

In the NUDIPU survey, it is possible to categorize the answers according to the respondents' personal characteristics. A general result is that respondents with higher education levels fear rejection less than those respondents with little or no education. Moreover, farmers and the hearing impaired are generally more pessimistic than other respondents. Finally, respondents who already have some experience with the services fear rejection less than respondents without any microfinance experience.[49]

Applying the AMFIU survey, we have studied the barriers to microfinance services from a staff perspective. In the AMFIU survey, the respondents—the staff members—were presented with 16 statements. For each statement, the answers were graded from 1 to 5, where 1 denoted "Fully disagree" and 5 "Fully agree." We categorized the statements according to the five barriers to microfinance.[50]

The data reveal that the staff generally disagrees with the statement that persons with disabilities lack the skills to run viable businesses. Nevertheless, most respondents believe that one could easily increase outreach to persons with disabilities through more personal efforts. The survey shows that the staff does not believe that exclusion by other members of credit groups is particularly widespread; however, data described earlier suggest that this barrier may be relevant. Furthermore, the staff strongly believes in motivating existing credit groups to take on disabled clients as a general means to increase outreach to the disabled. It is also worth mentioning that the respondents agree more or less unanimously that one should identify successful disabled customers and use those as examples on how to reach out to more disabled costumers.

In the AMFIU survey, there are generally few differences in the responses based on the respondents' personal characteristics. However, some interesting aspects are revealed. For instance, credit officers, the staff with direct contact with the costumers, appear less convinced that discrimination of persons with disabilities does not occur. Moreover, staff members with disabled relatives are more optimistic with respect to persons with disabilities' ability to run successful businesses. There is some evidence that younger staff members have a more positive attitude toward costumers with disabilities, whereas very few differences are found when the staff members' gender and length of work experience are investigated.

4. RECOMMENDATIONS FOR PRACTITIONERS AND POLICYMAKERS

This section outlines suggestions for practitioners and policymakers. The main focus is on policy recommendations to increase persons with disabilities' access and usefulness of microfinance services; however, we also present proposals for future research. Many of the suggestions follow more or less directly from the presented research, whereas other suggestions are based on subjective judgment because available research is still scarce.

The discussion is centered on persons with physical impairments. Mental impairments and access to microfinance and involvement in self-employment activities are, to the best of our knowledge, not discussed in the literature. Thus, the first suggestion for future research is to simply analyze to what extent persons with mental disabilities are involved in self-employment activities and to what extent they may benefit from microfinance services.

4.1 Borrowing for Self-Employment Activities

Financial capital is a necessary resource for self-employment but cannot stand alone in ensuring the viability of a business. Other capital, such as human and social capital, is necessary for the efficient use of financial capital. It is the combination of the different types of capital together with market opportunities that determines whether persons with disabilities' self-employment activities will succeed. Financial capital alone will often not improve the welfare of persons with disabilities, and in some cases, if a loan cannot be repaid or can only be repaid with great sacrifices, access to credit might actually be harmful for persons with disabilities. Figure 7.3 illustrates the importance of analyzing all types of capital before recommending the provision of credit to persons with disabilities for self-employment activities.

Disabled persons' organizations and policymakers advocating for better access to credit for persons with disabilities should keep in mind that the core of any business activity is normally not its financial capital, but the human

SITUATION TODAY	High level of human and social capital	Low level of human and social capital
Easy access to microcredit	Successful entrepreneurs that can be role models for others	Existing access to credit may have negative impact for the customer
Lack access to microcredit	Access to credit will often have immediate positive business impact	Need combined inputs of human, social and financial capital

Figure 7.3
The Importance of Human, Social, and Financial Capital for Enterprise Development[51]

and social capital of the microentrepreneur. The categorization suggested in Figure 7.3 is therefore an important exercise to be conducted before determining the most appropriate type of intervention when planning to improve the outcome of self-employment activities.

Our finding that earning levels differ considerably depending on the type of business in which the person with disabilities is involved[52] should motivate DPOs and others involved in livelihood projects to better assess potential income levels before recommending business ideas. In particular, the finding that persons whose primary income is from farming have a considerably lower income than others should lead livelihood project designers to consider off-farm opportunities for income generation.

Although this section deals with borrowing for self-employment activities, it should be emphasized that borrowing should not always be restricted to business loans only. In particular, loans for home improvement can be important for persons with disabilities. For example, many persons with disabilities need houses adapted to their needs. Moreover, as indicated by Collins and coworkers, poor people often need loans to cover medical or other precarious needs.[53] Such loans should be granted, on the condition that the person has the requisite repayment capacity.

4.2 The Importance of Savings

Our past work finds that economic activities often start with savings; in fact, 50% of the respondents of the study state that they use savings as their start-up capital. Another 43% obtained their start-up capital from sales of assets or from family members. Only 7% started their business with the help of a loan.[54] This result illustrates that disabled microentrepreneurs are similar to other entrepreneurs. It is well known in the entrepreneurship literature that personal savings as well as help from family members and others are the financial capital used to initiate new business activities. The Ugandan data confirm, once again, that loans are a minor source of funding for new self-employment activities. The reasons for this finding are, first, that survival rates of new enterprise ventures are seldom above 50% and that banks cannot take such high risks, and second, that the chance of success in business is higher if the entrepreneur's own money is at stake. This latter finding is also observed in the study of Handicap International; providing grants to help persons with disabilities to become self-employed often leads to a dependency on grants and not a successful business activity.[55] Moreover, because lending methodologies are normally conditioned on applicants having some existing savings, a demonstrated savings capacity is actually a prerequisite to receive a loan. Taken together, DPOs and policymakers interested in improving persons with disabilities' outcome from self-employment activities should focus on the importance of savings, not only loans.

Another reason for focusing on savings is related to consumption smoothing. As mentioned, a major challenge for poor persons is the high variation of incomes and expenses. Access to savings is what can best help balance uneven incomes and expenses and thus ensure that basic needs can be met on a daily basis. Many may argue that persons with disabilities are too poor to save; however, we have documented in past research that a vast majority of persons with disabilities do save.[56] The fact that poor people save (although often not in formal bank accounts) is now well documented in the literature and should be considered in development projects aiming to improve persons with disabilities' entrepreneurial activities.[57] Moreover, projects promoting savings among poor people should keep in mind the title of the study by Eggen and Mersland, "We Cannot Save Alone."[58] Good project design thus combines individual savings with group structures.

4.3 Informal Financial Structures Should Be Appreciated

One of our past studies reports that persons with disabilities are often involved in informal savings and credit groups.[59] Disability policymakers are often not familiar with such groups and do not sufficiently appreciate their existence. An interesting effect of the NUDIPU survey was that NUDIPU and their donor, the Norwegian Association of the Disabled, decided to design a new project to promote savings and credit groups among persons with disabilities. Initial results from this project, called We Can Manage, indicate that much higher numbers of persons with disabilities than expected are being mobilized and that the saving capacity is higher than traditionally assumed.

For the enhancement of the livelihoods of persons with disabilities, the promotion of savings and credit groups can be of particular importance because these schemes can allow for a more flexible and integrated approach. Compared with MFIs, the savings and credit group methodology can reach poorer target groups and help enhance social and human capital.[60]

4.4 Ensuring Access for Persons with Disabilities in Mainstream Microfinance Institutions

In much of the research on microfinance and disability, the importance of incorporating persons with disabilities in *formal* mainstream microfinance institutions has been emphasized. The background of this recommendation is that access to microfinance needs to be permanent and not a one-time event. The problem with many development efforts and ad-hoc programs is that they are not financially sustainable and tend to disappear after a few years. Thus, mainstream institutions represent the preferred alternative, and we agree with the recommendation that the provision of credit by nonspecialist providers should be discontinued.[61]

4.5 Breaking Down Barriers Hindering Persons with Disabilities' Access to Microfinance

Regarding ensuring access to mainstream microfinance institutions, the five barriers explained earlier have proved useful for both practitioners and researchers to better understand the mechanisms hindering access for persons with disabilities. We thus recommend the continued use of this theoretical framework.

4.5.1 Staff Barrier

To date, there has been a considerable focus on the staff barrier in the literature, and there appears to be agreement that staff prejudice and stigmatization is a major explanation for why persons with disabilities often do not access microfinance services.[62] We thus recommend a continued focus on training and awareness-creation among MFI staff. This recommendation also follows directly from our past work, in which MFI staff strongly believed that they could easily increase outreach to clients with disabilities if they were more motivated and exerted increased personal efforts.[63]

Nevertheless, it is important to note that, on a detailed level, there is little or no research on the nature of discrimination and how it is conducted. After all, a rejection of a loan application for a disabled person is not discrimination if it is based on an analysis demonstrating lack of repayment capacity. Thus, to better understand how, when, and why discrimination occurs, future research should continue focusing on barriers at the staff level of microfinance.

4.5.2 Credit and Service Design Barrier

Exclusion by credit design typically has not been a frequently discussed barrier in prior research. Nevertheless, our past work finds that the disabled themselves consider this barrier to be by far the most important obstacle; almost half of the sample fears that the loan conditions may not suit their needs.[64] A weakness of the study is that it does not disentangle the interest rate level from other loan conditions. Nevertheless, considering the fact that two thirds of the respondents state that they are willing to pay the same interest rates as nondisabled clients, there is reason to believe that other loan conditions play an important role.

As noted by Beisland and Mersland, unfavorable credit design is a general problem in the microfinance industry, and design improvements could potentially benefit all customers.[65] Thus, a useful recommendation may be to adapt products to serve the needs of persons with disabilities, because this adaptation would often be a test to ensure that the product would be friendly for *all* customers. For instance, less frequent repayments could be beneficial for all persons living in remote areas, not only those with disabilities.

The problem regarding credit and service design is that we know little about what design issues are particularly troublesome for persons with disabilities. Generally, MFIs struggle in designing customer-friendly products; thus, we do not know whether customers with disabilities are less satisfied than other customers. Another challenge is related to the heterogeneity within the disability group. The needs of persons with hearing impairments differ greatly from those of persons with mental health impairments. Thus, designing special microfinance products for all customers with disabilities could lead to many different types of products. However, Banco D-MIRO in Ecuador experienced that these adaptations are not necessarily required to increase the outreach to persons with disabilities. In this bank, they decided to specifically target the disability segment and started with sensitivity training for their staff together with targeted marketing efforts, including partnering with local DPOs. Customers with disabilities were offered exactly the same products as other customers. Within one year, the number of customers with disabilities tripled. Banco D-MIRO also found that using existing customers with disabilities to reach potentially new customers with disabilities was one of the most efficient marketing channels.

Many people, including staff, appear to believe that persons with disabilities need more favorable loan conditions than others.[66] There is also evidence to suggest that some persons with disabilities expect better conditions.[67] However, whether better conditions would influence the supply of or demand for microfinance is an unsolved issue.

4.5.3 Other Group Members

It is difficult to address local stigmatization and discrimination that lead to the exclusion of persons with disabilities from credit groups and saving associations. Eggen and Mersland explain the importance of letting groups be autonomous regarding the selection of members.[68] Policymakers, DPOs, MFIs, and others thus need to continue raising awareness about the rights of persons with disabilities. In addition, current trends in the microfinance industry might be beneficial for persons with disabilities. As competition in the industry increases, MFIs are lowering their prices, improving their services, and targeting new market segments, including persons with disabilities. In addition there is now a strong shift away from group methodologies toward individual methodologies,[69] which in most cases are preferred by persons with disabilities.

4.5.4 Self-Exclusion

Although our past studies find that, according to persons with disabilities themselves, self-exclusion stemming from low self-esteem is not the major problem,[70] we suggest maintaining a focus on this exclusion barrier. Similar to others who have experienced exclusion, stigmatization, and discrimination, some persons with disabilities avoid seeking out new opportunities. Disabled persons' organizations are most likely those best suited to address these challenges; however, MFIs and others should be aware of the challenge and ensure respectful customer service.

One important type of self-exclusion is the fact that many persons with disabilities (as many other vulnerable persons) are not informed about available services. This finding is also documented in recent research suggesting that persons with disabilities do not approach microfinance services simply because they are not aware that they would be eligible for such services.[71] Increased and targeted marketing efforts as exemplified by Banco D-MIRO are needed.

Finally, there is an often-neglected effect of financial services; being trusted by a credit company or having been able to steadily save money can completely change a person's self-respect. We thus welcome systematic project efforts as well as rigorous research to study the self-esteem effect from accessing microfinance.

4.5.5 Physical and Informational Barriers

Unfortunately, most countries in which MFIs operate are weakly equipped regarding ensuring equal opportunities for persons with disabilities. Information available in Braille language, sign interpreters, or wheelchair ramps are theoretical, unrealistic solutions. Even if microfinance information were available in Braille, there are few persons with visual impairments who can read it; similarly, there are few persons with hearing impairments who practice sign language. Because the microfinance industry is a very international industry with significant donor support, we recommend that this industry take the lead in demonstrating that reducing physical and informational barriers for persons with disabilities is also possible in low- and middle-income countries. Some solutions are obvious, for example, not locating MFIs in premises that require persons with disabilities to climb steep and narrow staircases.

4.6 Microfinance and Education

Prior research suggests a strong relation between the use of microfinance and the level of education and between the level of income and the level education. As the education level increases, there is a corresponding increase in income and in the use of microfinance services.[72] Moreover, there is far less fear of the various barriers to microfinance if the education level is high.[73] Thus, even though education is important by itself, it is also important as a means to improve income levels and to improve access to private and public services, in this case, microfinance services. We cannot emphasize enough that the best way to ensure better employment opportunities for persons with disabilities is to provide better education for children with disabilities.

5. CONCLUSION

An implicit assumption of this chapter is that access to microfinance services is advantageous to persons with disabilities. It has typically been accepted that by giving poor people access to such services, they will experience economic development. In fact, most studies conclude that access to microfinance, whether loans or savings, has a positive impact on poor people's economic activities and lives;[74] however, it is important to note that this general belief is challenged by recent studies.[75] Collectively, there is a reasonable degree of consensus that access to savings is positive in the fight against poverty and that access to loans can be useful to ensure consumption smoothing.[76] However, whether access to loans increases poor people's income is still being debated, and recent studies applying randomized control trials have resulted in different findings.[77] Very often, the microcredit effect may be difficult to isolate for individual households and small enterprises. For instance, loans from MFIs are often given for consumption smoothing, and the usefulness of such smoothing is difficult to estimate empirically.

In general, findings on the effects of microfinance cannot necessarily be extrapolated to the disability community. Because an overwhelming majority of persons with disabilities are self-employed,[78] access to capital is important, possibly more important than for the average citizen of a low- or middle-income country. Moreover, although improvements in incomes and assets obviously are important, access to microfinance may also influence persons with disabilities' self-esteem and general integration into society.[79] Thus, there may be reason to believe that the (positive) development effects of microfinance on average are larger for persons with disabilities than others.

Nonetheless, the microfinance industry recently has come under a certain amount of public and media pressure. There has been a critical focus on interest rates and collection methods, and the major question has been whether microfinance truly helps to bring persons out of poverty. Unfortunately, we are unaware of rigorous academic research that has been able to document the welfare impacts of microfinance services for persons with disabilities. Thus, we conclude this chapter with a caveat: We cannot rule out the possibility that microfinance under specific circumstances can be detrimental to a disabled person's standard of living. However, in general, we agree with those who claim that access to microcredit should be a priority in pro-disability policies.[80] In particular, we strongly support the recent United Nation Convention of the Rights of Persons with Disabilities, which clearly indicates that persons with disabilities have the right to equal opportunities, including equal access to microfinance services.

ACKNOWLEDGMENTS

Roy Mersland has worked as a consultant for the Norwegian Association of the Disabled in their efforts in Uganda and elsewhere, and some results reported throughout the text come from his personal contact with the project officers and donor representatives. Roy Mersland is also a board member at Banco D-MIRO.

NOTES

1. Cramm, J.M., & Finkenflugel, H. (2008). Exclusion of disabled people from microcredit in Africa and Asia: A literature study. *Asia Pacific Disability Rehabilitation Journal, 19*(2), 15–33.
2. Martinelli, E., & Mersland, R. (2010). Microfinance for people with disabilities. In T.Barron (Ed.), *Poverty and Disability* (London, United Kingdom: Leonard Cheshire International).
3. Bwire, F.N., Mukasa, G., & Mersland, R. (2009). Access to mainstream microfinance services for persons with disabilities—lessons learned from Uganda. *Disability Studies Quarterly 29*(1), 4. Retrieved January 29, 2013, from: http://dsq-sds.org/article/view/168/168.

4. For a summary of the microfinance impact research, see Duvendack, M., et al. (2011). *What is the evidence of the impact of microfinance on the well-being of poor people?* London, United Kingdom: EPPI-Centre.
5. Imai, K.S., Gaiha, R., Thapa, G., & Annim, S.K. (2012). Microfinance and poverty—a macro perspective. *World Development 40*, 1675–1689.
6. Collins, D., Morduch, J., Rutherford, S. & Ruthven, R. (2009). *Portfolios of the poor: How the World's poor live on $2 a day.* Princeton, NJ: Princeton University Press.
7. Beisland, L. A., & Mersland, R. (2012). The use of microfinance services among economically active disabled people: Evidence from Uganda. *Journal of International Development 24*, S69–S83.
8. International Labour Organization (2002). *Disability and Poverty Reduction Strategies—How to ensure that access of persons with disabilities to decent and productive work is part of the PRSP process.* Geneva, Switzerland: ILO.
9. United Nations. (2008). *Convention on the rights of persons with disabilities.* New York: United Nations.
10. Handicap International. (2006). *Good practices for the economic inclusion of people with disabilities in developing countries.* Paris, France: Handicap International, 6.
11. United Nations. (2008). *Convention on the rights of persons with disabilities.*
12. Handicap International. (2006). *Good practices.*
13. Cramm & Finkenflugel (2008). Exclusion of disabled people; Martinelli and Mersland (2010). Microfinance for people with disabilities.
14. Simanowitz, A. (2001). Thematic report No. 4: Microfinance for the Poorest—A review of issues and ideas for contribution of Imp-Act. *Improving the impact of microfinance on poverty Imp-Act.* Brighton, United Kingdom: Institute for Development Studies.
15. Bwire, Mukasa, & Mersland (2009). Access to mainstream microfinance.
16. Ibid.
17. Martinelli & Mersland (2010). Microfinance for people with disabilities, 249.
18. Labie, M., Meon, P. G., Mersland, R., & Szafarz, A. (2010). Discrimination by Microcredit Officers: Theory and Evidence on Disability in Uganda. Working paper N°11-06.RS, Universite Libre de Bruxelles. Retrieved March 31, 2013, from https://dipot.ulb.ac.be/dspace/bitstream/2013/87194/1/11-06Discrimination_by_Microcredit_Officers_May%202011.pdf
19. Bwire, Mukasa, & Mersland (2009). Access to mainstream microfinance.
20. Martinelli & Mersland (2010). Microfinance for people with disabilities.
21. Ibid.
22. Bwire, Mukasa, & Mersland (2009). Access to mainstream microfinance.
23. Ibid.
24. International Labour Organization (2002). *Disability and Poverty Reduction Strategies.*
25. Thomas, M. (2000). Feasibility of integrating people with disabilities in savings and credit programmes in Bangladesh. *Asia Pacific Disability Rehabilitation Journal, 11*, 27–31.
26. Handicap International. (2006). *Good practices.*
27. Ibid.
28. Ibid.
29. Ibid., 108.

30. de Klerk, T. (2008). Funding for self-employment of people with disabilities. Grants, loans, revolving funds or linkage with microfinance programmes. *Leprosy Review, 79*, 92–109.
31. Thomas, M. (2000). Feasibility of integrating people with disabilities
32. Ibid.
33. Ibid.
34. Bwire, Mukasa, & Mersland (2009). Access to mainstream microfinance.
35. Labie, Meon, Mersland, & Szafarz (2010). Discrimination by Microcredit Officers.
36. Lewis, C. (2004). Microfinance from the point of view of women with disabilities: lessons from Zambia and Zimbabwe. *Gender and Development 12*, 28–39.
37. Ormazabal, I. (2010). *Microfinance and Disability: do persons with disabilities contribute to the double bottom line of MFIs? Key factors for success stories—a case study in Bamako.* Master's Thesis. Brussels, Belgium: Solvay Brussels School of Economics and Management.
38. Ahmad, M., & Ahmad, M.M. (2011). Measuring Support Provisions for People Living With Disabilities in South Asia: An Accessibility Index. *Journal of Social Service Research 37*, 439–455.
39. Beisland, L.A., & Mersland, R. (2012). Barriers to microcredit for persons with disabilities: Evidence from economically active persons in Uganda. *Enterprise Development and Microfinance Journal 23*, 11–24; Beisland, L.A., & Mersland, R. (2012). Barriers to microfinance services for persons with disabilities: The staff perspective. Working Paper. Agder, Norway: University of Agder; Beisland, L.A. & Mersland, R. (forthcoming). Income Characteristics and the Use of Microfinance Services: Evidence from Economically Active Persons with disabilities. *Disability & Society*. Agder, Norway: University of Agder; Beisland & Mersland (2012). The use of microfinance services.
40. Beisland & Mersland (2012). The use of microfinance services.
41. In a ROSCA, a group of 15-30 people pool their savings weekly or monthly. These savings are distributed as grants or loans among the members in a rotating system. ROSCAs have been around for centuries and exist in virtually every developing country including Uganda.
42. Beisland & Mersland (2012). The use of microfinance services.
43. Ibid.
44. *Source:* Beisland and Mersland (2012). The use of microfinance services.
45. Beisland & Mersland (forthcoming). Income Characteristics and the Use of Microfinance Services.
46. Ibid.
47. Beisland & Mersland (2012). Barriers to microcredit for persons with disabilities.
48. Source: Beisland & Mersland (2012). Barriers to microcredit for persons with disabilities.
49. Beisland & Mersland (2012). Barriers to microcredit for persons with disabilities.
50. Beisland & Mersland (2012). Barriers to microfinance services.
51. Martinelli & Mersland (2010). Microfinance for people with disabilities.
52. Beisland & Mersland (forthcoming). Income Characteristics and the Use of Microfinance Services.
53. Collins, Morduch, Rutherford, & Ruthven (2009). *Portfolios of the poor.*
54. Beisland and Mersland (2012). The use of microfinance services.

55. Handicap International. (2006). *Good practices*.
56. Beisland & Mersland (2012). The use of microfinance services.
57. Collins, Morduch, Rutherford, & Ruthven (2009). *Portfolios of the poor*.
58. Eggen, Ø., & Mersland, R. (2007). *You Cannot Save Alone—Financial and Social Mobilisation in Savings and Credit Groups. NORAD Report.* Oslo, Norway: NORAD.
59. Beisland & Mersland (2012). The use of microfinance services.
60. Eggen & Mersland (2007). *You Cannot Save Alone*.
61. For a more comprehensive discussion of the preferred types of microfinance providers, see Handicap International. (2006). *Good practices*; and Martinelli & Mersland (2010). Microfinance for people with disabilities.
62. Cramm & Finkenflugel (2008). Exclusion of disabled people; Labie, Meon, Mersland, & Szafarz (2010). Discrimination by Microcredit Officers.
63. Beisland & Mersland (2012). Barriers to microfinance services.
64. Beisland & Mersland (2012). Barriers to microcredit for persons with disabilities.
65. Ibid.
66. Beisland & Mersland (2012). Barriers to microfinance services.
67. Beisland & Mersland (2012). Barriers to microcredit for persons with disabilities.
68. Eggen & Mersland (2007). *You Cannot Save Alone*.
69. Mersland, R. & Strøm, R.Ø. (2012). The past and future of innovations in Microfinance. In D. Cumming (Ed.). *The Oxford Handbook of Entrepreneurial Finance* (New York: Oxford University Press), 859–892.
70. Beisland & Mersland (2012). Barriers to microcredit for persons with disabilities.
71. Bwire, Mukasa, & Mersland (2009). Access to mainstream microfinance; Lewis (2004). Microfinance from the point of view of women with disabilities.
72. Beisland & Mersland (forthcoming). Income Characteristics and the Use of Microfinance Services; Beisland & Mersland (2012). The use of microfinance services.
73. Beisland & Mersland (2012). Barriers to microcredit for persons with disabilities.
74. See, for example, Goldberg, N. (2005). *Measuring the impact of microfinance: Taking stock of what we know*. Washington D.C.: Grameen Foundation USA.
75. Duvendack et al. (2011). What is the evidence of the impact of microfinance.
76. Rosenberg, R. (2010). *Does microcredit really help poor people?* Washington D.C.: Focus Note, CGAP.
77. Ibid.
78. Handicap International. (2006). *Good practices*.
79. Cramm & Finkenflugel (2008). Exclusion of disabled people.
80. For example, Handicap International. (2006). *Good practices*; Cramm & Finkenflugel (2008). Exclusion of disabled people.

A Life-Course Approach and Beyond

CHAPTER 8

Transition from School to Work

New Directions for Policy and Practice

FRANK R. RUSCH, JOHN DATTILO, ROBERT STODDEN,
AND ANTHONY J. PLOTNER

1. INTRODUCTION

With the evolution of society's views of disability and an increasing collective commitment to human rights and inclusiveness for all human beings, is it time to rethink special education as the primary vehicle for the delivery of educational services and supports to students deemed to have a disability? Clearly, special education has enjoyed unprecedented gains in providing learning opportunities for a diversity of students with disabilities in the United States and among members of the Organization for Economic Co-operation and Development. However, a question arises: have the results of participating in special education resulted in individuals acquiring better jobs, experiencing a higher quality of life, and encountering new opportunities for membership in the mainstream of society? After 35 years of providing special education services, the US Department of Education, for example, recently reported that more youth are:

- Graduating from high school with a diploma
- Attending postsecondary education programs
- Employed as a result of their participation in special education programs[1]

The tone of the US Department of Education's message is clearly a positive one, and few would argue with the growth of special education services over the past 35 years in the United States.[2] Fewer yet would argue against its positive impact on schools and students. Indeed, two of the most dramatic areas of growth have been among young children who have been deflected from special education altogether as a result of their receiving early childhood special education, and also among young students who have participated in early identification and directed instruction that diverts underachieving and minority status early learners away from special education as a result of their response to instruction.

The outcomes associated with youth with disabilities are not as positive. Although transition-related services have proliferated in US high schools since 1983, outcomes associated with US high schools are mixed. For example, postsecondary enrollments are at an all-time high, but arrests have increased and employment has stagnated among youth in transition.[3]

This chapter reviews these transition-related outcomes and suggests that new directions for transition policy and practice in the United States may be warranted. Our review of transition-related outcomes suggest that: (1) elementary schools must be held accountable for preparing students to meet grade-level expectations in core curriculum areas (e.g., reading and math) before they enter middle schools; (2) middle schools must be held accountable for ensuring that students learn to be active participants in planning their curriculum, including their curriculum goals and high school studies so that these goals and studies complement their eventual post-high school aspirations; and (3) high schools must play a leadership role in providing a meaningful curriculum, including coordinating resources and developing community support for postsecondary education participation and employment opportunities after departing high school, including developing dropout prevention and recovery programs that focus on as many as 50% of youth who depart from high schools before they graduate.

The fact that the US Department of Education's 35-year report indicated that more youth are graduating from high schools, enrolling in postsecondary education, and finding employment suggests that transition services have been successful in meeting high school students' goals after participation in transition services.[4] However, additional data suggest that these outcomes are associated with a smaller population of students who either remain in school to eventually attend higher education or remain in school because they represent the hardest to teach and their choices are limited.

This chapter begins with an overview of transition "best practices" that have emerged over the past 30 years, practices that one would expect would lead to better outcomes associated with high schools who endorse these practices. Following this discussion, we present outcomes that served as the springboard for transition legislation introduced more than three decades ago and compare these outcomes with those that have been reported more recently. This comparison is important because it suggests that transition-related outcomes today are similar to those described more than 30 years ago, which were the very impetus for change. Unfortunately, it appears that large numbers of transition-age youth with disabilities are continuing to fail to make the transition from being a youth to becoming a young adult with a future, despite 30 years of transition-related activities that resulted from legislation passed in the early 1980s.

This chapter is situated in the belief that our educational system is not providing a context that facilitates goal achievement for most of these students. We are concerned about the largely untold stories of the extent to which students enter middle school unprepared for the academic challenges they experience and eventually drop out of high school. Unfortunately, for many students their high school curriculum is not tailored to meet their post-high school goals, which is often followed by unemployment and the dire outcomes associated with unemployment, including lowered self-esteem, isolation, loneliness, and a 30% chance of being arrested.[5] We review recent data that appear to support as well as challenge the effectiveness of secondary special education and transition-related services, suggesting new directions for policy and practice as a result of our apparent failure to design transition services to meet individuals' unique needs.

Recent research and growth in transition services and goals for youth with disabilities have not resulted in major life changes associated with (1) school retention, (2) employment and poverty, (3) postsecondary education, and (4) incarcerations. Therefore, we outline three new directions for policy and practice that rely on data largely available in the United States. These recommendations suggest that the solutions to some of the problems that confront youth in transition may originate early in their school experience and these problems are complicated by our failure to promote students with disabilities to becoming more self-reliant and self-determined. Further, based on best available evidence we believe that more than 50% of youth who enter middle school do not finish high school, which suggests that our high schools need to fundamental realign with their communities in providing better jobs after graduation and provide a better high school experience that better prepares these youth for postsecondary education. Because so many youth appear to drop out of our schools prior to completing their education, we also suggest establishing dropout recovery programs designed to meet the explicit needs of youth.

2. OVERVIEW OF TRANSITION BEST PRACTICES

Evidence-based practices in schools are essential in the area of transition as the number of students with disabilities requesting transition services is increasing.[6] With the growing number of students requesting transition services, transition professionals have been pressed to promote the development of work-related skills in order to evolve with the field of transition service delivery.[7]

The reauthorization of No Child Left Behind (2001) and the Individuals with Disabilities Education Act (2004) mandate that teachers use proven practices to guide instructional decision making for students with and without disabilities. Unfortunately, the effectiveness of services and programs that define transition service delivery has been questioned,[8] and research that discusses the use of evidence-based practice remains sparse if not nonexistent. Converting research findings into educational practices is a critical component often missing from transition service delivery.[9] Researchers have found that (1) special education teachers do not use evidence-based practices to successfully instruct students with disabilities and (2) inservice professional development opportunities are often needed to meet the needs of these students.[10]

Researchers began to identify the skills needed for personnel providing transition services in the 1980s.[11] In 1983, the federal government began authorizing funds for personnel preparation projects focusing on transition.[12] In 1987, the Office of Special Education and Rehabilitation Services founded 13 programs for preparing transition personnel. As a result, over the last 25 years, teacher competencies and transition practices believed to be related to better transition planning and supports have emerged; however, the field has continued to suffer from poor reports associated with retention and employment.

Based on the findings of emerging studies suggesting rising unemployment, dropping out, and poor social engagement among students with disabilities, the Division on Career Development and Transition of the Council for Exceptional Children developed a set of competency areas needed by transition specialists to be more effective at their jobs.[13] Further, Kohler published a review of best practices in transition services after identifying 49 documents from the years 1985 to 1991,[14] which ultimately led to the Taxonomy for Transition Programming.[15]

More recently, Landmark, Ju, and Zhang updated Kohler's study by reviewing 18 new documents and 11 reviewed by Kohler in 1993 to substantiate best practices. Landmark and colleagues utilized the same empirically substantiated criteria used by Kohler: (1) Samples consisted of secondary students with disabilities; (2) outcome variables included postsecondary employment, postsecondary education, or postsecondary independent living; (3) dependent variables that educators could influence were investigated versus demographic variables (e.g., age, gender, disability); and (4) the study used quantitative or qualitative analysis to link dependent and outcome variables.[16]

Landmark and coworkers found that the following eight practices were mentioned most by investigators as meeting minimal criteria associated with being "best practices:"

1 Paid or unpaid work experience
2 Participating in an employment preparation program
3 Participating in general education vs. segregated special education

4 Family involvement
5 Social skills training
6 Daily living skills training
7 Self-determination training
8 Community or agency collaboration[17]

Many of the best practices identified by Landmark and colleagues are supported by Mazotti, Test, and Mustian, who identified 16 predictors of post school outcomes across 22 studies that met their quality indicator criteria.[18]

3. OVERVIEW OF YOUTH OUTCOMES IN THE UNITED STATES

Secondary special education and transition-related services have enjoyed much attention and funding since the mid 1980s;[19] however, as noted above, outcomes associated with transitioning youth in the United States appear to have lagged behind expectations associated with the attention and funding provided. Indeed, according to Rusch,[20] statistics reported by the federally-funded National Longitudinal Transition Study (NLTS) Parts 1 and 2[21] appear to contradict the 35 Years of Progress Report.[22] After reviewing NLTS data, Rusch suggested a different story associated with youth in transition. Specifically, he concluded the following:

- After entering the ninth grade, students with disabilities drop out of school at alarming rates before they turn 18 years old. They do not graduate.
- Youth with disabilities are likely to experience a life of poverty. They are unemployed or underemployed.
- Almost 30% of youth with disabilities appear to pursue postsecondary education and training; however, retention rates, if they follow patterns of students without disabilities, would suggest that most do not complete postsecondary education.
- Arrest rates increase over time, with more than 30% of all youth with a disability reportedly being arrested at some point within three years after leaving high school. A criminal record reduces one's chances to attain a job and eventually meaningful employment.[23]

These outcomes are similar to those reported by Will[24] and others[25] almost three decades ago and they are confusing in light of the US Department of Education's 35-year report mentioned previously. More recent data supplied by the US Department of Education suggest a more positive story. The following section reviews transition-related findings, paying particular attention to corroborating research on selected outcomes, including dropout and arrest rates, poverty levels, employment, and postsecondary enrollments. These data are considered when making recommendations for improving youth-related outcomes in the United States, shifting the responsibility to include a focus on elementary and middle school practices that would complement secondary special education and transition-related services.

3.1 School Retention

The dropout population among students with disabilities in the United States has not been studied extensively.[26] Among existing studies, Rusch analyzed nine consecutive Annual Reports to Congress (1993–2001) and found that an average of 422,540 students participated in special education when they are 14 years old; this total appears to drop significantly over time. Rusch estimated that more than 50% of high school ninth graders with a disability depart special education for a variety of reasons before age 19. By the age of 18, just over 170,000 students with disabilities appear to participate in special education, with over 60,000 of these students dropping out of school before they reach 19 years of age. By age 18, a little more than 170,000 students appear to participate in special education programs. Most of approximately 400,000 14-year-old students who participate in special education leave special education, with the largest group dropping out of high school. After age 18, the number of students enrolled in high school drops by more than two thirds to 55,425 (age 19), followed by more than half leaving special education between ages 19 and 20, and yet another 50% reduction after age 20. According to Rusch, the primary reasons students leave special education is earning a diploma (20% of total exits). A further 3% leave special education after obtaining a certificate of attendance, and 12% leave because they return to general education. At the same time, however, 15% of all exits from special education are due to the student dropping out.[27]

The number of diplomas awarded is higher after the students' 16th year, with a spike in diplomas awarded at age 18, an age that accounts for almost half of all diplomas awarded, followed by graduating with a diploma at age 19, which accounts for a further quarter of all diplomas awarded. The awarding of certificates of attendance follows a similar pattern.[28]

The same holds true, however, for dropping out of school. Half of the students with a disability that drop out do so in their junior and senior years. The numbers of students who drop out doubles from age 14 to age 15, and keeps increasing to the point that almost 3 in 4 dropouts occur during the remaining high school years.[29]

Rusch also indicated that the number of students without a disability between the ages of 14 and 18 (a five-year span) served in general education reaches about 16 million in any given year. By comparison, the number of students in the same age range served in special education totals just over 1.6 million, and the percentage of general versus special education students who drop out after age 16 is almost identical (11.25% and 10.17%, respectively).[30]

Among students without a disability, dropping out of the general education curriculum is associated with increased absenteeism from school, lower grades, diminished parental control, and increased use of tobacco and alcohol;[31] however, a major reason why students with disabilities drop out appears to relate to their academic performance. The Consortium on Chicago School Research suggested that course performance and higher absentee rates are strong predictors of five-year graduation rates of youth with disabilities. Specifically, this report indicated that *if students with a disability entered high school two or more years below grade level, they were more likely to drop out.*[32] Moreover, attempts to increase their ability to catch up to their peers without a disability were not successful, suggesting that early efforts to maintain grade level performance among students with disabilities is essential before these students reach later elementary years and are at the threshold of entry into middle school. Poor performance in middle school results in students with disabilities attending school less, which further complicates their educational progress. Eventually, school becomes less rewarding.

3.2 Employment and Poverty

Since transition became a national priority,[33] employment of youth with disabilities has been considered in most studies focused on how well they fare after high school. In the 1980s, for example, the US Commission on Civil Rights reported that the unemployment of people with disabilities was 50% to 75%. Describing the results of a 1987 Harris Telephone Survey, Rusch and Phelps noted that 67% of people with a disability (N = 1,000) (ages 16–64) were not working and that those employed were primarily working part-time.[34]

Further, Wagner found that 46% of a nationally representative sample of 8,000 students was employed within two years of departing high school.[35] In contrast, the National Organization on Disabilities indicated that 70% of respondents from a national sample of 1,000 people with a disability were not working compared with almost 20% of their peers without a disability.[36]

Fifteen studies conducted between 1985[37] and 1995[38] provide compelling data that the employment rate among people with disabilities is dire and may actually be worsening. In fact, information obtained from the Current Population Survey indicated that between October 2008 and June of 2010, the number of job losses among employees with disabilities far exceeded those of workers without disabilities; the 18- to 39-year-old working-age adult population employment rate dropped by 14.8%.[39]

Blanchett and Fremstad argued that attempts to make reductions in poverty among individuals with disabilities must originate in our understanding of the interconnectedness of disability and poverty, and that any effort to reduce the incidence of poverty among our youth must begin in high school. Better trained and educated youth should result in better employment opportunities;[40] however, as pointed out above, most youth with disabilities appear to drop out of school before they graduate and/or benefit from training. Hughes and Avoke connected unemployment among young adults with disabilities and poverty, suggesting that students who attend high-poverty-area schools spend "less time participating in school-based job training";[41] school-based job training has been suggested a strong predictor of future employment.[42]

Large numbers of US high school students with disabilities drop out of high school, which results in fewer opportunities for employment training, which in turn results in corresponding losses in competitive wages. Our failure to retain youth with disabilities in high school contributes to exiting youth living in poverty. For individuals with disabilities, Newman, Wagner, Cameto, Knokey, and Shaver reported that employment among all youth with disabilities fell for the 15-year period from 1990 to 2005 (62% vs. 56%), as did the number of hours worked (38 hours vs. 35 hours) and their benefits such as paid vacation or sick leave (60% vs. 38%).[43] Clearly, lower wages among young adults with disabilities only increases their exposure to poverty.

Alternative employment opportunities such as employment in sheltered workshops have historically been associated with poor earnings. In 1998, for example, young adults entering a sheltered workshop averaged an hourly wage of $2.64 and worked an average of 28 hours per work week, with 12% receiving benefits.[44] These figures suggest that sheltered workshop participants earned, at most, $3,700 annually for 52 weeks of work; alternatively, if they entered competitive employment and worked 40 hours a week at minimum wage, they would have earned well above $15,000.[45] Both earning figures are considered to be at or below the poverty level.

3.3 Postsecondary Education

Postsecondary education has been a bright spot for youth with disabilities; however, to date there are no data on retention rates. Using high school grades as a predictor variable, Astin suggested that an A– student has a 67% chance of completing college in four years. By comparison, a C student has a 20% chance of completing the same college within the same four-year time period.[46] Although no formulas exist for predicting college completion for youth with disabilities, predictions can be estimated by utilizing similar-aged youth without disabilities, although these estimates should be cautiously considered as they most likely are overestimates.

College enrollment among youth with disabilities is at an all-time high.[47] Newman and coworkers reported that 46% of youth with disabilities in their 2005 cohort entered a postsecondary institution within four years of leaving high school compared with 26% of a similar 1990 cohort.[48] Yet, it is important to note that, in the United States, only half of all college entrants irrespective of disability status complete college. If these attrition rates are the same for college entrants with disabilities, which they probably are not, at least half of students with disabilities may not complete college.

Students with intellectual and developmental disabilities historically have not been afforded opportunities to attend college; however, an outcry for better education opportunities for this population has recently resulted in the emergence of postsecondary education programs for these youth. In October of 2010, the Office of Postsecondary Education awarded 11 million dollars to 27 institutions of higher education for development and support of these postsecondary programs. As a result, in the near future we can expect to see new predictive models for enrollment and completion among this population, which should lead to new models emerging for youth with other disabilities and eventually better retention data.

3.4 Incarcerations

Newman and coworkers suggested that, in terms of graduation and postsecondary enrollment, the status of youth with disabilities improved between 1990 and 2005 in comparison with their peers without disabilities. However, one area was an important exception—more youth with disabilities were arrested in 2005 than in 1990.[49] Although scant research is available to help us understand arrest records,[50] some data suggest that a potential contributor to arrests and/or adjudications is confusion associated with youth with behavioral and emotional problems. For example, Doren, Bullis, and Benz reported that students with behavioral and emotional problems (including aggressive behaviors) are 13 times more likely to be arrested and that males with disabilities are 2.4 times more likely than females with similar disabilities to be arrested.[51]

Estimates of incarcerated youth with disabilities range from 30% to 50% of all youth in correctional facilities,[52] which represents an increase from estimates made more than 15 years earlier.[53] Wagner and coworkers reported arrest rates of dropouts with disabilities as high as 56%, compared with 16% of youth with disabilities who graduate from high school and 10% of youth who "age out" of school; in addition, arrest rates among youth with serious emotional problems has been identified as high as 73%.[54] Although the exact numbers of youth with disabilities who are arrested is not clear, arrest and adjudication is a serious and costly problem.

3.5 Summary

When considering dropout rates, employment and poverty, postsecondary enrollment, and arrests, a question arises: *Why are the outcomes for youth with disabilities so poor after several decades of attention focused on improving secondary special education and transition services?* According to the National Disability Rights Network (NDRN), poor outcomes associated with youth with disabilities may relate to our tendency to "isolate and segregate individuals with disabilities" and to provide "a history of purposeful unequal treatment."[55] Indeed, the NDRN released an incendiary exposé of legislation that relegated people with disabilities to being paid subminimum wages, in segregated settings, with little chance to earn a wage that provides a route to escape poverty or even to avoid debilitating expectations from the general public as a "powerless minority in our society."[56]

Educating youth with disabilities apart from their peers without disabilities has been a long-standing practice in special education. Historically, this practice was supported by educators as important to the early learning gains made by students in special education.[57] Yet, the dropout rate of youth with disabilities may, disputably, be tied to the failure of separate education to prepare these children to the academic standards of their peers without disabilities before they enter high school. However, special education appears to be failing more than 50% of all children and youth served. Based on our data, if you are a young man or woman with a disability you typically enter high school unprepared for the academic challenges that face you, which will likely lead to you (1) being less interested in attending high school, (2) likely dropping out, (3) being arrested, (4) not finding work, and (5) living in poverty.

4. NEW DIRECTIONS FOR POLICY AND PRACTICE

Our recommendations for policy and practice point to the need to move current special education practices to coincide with new goals for receiving special education services—goals that focus on elementary schools, middle schools, and high schools engaging in meeting higher academic standards, higher expectations related to empowering this population of youth, and better coordination of secondary and postsecondary services that support youth goals and desirable outcomes, respectively. There is a fundamental need for a policy of full inclusion in our schools and in our communities with the realization that an entire segment of our society is impoverished, segregated, and devalued, and that practices exist that continue the status quo at every level of service delivery. And schools, including high schools, are not being held accountable.

Our policy recommendations are not entirely new. In fact, they are similar to recommendations issued almost 35 years ago, and relate to recommendations made more recently by Rusch, Hughes, Martin, and Agran.[58] Briefly, "new bridges" need to be constructed between elementary schools and middle schools, between our middle schools and our high schools, and between high schools and agencies established to offset the disincentives that face youth in transition from school to community participation.

Our elementary schools must better prepare children to be competent learners before they enter middle school. Among students without a disability, for example, recent evidence suggests that early warning signs of dropping out of high school include chronic absences, poor behavior, and failing math or language classes. As presented above, these same warning signs exist among students with disabilities. Recent research by Hernandez indicated that third-grade reading ability appears to be linked to high school graduation. Specifically, Hernandez found that 88% of his sample of poor third-grade readers did not complete high school at age 19.[59] It makes sense to suggest that if a third grader with a disability is a poor reader, that student most likely will struggle with learning, which will result in finding education not to be useful in their daily lives. Our first policy recommendation, therefore, is focused on *ensuring that students with a disability meet grade-level expectations and equal the academic progress of children without a disability*.

Our second policy recommendation relates to *establishing the positive relationship between students with disabilities being meaningful participants in their transition planning and post-high school outcomes*.[60] These postschool outcomes include improved employment status[61] and increased levels of participating in postsecondary education.[62] Agran and Hughes presented evidence that middle school students can form strong opinions about their education and become active in planning their transition-related program of instruction.[63] Middle schools should provide instruction that helps students with disabilities direct their own programs of study, making school a more meaningful experience. Specifically, students must become competent in convening their own education meetings, identifying their career goals, and evaluating effects of these decisions to make meaningful adjustments during their high school education and planning.

Our third and final policy-related recommendation is *developing expectations within communities that include dropout prevention*. Preventing transition-age youth from dropping out has received much attention, especially following decreasing graduation rates throughout the 1990s and increasing demands for a highly skilled, highly trained workforce.[64] Whereas prevention efforts are growing and are based on a foundation of evidence-based practices, second-chance education and training programs have received limited attention, especially pertaining to students with disabilities. According to Anne Lewis of "Direct from Washington," in 2006 at the federal level, three times fewer dollars were spent on efforts to recover out-of-school youth with a disability than were spent in the 1970s. Furthermore, beyond a few studies, much of the information regarding reengagement in education is anecdotal. Evidence that is available about successful recovery programs consistently supports the combination of education and career training (i.e., Career and Technical Education). High schools must attempt to reengage youth who have dropped out through various methods supported by research and to develop innovative ways to reengage transition-age youth.

Importantly, high schools must become places where youth can expect and enjoy a meaningful education, which includes opportunities to better prepare them for postsecondary education as well as employment after graduation. Establishing the expectation among this population of learners that their education is designed to engage them in academic instruction at an early age that results in their being able to engage those around them in planning an education that results in their attaining their goals will provide new opportunities to rethink the importance of school engagement, reducing the chances of their dropping out. Employment and community participation are long-held goals of youth in transition, including youth with disabilities.

ACKNOWLEDGMENTS

1 This paper was funded in part by the National Institute for Disability Rehabilitation Research, U.S. Department of Education, Grant # H133F100005.

NOTES

1. United States Department of Education, Office of Special education and Rehabilitation Services (2010). *Thirty-five years of progress in educating children with disabilities through IDEA.* Washington, D.C.: U.S. Department of Education.
2. Lamb, P. (2007). Implications of the summary of performance for vocational rehabilitation counselors. *Career Development for Exceptional Individuals* *30*(1), 3–12.
3. Rusch, F. R. (Ed.). (2008). *Beyond high school: Preparing adolescents for tomorrow's challenges* (2nd ed.). Columbus, OH: Pearson Merrill Prentice Hall.
4. United States Department of Education (2010). *Thirty-five years of progress.*
5. Newman, L., Wagner, M., Cameto, R., Knokey, A. M., & Shaver, D. (2010). *Comparisons across time of the outcomes of youth with disabilities up to 4 years after high school. A report of findings from the National Longitudinal Transition Study (NLTS) and the National Longitudinal Transition Study-2 (NLTS-2).* Menlo Park, CA: SRI International.
6. Hayward, B. J., & Schmidt-Davis, H. (2000). Longitudinal study of the vocational rehabilitation service program. *Fourth Interim Report: Characteristics and Outcomes of Transitional Youth in VR.* Research Triangle Institute. Retrieved Feberuary 18, 2013, from http://www.ed.gov/policy/speced/leg/rehab/

eval-studies.html#vr; Plotner, A. J., Trach, J., & Strauser, D. (2012). Vocational rehabilitation counselors. *Rehabilitation Counseling Bulletin 55*(3), 135–143; Lamb (2007). Implications of the summary of performance.

7. Plotner, A. J., Shogren, K., & Strauser, D. (2011). Analyzing the emphasis on transition in rehabilitation counseling journals: A content analysis. *Journal of Applied Rehabilitation Counseling 42*(4), 27–32.

8. Sitlington, P. L., Clark, G. M., & Kolstoe, O. P. (2000). *Transition education and services for adolescents with disabilities* (3rd ed.). Boston, MA: Allyn & Bacon; Test, D., et al. (2009). Evidence-based practices in secondary transition. *Career Development for Exceptional Individuals 32*(3), 115–128.

9. Greenwood, C., & Abbott, M. (2001). The research to practice gap in special education. *Teacher Education and Special Education 24*(4), 276–289; Test, D. W., et al. (2009). Evidence-based secondary transition predictors for improving post-school outcomes for students with disabilities. *Career Development for Exceptional Individuals 32*(3), 160–181.

10. Boardman, A. G., Argüelles, M. E., Vaughn, S., Hughes, M. T., & Klingner, J. (2005). Special education teachers' views of research-based practices. *The Journal of Special Education 39*(3), 168–180; Burns, M. K., & Ysseldyke, J. E. (2009). Reported prevalence of evidence-based instructional practices in special education. *Journal of Special Education 43*(1), 3–11.

11. Bull, K. S., Montgomery, D., & Beard, J. (1994). Teacher competencies for transition programs as reported by state directors of special education. *Rural Special Education Quarterly 13* (4), 10–16.

12. Baker, B. C., & Geiger, W. L. (1988). *Preparing transition specialists: Competencies from thirteen programs.* Little Rock, AR, and Washington, D.C.: University of Arkansas and Office of Special Education and Rehabilitation Services, Division of Personnel Preparation.

13. Division on Career Development and Transition. (2000). *Transition specialist competencies: Fact sheet.* Retrieved February 18, 2013, from http://www.dcdt. org/wp-content/uploads/2011/09/DCDT_Fact_Sheet_Compentencies_3.pdf

14. Kohler, P. D. (1993). Best practices in transition: Substantiated or implied? *Career Development for Exceptional Individuals 16*(2), 107–121.

15. Kohler, P. D. (1996). Preparing youths with disabilities for future challenges: A taxonomy for transition planning. In P. D. Kohler (Ed.), *Taxonomy for transition planning: Linking research and practice.* Champaign, IL: University of Illinois at Urbana-Champaign, 1–62.

16. Landmark, L. J., Ju, S., & Zhang, D. (2010). Substantiated best practices in transition: Fifteen plus years later. *Career Development for Exceptional Individuals 33*(3), 163–177.

17. Ibid.

18. Mazzotti, V. L., Test, D. W., & Mustian, A. L. (2012). Evidence-based practices and predictors: Implications for policy makers. *Journal of Disability Policy Studies* published online before print, doi 10.1177/1044207312460888.

19. Stodden, R. A., & Roberts, K. (2008). Transition legislation and policy: Past and present. In F. R. Rusch (Ed.), *Beyond high school: Preparing youth for adult roles* (2nd Ed.). Columbus, OH: Pearson Merrill Prentice Hall Publishers, 24–54.

20. Rusch (Ed.). (2008). *Beyond high school.*

21. Wagner, M., et al. (2003). *The achievements of youth with disabilities during secondary school: A report from the National Longitudinal Transition Study-2.* Menlo Park: CA: SRI International; Wagner, M., Blackorby, J., Cameto, R., & Newman,

L. (1993). *What makes a difference? Influence on post-school outcomes of youth with disabilities: The third comprehensive report from the National Longitudinal Transition Study of Special Education Students.* Menlo Park, CA: SRI International.

22. United States Department of Education (2010). *Thirty-five years of progress.*

23. Rusch (Ed.). (2008). *Beyond high school.*

24. Will, M. (1983). *OSERS programming for adults with disabilities: Bridges from school to working life.* Washington, D.C.: Office of Special Education and Rehabilitative Services.

25. See for example Mithaug, D. E., Horiuchi, C. N., & Fanning, P. N. (1985). A report on the Colorado statewide follow-up survey of special education students. *Exceptional Children 51*(5), 397–404.

26. Grayson, T.E. (1997). Dropout prevention and special services. In F. R. Rusch and J. G. Chadsey (Eds.), *Beyond high school: Transition from school to work.* New York: Wadsworth Publishing, 77–98; Lamb (2007). Implications of the summary of performance.

27. Rusch (Ed.). (2008). *Beyond high school.*

28. Ibid.

29. Ibid.

30. Ibid.

31. Ianni, F. (1989). *A search for structure: A report on American youth today.* New York, NY: Free Press; Steinberg, L., & Dornbush, S. M. (1991). Negative correlates of part-time employment during adolescence: Replication and elaboration. *Developmental Psychology 27*(2), 304–313.

32. Gwynne, J., Lesnick, J., Hart, H.M., E.M. Allensworth (2009*). What Matters for Staying On-Track and Graduating in Chicago Public Schools. A Focus on Students with Disabilities.* Chicago, IL: Consortium on Chicago School Research.

33. Will, M. (1983). *OSERS programming for adults with disabilities.*

34. Rusch, F. R., & Phelps, L. A. (1987). Secondary special education and transition from school to work: A national priority. *Exceptional Children 53*(6), 487–492.

35. Wagner, M. (1991). *The benefit of secondary vocational education for young people with disabilities: Findings from the national longitudinal transition study of special education students.* Menlo Park, CA: SRI International.

36. National Organization on Disability (1998). *1998 N.O.D. Annual Report.* New York: National Organization on Disability.

37. See for example Mithaug, Horiuchi, & Fanning (1985). A report on the Colorado statewide follow-up survey.

38. See for example, Heal, L., & Rusch, F. R. (1995). Predicting employment for students who leave special education high school programs. *Exceptional Children 61*(5), 472–487.

39. Kaye, H. S. (2010). The impact of the 2007–09 recession on workers with disabilities. *Monthly Labor Review Online,* 133. Retrieved February 16, 2013, from http://www.bls.gov/opub/mlr/2010/10/art2exc,htm

40. Blanchett, W. J. (2008). We've come a long way but we're not there yet: The impact of research and policy on racially/ethnically and culturally diverse individuals with disabilities and/or those affected by poverty. *TASH Connections 34,* 11–13, 20; Fremstad, S. (2009). *Half in ten: Why taking disability into account is essential to reducing poverty and expanding economic inclusion.* Washington, D.C.: Center on Economic and Policy Research.

41. Hughes, C., & Avoke, S. K. (2010). The elephant in the room: Poverty, disability and employment. *Research and Practice for Persons with Severe Disabilities 35,* 3.

42. Benz, M. R., Lindstrom, L., & Yovanoff, P. (2000). Improving graduation and employment outcomes of students with disabilities: Predictive factors and student perspectives. *Exceptional Children 66*(4), 509–529.
43. Newman, Wagner, Cameto, Knokey, & Shaver (2010). *Comparisons across time.*
44. National Disability Rights Network. (2011). *Segregated and exploited: The failure of the disability service system to provide quality work.* Washington, D.C.: National Disability Rights Network.
45. Newman, Wagner, Cameto, Knokey, & Shaver (2010). *Comparisons across time.*
46. Astin, A. W. (1997). How "good" is your institution's retention rate? *Research in Higher Education 38*(6), 647–658.
47. Ewell, P., & Wellman, J. (2007). *Enhancing student success in education: Summary report of the NPEC Initiative and National Symposium on Postsecondary Student Success.* Washington, D.C.: National Postsecondary Education Cooperative.
48. Newman, Wagner, Cameto, Knokey, & Shaver (2010). *Comparisons across time.*
49. Ibid.
50. Rutherford, R. B., Bullis, M., Anderson, C. W., & Griller-Clark, H. M. (2002). *Youth with disabilities in the correctional system: Prevalence rates and identification issues.* Washington, D.C.: American Institutes for Research.
51. Doren, B., Bullis, M., & Benz, M. M. (1996). Predicting the arrest status of adolescents with disabilities in transition. *The Journal of Special Education 29*(4), 363–380.
52. Rutherford, Bullis, Anderson, & Griller-Clark (2002). *Youth with disabilities in the correctional system.*
53. Nelson, C. M., Rutherford, R. B., & Wolford, B. I. (1985). Special education for handicapped offenders. In J. E. Gilliam & B. K. Scott (Eds.), *Topics in emotional disturbance.* Austin, TX: Behavior Learning Center, 311–315.
54. Wagner, M., et al. (1992). *What Happens Next? Trends in Post-school Outcomes of Youth with Disabilities. The Second Comprehensive Report from the National Longitudinal Transition Study of Special Education Students.* Menlo Park, CA: SRI International.
55. National Disability Rights Network. (2011). *Segregated and exploited*, 10.
56. Ibid.
57. Fuchs, D., & Fuchs, L. S. (1994). Inclusive schools movement and the radicalization of special education reform. *Exceptional Education 60*, 294–309.
58. Rusch, F. R., Hughes, C., Agran, M., Martin, J. E., & Johnson, J. R. (2009). Toward self-directed learning, post-high school placement, and coordinated support: Constructing new transition bridges to adult life. *Career Development for Exceptional Individuals 32*(1), 1–7.
59. Hernandez, D.J. (2011). Double Jeopardy. *How Third-Grade Reading Skills and Poverty Influence High School Graduation.* Baltimore, MD: Annie E. Casey Foundation.
60. Wehmeyer, M., et al. (2007). *Promoting self-determination for students with developmental disabilities.* New York, NY: Guilford.
61. Wehmeyer, M. L., & Schwartz, M. (1998). The self-determination focus of transition goals for students with mental retardation. *Career Development for Exceptional Individuals 21*(1), 75–86.
62. Field, S., Sarver, M. D., & Shaw, S. F. (2003). Self-determination: A key to success in postsecondary education for students with learning disabilities. *Remedial and Special Education 24*(6), 339–349.

63. Agran, M., & Hughes, C. (2008). Asking student input: Students' opinions regarding their individualized education program involvement. *Career Development for Exceptional Individuals 31*(2), 69–76.
64. Association for Career and Technical Education. (2007). *Career and Technical Education's Role in Dropout Prevention and Recovery*. Alexandria, VA: Association for Career and Technical Education.

CHAPTER 9

Career Advancement for Young Adults with Disabilities

LAUREN LINDSTROM AND LAURIE GUTMANN KAHN

1. INTRODUCTION

Career development is the process of defining and refining occupational choices. Although career development is sometimes conceptualized as a one-time decision that is systematic, logical, and linear, for many individuals with disabilities the process is more likely to be multifaceted, discontinuous, and unpredictable.[1] Career decisions often unfold over time and are influenced by a multitude of factors including individual abilities and disabilities, career attitudes and behaviors, social supports, developmental opportunities such as higher education and training, and barriers and supports in the workplace.[2] For individuals with disabilities worldwide, career development is frequently constrained by misperceptions about disability, discrimination and prejudice in the labor market, and disincentives created by disability benefits systems.[3]

This chapter focuses on career advancement for young adults with disabilities, a component of career development that has been overlooked and understudied.[4] Career development for young adults with disabilities is especially critical due to a variety of vocational disparities that exist between individuals with disabilities and their nondisabled peers worldwide.[5] A study by Benshoff, Kroeger, and Scalia found that young adults with disabilities often take more time to enter the workforce, thus impacting their early career trajectories.[6] In addition, low expectations, low self-concept, and negative stereotyping can have significant implications for the career development of young adults with disabilities.[7] These barriers may limit career options, leading to underachievement and job dissatisfaction.[8]

Unemployment, underemployment, and poverty are significant indicators as well as contributors to the vocational inequalities that exist for young adults with disabilities in the early career years. The US Census Bureau found that for individuals with disabilities between the ages of 18 and 34, 31.3% were earning wages that placed them below the federal poverty line, as compared with only 18% of their nondisabled peers.[9] The World Health Survey, which includes results from 51 countries, confirms these disparities, reporting an overall employment rate of 52.8% for men with a disability, and 19.6% for women with a disability compared with 64.9% for nondisabled men and 29.9% for nondisabled women.[10] Much of this inequity is due to limited access to living wage jobs, lack of individuals with disabilities in higher-level (and higher paid) managerial positions, and inadequate opportunities for career advancement.[11]

This chapter summarizes and synthesizes information from the fields of career development, counseling psychology, disability policy, human resources, special education, and vocational rehabilitation to illuminate the multifaceted process of career advancement for young adults with disabilities worldwide. By examining the inequalities and barriers that exist for young adults with disabilities in the career advancement process, we can further develop and implement policies, interventions, and supports that will provide the structures needed for all individuals, regardless of disability status, to develop meaningful careers and earn living wages.[12]

2. EXAMINING THE ISSUES

Ultimately the judgment of successful outcomes must be looked at further down the vocational path in job maintenance, employment stability, career advancement and attainment of leadership roles.[13]

This section of the chapter is focused on exploring the complex issues that influence career advancement for young adults with disabilities entering the workforce. We know that it is not enough to simply get a job. Instead, young adults with disabilities need opportunities to grow on the job and advance into higher-wage, higher-skill employment opportunities. Below we describe early employment outcomes and career development for young adults with disabilities, beginning with an examination of the factors that influence patterns of initial employment. In addition, we present some of the major barriers to career advancement, including lack of career information and opportunities as well as the prevalence of disability discrimination in the workforce.

2.1 Early Career Outcomes: Entering the Workforce

Initial career development typically begins in late adolescence and extends through early adulthood. Developmental psychologists and career researchers often characterize this period as the "early career years."[14] These early years of career development are especially important in setting an overall trajectory for advancement because the biggest gains in salary and the largest advancement opportunities typically occur during the first 10 years of a career.[15]

There are a number of programs and supports that can be put in place to influence these early career trajectories. First, participation in high school transition programs can contribute to the early career development process. A study that examined the outcomes of students with disabilities in the twin-island Republic of Trinidad and Tobago found that young adults (ages 17–34) who participated in a combined program of academic and vocational education reported higher wages, more work hours, and more positive job characteristics than those who participated in solely academic or vocational education programs.[16] In the United States, data from the National Longitudinal Survey of Youth showed that involvement in specific elements of school-to-work programs was associated with more positive employment outcomes, including higher annual income, stable employment, and full-time work for a representative sample of 2,254 young adults with disabilities ages 20 to 24.[17] More specifically, young adults who enrolled in cooperative education, school-sponsored enterprises, career majors, or technical preparation programs were more likely to be employed in the early years after high school.[18] In addition, other researchers have documented that participation in work experience, community internships, and vocational training in high school leads to a greater likelihood of post school employment.[19] From these studies, it seems clear that future employment is highly dependent on previous employment—the number of work experience hours and the number of paid jobs in high school has consistently been associated with later employment success.[20]

Career researchers have also demonstrated the important role of the first job in supporting later career development opportunities for young adults with disabilities. In a study of 1,393 former special education students from 37 school districts in Alabama, Rabren, Dunn, and Chambers found that 87% of former students who were employed when they exited high school were also working one year later. In fact, the odds of having a job one year later were *3.8 times* greater for those who had a paying job at exit from high school.[21] Other longitudinal studies of young adults with disabilities have found that engagement in either employment or postsecondary training at high school exit is related to stability of employment as well as the ability to advance.[22] A World Bank global study found that although many programs have been developed to provide "second chances" in education and vocational training for those who were not employed at high school exit, or did not have adequate schooling, these programs often leave out young adults with disabilities, many of whom are not even given a first chance because of stigma and lack of educational and vocational opportunities.[23]

2.2 Career Trajectories: Barriers to Advancement

Individual and systemic barriers limit career advancement for individuals with disabilities worldwide.[24] After entering the labor market, early career employees with disabilities face numerous barriers that constrain their opportunities for advancement, promotion, and long-term satisfaction. Primary barriers to advancement include: (1) lack of access to career information, (2) restricted opportunities for training and development, (3) financial disincentives, and (4) discrimination and prejudice in the workplace.[25]

2.2.1 Limited Access to Career Information

For youth with disabilities, lack of exposure to early experiences in the workplace serves as a critical barrier to the process of career development and advancement.[26] These limited experiences in community-work settings limit the natural process of career exploration and self-discovery.[27] Without the opportunity to experience or observe a variety of jobs first-hand, many young adults with disabilities inadvertently foreclose a number of potentially meaningful career options. Constrained career and transition planning opportunities are especially salient for young women with disabilities, who have limited exposure to a range of employment opportunities and often work in low wage/low skill jobs with no benefits and very few opportunities for advancement.[28] Guided career exploration experiences such as job shadowing, employment site visits, and community based work experiences can help to expand options and shape career aspirations.[29]

2.2.2 Lack of Opportunities for Training and Development

Young adults with disabilities also may not have access to the specific skill training or postsecondary education needed to enter high wage jobs or advance in their careers.[30] For example, in Argentina, about 33% of individuals with disabilities have not completed elementary school, compared with only about 10% of the total population,[31] thus limiting their access to higher education and training options. In the United States, young people with disabilities are about half as likely as their peers without disabilities to attend college.[32] Approximately 30% of youth with disabilities engage in postsecondary education during the first two years after leaving high school, compared with nearly 70% of high school graduates in the general population.[33] In addition to these lower enrollment rates, students with disabilities are also less likely to complete a program of study than their peers without disabilities.[34] Without further training or postsecondary education, young people with disabilities may find their career options limited to entry level low-paying service industry jobs such as janitorial, housekeeping, and fast food work.[35]

Another important component that influences career development for all individuals is the opportunity to obtain on-the-job training and/or mentoring in order to advance into more challenging or higher paying career options.[36] On-the-job supervisors and experienced mentors can offer an entrée to key skills needed for advancement and continued growth. Yet, individuals with disabilities may not have access to the organizational or peer supports needed in the workplace. In a Canadian study of 76 young adults ages 20 to 30 with motor disabilities, Magill-Evans and colleagues found extensive evidence of the phenomenon of being "stuck" in an unsatisfying career without support to advance. Illustrating that point, young adults with motor disabilities who participated in the program expressed thoughts such as having "become 'stuck at the job I'm at' and being unable to 'increase my skill set to do more types of jobs than I can currently do.'"[37] Other studies have described the lack of mentors and role models in the workplace even for well-established and highly successful adults with disabilities.[38]

2.2.3 Financial Disincentives

Some government-sponsored programs designed to alleviate financial burdens for individuals with disabilities may inadvertently serve as a disincentive to career advancement.[39] Many government public assistance programs have explicit policies that once an individual's earnings exceed a certain threshold, they will no longer receive cash assistance. This predicament is often referred to as the "cash cliff" and can act as a significant barrier to meaningful long-term employment.[40]

In addition to financial assistance, eligible individuals with disabilities in some countries also receive health insurance as long as their earnings are below a certain limit. Many workers with disabilities fear that if their earnings reach the upper threshold, they will lose much-needed health coverage. Often, individuals with disabilities are not able to obtain private health insurance to reimburse services they may need to live independently such as prescriptions, personal assistance services, or equipment. In addition, some individuals with disabilities may be self-employed or work for small companies that may not provide health insurance. For example, in the United States 10.7% of people with disabilities are self-employed compared with 6.8% of people without disabilities.[41] With rising health care costs, many workers with disabilities may choose to drastically reduce their work hours or terminate their employment in order to maintain stable, high-quality medical benefits.[42]

Programs to reduce disincentives and replace government social insurance benefits with labor market participation have been successful in a number of countries. Hungary, Italy, the Netherlands, and Poland have instituted tighter requirements for employers to provide health services. Along with employer supports, these policies have helped transition many disability beneficiaries into the workforce.[43]

2.2.4 Discrimination in the Workforce

Finally, patterns of discrimination against people with disabilities in the labor market create additional, sometimes insurmountable barriers to career advancement.[44] For example, in Cambodia, the types of jobs available are divided into two categories. "Big jobs" are reserved for people with social and economic capital and "small jobs" are those that are not valued and tend to be in the informal sector. People with disabilities in Cambodia are typically considered only suitable for "small jobs."[45] Employers may discriminate because of misconceptions, lack of information, or stereotyped assumptions about people with disabilities.[46] One analysis of the major barriers to career development for individuals with disabilities noted evidence of employer bias and discrimination across all aspects of employment including selection, staffing, advancement, and promotion.[47] Jones documented two main types of discrimination that may impact individuals with disabilities: (1) *access discrimination*, which refers to barriers to gaining employment, and (2) *treatment discrimination* referring to unfair treatment on the job. Treatment discrimination can result in significant negative consequences including fewer opportunities for training, slower rates of promotion, unchallenging project assignments, and dead-end position assignments.[48]

Employer discrimination in the United States has also been documented through a review of complaints filed by individuals with disabilities under the Americans with Disabilities Act. Chan and colleagues examined 35,763 allegations of workplace discrimination filed by people with disabilities between July 1992 and September 2003.[49] This research team documented eight broad areas of on-the-job discrimination including: (1) discharge, (2) intimidation, (3) harassment, (4) failure to provide reasonable accommodations, (5) issues around terms and conditions of employment, (6) hiring practices, (7) promotion, and (8) wages. This study also found that overall negative attitudes from employers created invisible barriers to advancement and that "workplace prejudice and discrimination have a constricting effect on opportunities of people with disabilities to achieve important life goals."[50]

It is important to note that even highly successful professionals with disabilities who have advanced in their careers routinely encounter this sort of discrimination and stereotyping based on disability.[51] In a qualitative study of prominent, high-achieving women with physical and sensory disabilities, Noonan confirmed that all of the participants had experienced disability discrimination at one or more stages:

> These experiences of prejudice comprised some of the most influential events on the career development of the women in this sample and included restricted educational opportunities, discrimination in hiring, biased performance evaluations, job tracking, pay inequities, lack of support and mentoring, negative attitudes and chilly workplace climates, lack of accommodations, and general discouragement.[52]

3. STRATEGIES TO SUPPORT CAREER ADVANCEMENT

The majority of barriers are permeable (or semi-permeable) and many individual, structural and organizational impediments can be removed through education, technology and increased awareness about the varied experiences of individuals with disabilities.[53]

This section of the chapter provides specific information and concrete strategies to address many of the previously described barriers to career advancement. Utilizing a career development framework,[54] we consider career advancement to be a multifaceted process that is dependent on both individual characteristics and external supports.[55] Although it is clear that external barriers can constrain career options and opportunities for individuals with disabilities, environments are not immutable. Individual qualities and skills as well as systemic services and supports can and do have a part in influencing employment opportunities and career development for young adults with disabilities in high-, middle- and low-income countries.[56] We begin by describing individual attributes that lead to career advancement, incorporating lessons from highly successful individuals with disabilities. In addition, we provide a number of recommended services, supports, and policies for advancing career outcomes and promoting equity in the labor market.

3.1 Individual Strategies for Career Advancement

Advancing in employment settings requires a combination of individual skills and persistence as well as targeted access to supports. Drawing from research findings describing highly successful individuals with disabilities[57] we summarize key attributes and skills related to obtaining and maintaining positive employment outcomes over time. In addition, we describe specific supports that individuals with disabilities have accessed to bolster job retention and increase opportunities for advancement.

3.1.1 Personal Attributes and Skills

Previous studies have documented a number of individual characteristics and skills that play a role in supporting positive career trajectories over time. First, personal agency and a sense of control are key facets.[58] The International Study on Income Generation, which analyzed 81 self-employment projects worldwide, found that most successful self-employed individuals with disabilities were self-directed and independent. An American study of young adults with disabilities ages 21 to 25 found that those who were proactive and goal-oriented were more likely to earn higher weekly wages, express satisfaction with current employment, and have opportunities for ongoing training and advancement over time.[59] Gerber's study of adults with learning disabilities who were highly successful in the workforce also confirms the interconnection of personal agency and vocational achievement.[60] More than half of the sample in this ethnographic study completed either a Ph.D. or M.D., and 50% reported yearly incomes of over $100,000. For these high-achieving individuals with disabilities, the ability to take charge of both internal decisions and external environments was crucial. Gerber noted,

> Control was the key to success for adults with learning disabilities. This was obvious across the entire sample. Control meant making conscious decisions to take charge of one's life (internal decisions) and adapting and shaping oneself to move ahead (external manifestations). Control was the fuel that fired their success.[61]

Motivation and persistence in the face of adversity are other traits commonly displayed by highly achieving individuals with disabilities in the workforce.[62] In a study of young adults with disabilities ages 25 to 29 who were employed in living wage occupations seven to ten years after high school, Lindstrom and colleagues found that ongoing career advancement was influenced by a set of personal attributes, including persistence and coping skills.[63] Noonan's study of highly achieving women with physical and sensory disabilities provides additional evidence of the critical role of perseverance. The women with disabilities in this study worked in a variety of prominent occupations in education, law, science, politics, and business. In order to advance in their fields, participants displayed high levels of motivation and utilized a variety of coping skills to address and overcome barriers on the job.[64] For example, many participants utilized stress management and self-care strategies to cope with difficult situations including: exercising and eating well, accessing support from others, and maintaining humor and optimism.

In addition to self-agency and persistence, individuals with disabilities who have successfully advanced in their careers also display a set of concrete skills that assist in meeting the challenges inherent in achieving job stability and retention. These skills include: problem-solving, goal-setting, time management, prioritization, effective relationships with peers and supervisors, and the ability to adapt to new and/or changing work environments.[65] Mastery of required occupational skills and the ability to adapt by reframing negative experiences as challenges are other abilities that have been linked to long-term vocational success.[66]

Finally, disability knowledge and awareness are significant attributes that influence career development and employment outcomes over time.[67] One study that examined career development for high school and college women with disabilities, found that many participants lacked knowledge of their disabilities and were unaware of the accommodations and supports needed to succeed in higher education or the workforce.[68] Researchers in the United States and Canada have documented the need for individuals with disabilities to be able to clearly describe their specific disability, know the associated functional limitations, and advocate for the accommodations they need to perform on the job.[69] In a survey of 156 workers with disabilities from England, Scotland, and Wales, Roulstone and colleagues found that one of the most commonly used strategies to promote job retention and career advancement was being assertive and direct with coworkers and supervisors about the nature of the disability and associated accommodations needed to perform successfully. "Being direct, confident and assertive early on was seen as important by many disabled workers in getting changes at work, resolving access issues, and being accepted as a colleague."[70]

Post School Achievement Through Higher Skills (PATHS) is a career development curriculum that addresses many of the individual skills and attributes that have been linked to career advancement and success, including self-advocacy, problem-solving, goal-setting, disability knowledge, and awareness. Post School Achievement Through Higher Skills was designed specifically to improve educational and career outcomes for high school girls with disabilities.[71] Initial findings from a pilot test showed that girls who participated in the PATHS class made gains in the areas of vocational self-efficacy, career outcome expectancy, autonomy, and self-advocacy, as well as gender and disability knowledge. Girls in the comparison group did not make similar gains and their skills actually decreased over time in many of these areas.[72]

3.1.2 Individual Supports

Individuals with disabilities who have advanced in the workforce are able to access a variety of social, emotional, and tangible supports.[73] Support networks can increase the likelihood of job retention while facilitating opportunities for advancement in the workplace. One longitudinal study of working adults with learning disabilities demonstrated that a key distinction between "highly successful" versus "moderately successful" individuals was the willingness to seek out and accept support throughout all stages of their careers.[74]

Individual support for career advancement can be provided through a number of different sources depending on the unique needs and social ecology of the individual with a disability.[75] For some, family, friends, and significant others may offer crucial advocacy and guidance.[76] Other successfully employed adults with disabilities have been able to build peer and coworker networks, enabling them to access career knowledge and skills as well as understand the paths to promotion within an organization.[77] Another effective strategy has been to utilize support staff or other outside experts to help with organization and management of specific tasks that may be challenging.[78]

Last, the ability to access mentorship from either disabled or nondisabled colleagues promotes opportunities for career advancement. Positive individual relationships with stable, successful mentors can help build self confidence, provide career direction and guidance, and offer specific feedback to enhance employee's effectiveness and development.[79] Dix and Savickas created a career coaching/mentoring model to enhance career adaptability for individuals with disabilities. This model includes 31 classes focused on coping responses, which are operationalized into concrete behaviors. For example, one of the topics discussed in the class about organizational adaptability is the coping skill of "learning from experts" which includes "listening to advice" and "querying experts."[80] The Pathways to Work Program is another employment skills building model. Developed in the United Kingdom, Pathways to Work provides a number of services including personal advisors who are assigned to individuals with disabilities. These personal advisers assist individuals with accessing employment or career-related training, and also provide support for managing disabilities or other health conditions on the job. Initial findings from the Pathways to Work Program demonstrated a 7.4% increase in employment rates for individuals with disabilities.[81]

3.2 System Approaches and Interventions

Although individual skills and supports may be somewhat effective in enhancing career opportunities, it is vital to address system-level issues in order to truly ensure equal opportunities in the workforce for young adults with disabilities. This section offers a number of concrete recommendations for strategies, supports, programs, and policies designed to alleviate existing barriers while enhancing opportunities for job retention, promotion, and advancement. These system approaches and interventions are organized into four key areas: (1) entering the labor market, (2) growing on the job, (3) building skills, and (4) changing the workplace.

3.2.1 *Entering the Labor Market: Finding the First Job*

As noted earlier in this chapter, the type of initial employment obtained is a crucial element in predicting future employment stability and enhancing opportunities for later career advancement.[82] In a critical review of issues affecting advancement opportunities for individuals with disabilities, Jones noted that this initial foray into the workforce often "sets the stage for a career of lifelong earning capabilities."[83] Unfortunately, many young adults with disabilities are either not competitively employed after leaving school or transition from school into entry-level, unskilled, low wage positions without benefits.[84] In the United States, having a job with benefits typically implies that, in addition to a salary, an employer will provide some combination of paid sick leave, vacation pay, health insurance, and retirement benefits. These benefits can be especially critical for individuals with disabilities who often experience higher costs of living related to their disability. Employer benefits can offer critical resources to pay for medication, personal assistance services, or other costs associated with disability management.[85]

Career exploration and planning services can help increase occupational aspirations and potentially expand the variety and quality of initial job placements.[86] Online vocational exploration, career assessments, job shadowing, and job site visits are concrete strategies that help provide early exposure to a range of potential occupations. Vocational exploration tools and career assessments can provide initial information about possible career options, as well as detailed reports documenting individual strengths, interests and preferences that are useful for initial career planning and job matching.[87] Some computer-based career exploration and assessment programs also include resource information about education requirements and other training needed to prepare for specific careers.[88]

Job shadowing is a commonly used introductory work-based learning activity. A job shadow provides an opportunity for a young adult who is exploring careers to spend an extended period of time, such as a full work day, with someone who is actually performing that job.[89] For example, an individual with a disability who is interested in a medical career may spend a day at a hospital shadowing a physician, nurse, or medical technician, and observing the work performed in various departments.

Internships are another strategy for increasing access to higher-wage career options.[90] Sometimes referred to as "cooperative work experiences" or simply "work experiences," internships are paid or unpaid placements in community employment settings that can provide longer-term, structured job experiences in an established business setting.[91] Internships are dependent on successful partnerships with community employers and can also be enhanced by collaboration with local agencies such as vocational rehabilitation or other government-sponsored job training programs. Structured internships also offer a mechanism for placing women and individuals from diverse groups into on-the-job experiences that may lead to higher wage employment over time.[92]

There are a number of successful programs that have expanded vocational options by offering career exploration and community work experience as a bridge to initial job placement. The Marriot Foundation's Bridges From School to Work Program, which has served over 10,000 youth in six major urban locations across the United States, includes career counseling, paid community work experience, and follow-along support to assist in navigating the complexities of the workplace.[93] The Bridges program has documented positive employment outcomes for young adults with disabilities including youth of color and those with learning disabilities and emotional/behavior disabilities.[94] Using a logistic regression analysis, Fabian analyzed employment outcome data for 4,751 students who participated in the Bridges program between 2000 and 2005. Results from this study documented a 68% employment rate. Those youth who had some type of previous work experience were significantly more likely to get a job than those who did not.[95]

The Youth Transition Program (YTP) is another model program that teaches career development skills to young adults with disabilities. Students participating in the YTP receive (1) individualized planning, focused on post-school goals and self-determination, and help to coordinate school plans with relevant community agencies; (2) instruction in academic, vocational, independent living, and personal social skills and help to stay in and complete high school; (3) career development services including goal-setting, career exploration, job search skills, and self-advocacy; (4) paid employment including connections with local employers, on-the-job assessments, placement and training; (5) support services such as individualized mentoring and support or referrals for additional specific interventions; and (6) follow-up support for one year after leaving the program to assist in maintaining positive outcomes in employment or postsecondary settings.[96]

Outcomes for over 20,000 youth who have participated in the YTP have been consistently positive over time.[97] Several studies have documented increased collaboration and referrals to vocational rehabilitation, improvements in high school graduation rates, positive employment outcomes (e.g., wages, hours worked per week) and 75% to 80% rates of engagement in either competitive employment or career-related post-school training at exit, 6 months, and 12 months after completing the program. When compared with students with disabilities who did not participate in the YTP, these studies also found that YTP students were more likely to earn higher average hourly and weekly wages, and still be in their highest-paying job one year after leaving high school.[98]

Vocational Rehabilitation (VR) is another service delivery model that focuses on reducing barriers and increasing initial access to employment for individuals with disabilities.[99] It is a cooperative federal state program that operates in all 50 states of the United States, the District of Columbia, and US territories. Vocational Rehabilitation agencies can provide a number of services including: (1) assessment to determine eligibility for services, (2) vocational counseling and guidance, (3) vocational and on the job training, (4) personal assistant services, (5) rehabilitation technology to assist with on the job accommodations, and (6) job placement services.[100] Through the development of an individualized plan for employment, VR counselors can assist in the process of matching individuals to productive and satisfying careers. This congruence or "person-environment fit" results in greater personal satisfaction and the ability to succeed on the job long term.[101] In some countries, private nonprofit community rehabilitation agencies may also provide similar services to increase employment access and support career advancement over time.[102] For example, Perspektiva, a Russian NGO, encourages young people with disabilities to become career-ready through organizing job fairs and trainings on vocational skills as well as educating the public about disability discrimination.[103]

3.2.2 Growing on the Job: Career Adaptability

Career adaptability is the process of adapting to, performing, and sustaining a career over time. Career adaptability is an essential skill for job retention and has been linked to career advancement.[104] In this phase of career development, young adults with disabilities must be able to adjust to work demands and at the same time work environments may need to be adjusted to better support the individual. Beveridge and colleagues note some of the challenges inherent in this process,

> Despite the enormous amount of time and energy spent imagining, gathering information, analyzing job tasks, and choosing and obtaining an occupation, the reality of the workplace may require *unforeseen adaptations*. The individual must have a carefully developed plan for disability management that takes into consideration such issues as transportation, time management, medication management, and physical, cognitive, and emotional endurance.[105]

There are a number of strategies to enhance career adaptability and help prepare early career workers to cope with these unforeseen circumstances on the
job. First, young adults with disabilities can receive instruction in specific skills
that enhance job retention and increase career maturity. Career development
researchers have identified a number of alterable skills that can be taught and
learned, including problem-solving, goal-setting, decision-making, self-advocacy, and pro-social coping skills.[106] Instruction in these career adaptability
skills could potentially be offered through vocational rehabilitation programs
or human resources departments within businesses.[107] American Job Service
Centers are another potential setting to offer instruction in skills for employability. These centers are federally funded programs in the United States
created by the Workforce Investment Act of 1998 that provide resources to
anyone who needs help locating employment in the community.[108]

The Work Advancement and Support Center (WASC) in Fort Worth, Texas
was part of a model demonstration program designed to help low-wage workers improve their employability skills and increase their potential for advancement.[109] Although this program was not designed specifically for individuals
with disabilities, it offers an innovative training strategy to address workforce
development issues for a number of disadvantaged groups that are often
employed in low-wage jobs. The services of WASC are provided on the job site.
They include customized group instruction in language and other technical
skills, and individual job coaching sessions with employees to provide support
and information about employer policies and potential paths to advancement.
Initial studies of this program are promising, with evidence that employers
increased their capacity to train and support entry-level workers after participating in WASC.[110]

Peer-support groups are another viable strategy to increase opportunities for career advancement. Often based in large corporate settings, women
and minority groups have successfully used such "affinity groups" to support
professional growth, gain leadership skills, and promote advancement. The
role of employee support groups is to offer an informal opportunity to discuss
problems and solutions at the workplace on a regular basis. Groups are often
facilitated by more experienced coworkers with disabilities and address gaps
in knowledge about accommodations, community supports, and disability
management.[111] These peer-support systems are also an ideal venue to address
discrimination issues or attitudinal barriers in the workplace.[112]

Finally, supportive relationships with a mentor have been shown to play
a vital role in career development for many individuals with disabilities who
have advanced in their careers.[113] Although mentorships are often informal
relationships established by individuals, more formal mentorship programs
can also be developed and implemented by organizations or government
agencies.[114] Effective mentors can be individuals with or without disabilities
who offer an ongoing source of support for their less experienced protégés.

More specifically, mentors can provide career-enhancing functions such as sponsorship, coaching, visibility, and access to challenging assignments, as well as psychosocial functions such as role modeling, informal counseling, and friendship.[115] Mentors are important for all career trajectories, but are often even more crucial for the advancement of historically marginalized groups such as women, people of color, and those with disabilities.[116]

3.2.3 Building Advanced Skills: Postsecondary Education/Vocational Training

For individuals with and without disabilities, access to higher education is necessary to prepare for the demands of an increasingly technological and global economy.[117] Completion of postsecondary education, including short-term occupational training, significantly improves the chances of securing employment and achieving greater levels of financial independence.[118] In an evaluation of a program in Northern Ireland, researchers found that young adults with disabilities who received continuous classroom and study support in higher education or employment skills training achieved higher qualifications for employment and acquired critical skills needed for the world of work.[119] In the United States, individuals with disabilities who enroll in some level of postsecondary education are employed at twice the rate of those with only a high school diploma.[120] However, postsecondary participation rates for individuals with disabilities are still quite low compared with their same-age peers.[121] And although increasing number of students with disabilities are enrolling in higher education, they have met with limited success due to a number of individual and systemic barriers.[122]

University and four-year college programs provide direct pathways to career advancement. Participation in higher education and completion of advanced degrees such as bachelors or masters degrees are associated with higher levels of employment. In a US survey of 500 college graduates with learning disabilities, Madeus reported that 75% were employed full-time, and that 85% of employed participants were receiving full job benefits. These employment rates as well as levels of income and benefits were comparable to nondisabled peers in the workforce.[123] Lindstrom and colleagues also found that participation in postsecondary education over time was linked to higher wages and improved self-confidence.[124]

Community colleges and vocational training programs offer a viable but often underutilized option for individuals with disabilities who are not enrolled in other postsecondary education and who are seeking to build employment skills and gain access to higher wage career options.[125] In addition to academic programs and transfer degree options, many community colleges offer occupationally-specific, short-term training programs.[126] These programs have different labels, but they share several core characteristics, including: (1) a focus on specific occupations, (2) a curriculum that can be completed within one year or less, and (3) hands-on instruction and/or worksite-based training. The employment focus of these community college programs can provide an ideal service delivery structure to meet the needs of young adults with disabilities who are not attending a university. One study of adults with disabilities entering the labor market found that completion of a community college skills-training program significantly improved employment outcomes in the areas of wages, hours worked, and quarters worked.[127]

In India, the Leprosy Mission coordinates vocational training centers for young adults with leprosy and other disabilities. In these centers, students can learn a variety of occupational skills including: car repair, welding, tailoring, radio and television repair, offset printing, and computing. Business management skills, and critical interpersonal skills such as goal-setting, problem-solving, decision-making, and time management are also part of the core curriculum. Participants also have access to bank loans to support their business and education. Upon completion, Leprosy Mission students have a 95% job placement rate.[128]

4. CHANGING THE WORKPLACE: INCREASING EQUAL ACCESS

Increasing meaningful participation in the labor market and ensuring equal access for individuals with disabilities requires fundamental changes to workplace environments. Changes need to be made at the individual, organizational, and policy levels to influence recruitment, hiring, retention, and advancement opportunities.[129] Successful workplace reform is also dependent on multiple strategies to address environmental, logistical, and attitudinal barriers.[130]

4.1 Access and Accommodations

At the individual level, workers with disabilities in the United States, Canada, and many countries in the European Union are entitled to have their on the job needs accommodated as long as this does not create an undue hardship for the employer.[131] A workplace accommodation in the United States is typically defined as "any reasonable adjustment to the workplace that allows the person to perform at full capacity."[132] The EU does not have an operational definition of accommodation because they allow each country to define "reasonable" as they see fit. Examples of reasonable accommodations include: making facilities accessible, purchasing or adapting equipment or devices, transportation, modifying jobs or work schedules, adapting training materials or policies, and providing readers or interpreters. Employees must disclose their disabilities in order to receive reasonable accommodations.[133]

Given that reasonable accommodations can allow access to jobs that may have previously been unattainable for early career workers with disabilities, negotiating needed accommodations is a critical aspect of career advancement. Although employers may be wary of the financial drain associated with hiring and retaining an individual with a disability, the majority of individual accommodations are inexpensive and sometimes free.[134] The Job Accommodation Network interviewed more than 1,600 employers in the United States and found that 56% of employers had no associated costs for hiring someone with a disability, whereas the rest of the accommodations typically cost $500 (as compared with a hiring investment of approximately $343 for an employee without a disability). Of the accommodations with associated expenses, 38% of employers experienced a one-time cost and only 4% reported that the cost was annual.[135] Similarly, one large American retail chain reported that over a fifteen-year period 69% of accommodations provided for workers with disabilities involved no costs and only 3% cost more than $1,000.[136]

4.2 Resources for Employers

Currently, there are insufficient support services available in many countries to provide information and training to employers about relevant career development topics such as vocational assessments, job matching, reasonable work accommodations, and training opportunities.[137] In addition, a lack of individuals with disabilities at the managerial level in the public and private sectors may lead to workplace policies that do not take into consideration the unique needs of employees with disabilities, thus perpetuating the stigmatization, stereotyping, and other psychological barriers that can hinder career advancement.[138]

Despite these barriers, some employers have developed programs and procedures designed to increase access and advancement opportunities for individuals with disabilities. In their review of strategies for including people with disabilities in the workforce, Green and Brook offer several recommendations for human resources personnel and managers. First, recruiters and human resources personnel need to demonstrate to organizational leaders the economic case for hiring people with disabilities who are an "untapped talent pool" that can contribute to overall workplace functioning. In addition, corporate supports such as a centralized budget for workplace accommodations, funding for recruitment efforts, and employee mentoring programs can help to attract and retain highly-qualified workers with disabilities.[139] Employer training is another strategy to increase knowledge and skills in working with employees with disabilities as well as directly addressing issues of disability discrimination. Training should include a number of key topics including: (1) common misperceptions about individuals with disabilities; (2) laws and policies impacting hiring, retention, and promotion; (3) examples of assistive technology and workplace accommodations; and (4) information about on the job support strategies.[140]

Workplace access has also been addressed by the Business Disability Forum (BDF). Established in the United Kingdom, the BDF provides employers with resources to support the human rights of people with disabilities.[141] The BDF promotes antidiscrimination laws, helps companies assess their performance standards in regards to disability, and has also designed a systematic method to support recruitment, accommodation, and retention of employees with disabilities. The BDF includes over 100 global companies and works with employer networks all over the world to create a more equal and accessible workforce for people with disabilities.[142]

4.3 Policies and Legislation

Government-funded incentive programs can also help to increase employment options for workers with disabilities. In the United States, the Ticket to Work and Work Incentives Improvement Act created a variety of programs that expanded vocational rehabilitation services and offered financial incentives to employers. This act also reduces economic disincentives to work for individuals with disabilities by providing continuing health care and income subsidy during the initial period of employment. Other governments have developed specific measures, such as quotas, in order to improve access to the formal economy for people with disabilities.[143] Germany has a quota stipulating that all companies employing more than 20 workers must meet a 5% quota of severely disabled individuals.[144] In governmental organizations in South Africa, 2% of the workforce must be made up of individuals with a disability.[145]

Last, civil rights and antidiscrimination policies offer protection and support to individuals with disabilities in the workforce. In 1996, the United Nations officially ratified the Convention on the Rights of Persons with Disabilities (CRPD). The recommendations from the CRPD state that individuals with disabilities have equal rights to accessibility and accommodation in education, cultural life, economic and financial systems, as well as to employment. More specifically, Article 27 stresses the need for people with disabilities to have equal rights and inclusion in the labor market and access to opportunities for advancement. Article 27 includes the prohibition of discrimination on the basis of disability including recruitment, harassment, educational training, union rights, self-employment, hiring, career advancement, reasonable accommodations, and wages.[146]

Other countries have adopted antidiscrimination legislation to protect the rights of individuals with disabilities. Passed in 1990, the Americans with Disabilities Act prohibits discrimination against qualified employees with disabilities in all phases of employment including hiring, advancement, compensation, and training.[147] In 1995, the United Kingdom adopted the Disability Discrimination Act, which specifically addressed unreasonable discrimination in the workforce for individuals with disabilities, including recruitment, working conditions, training and promotion.[148] More recently, the United Kingdom replaced the Disability Discrimination Act with the Equality Act of 2010 that merges policies prohibiting discrimination on the basis of disability, race, gender, religion, age, or sexual orientation.[149] The Equality Act of 2010 calls for equal accessibility to employment as well as public and private services. In 2003, Kenya implemented the Persons with Disabilities Act, which was the first legislation in the country's history to specifically address inequality issues for people with disabilities.[150] This act called for the establishment of the National Council for Persons with Disabilities to develop national policies and services pertaining to education, employment, and social equality.[151]

5. RECOMMENDATIONS/FUTURE DIRECTIONS

There has been remarkable consensus across social theory and government policy that paid employment is central to social inclusion.[152]

Career advancement for individuals with disabilities is a social justice issue worldwide. Although young adults with disabilities are increasingly entering the labor market, they have not realized the full benefit of access to high wage careers, opportunities for personal growth, and economic independence. Early career trajectories have been limited by constrained occupational aspirations, restricted opportunities for work experience and training, disability discrimination, policy disincentives, and other barriers in the workplace. In order to address socioeconomic inequities and increase opportunities for independence and productive careers for all individuals with disabilities, we offer the following recommendations.

To achieve more equitable employment, career opportunities and options need to be expanded for young adults with disabilities worldwide. Interventions should promote the belief that young adults with disabilities can work effectively and efficiently, if provided with appropriate supports or accommodations, which can often be provided at very low or no cost.[153] Another key element is to offer supports for entrance into the workforce, as early work experience and placement into the first job is a predictor of later career advancement.[154] Supports for entrance into the labor market could include providing job matching or job search services as well as connections to social and occupational networks. Once on the job, there is a need for a successful fit between the person and job environment to promote the ability to succeed.[155] Programs based around career adaptability have proven successful, and additional training, especially at the postsecondary level, has emerged as key for workers with disabilities to advance in their careers.

On the employer side, companies worldwide need to implement programming in order to ensure the full inclusion of individuals with disabilities in the workforce. This may include training to increase disability awareness, address workplace discrimination, and increase employers' ability to provide reasonable accommodations and workplace supports.[156] Mentoring programs that provide support and career-related skill development can also be established to teach specific job-related technological or managerial skills and offer support for communication and self-advocacy.[157]

In addition to these individual approaches, career advancement for young adults with disabilities needs to be addressed at the organizational and legislative level. Individuals with disabilities must be included on all levels of the decision-making processes concerning employment for people with disabilities in order to create career opportunities with upward mobility and leadership potential.[158] National and international policies need to be developed, monitored, and enforced concerning the hiring and advancement of individuals with disabilities. Antidiscrimination laws strongly support the career advancement of young adults with disabilities[159] by framing the issue as an investment in human potential rather than charity or a mandate.[160] Last, across all of these recommendations, we believe it is vital to pay careful attention to the unique career needs of young adults with disabilities from marginalized groups, including people of color, women, and those from low-income families.

There is no single policy, program, or intervention that will remove all of the barriers for young adults with disabilities entering the workforce. Each country and culture must approach creating access and equal opportunity within their unique cultural, political, economic, and social context. However, by gaining a comprehensive understanding of the trends, policies, and experiences of the international disability community, we can develop more effective programs and policies that support equal access and promote career development worldwide.

NOTES

1. Beveridge, S., Heller Craddock, S., Liesener, J., Stapleton, M., & Hershenson. D. (2002). Income: A Framework for Conceptualizing the Career Development of Persons with Disabilities. *Rehabilitation Counseling Bulletin 45*(4), 195–206; Szymanski, E., & Parker. R.M. (2010). *Work and Disability: Contexts, Issues, and Strategies for Enhancing Employment Outcomes for People with Disabilities*. Austin, TX: Pro-Ed.

2. Lindstrom, L. (2008). Career Development: Improving Options and Opportunities for Women with Disabilities. *Impact: Feature Issue on Employment and Women with Disabilities 21*(1), 32–33; Noonan, B.M., et al. (2004). Challenge and Success: A Qualitative Study of the Career Development of Highly Achieving Women With Physical and Sensory Disabilities. *Journal of Counseling Psychology 51*(1), 68–80.

3. Krahn, G. (2011). WHO World Report on Disability: A review. *Disability and Health Journal 4*(3): 141–142.

4. Jones, G. (1997). Advancement Opportunity Issues for Persons with Disabilities. *Human Resource Management Review 7*(1), 55–76. Feldman, D.C. (2004). The Role of Physical Disabilities in Early Career: Vocational Choice, the School-to-Work Transition, and Becoming Established. *Human Resource Management Review 14*(3): 247.

5. Horvath-Rose, A.E., Stapleton, D.C., & O'Day, B. (2004). Trends in outcomes for young people with work disabilities: Are we making progress? *Journal of Vocational Rehabilitation 21*(3), 175–187; Krahn (2011), WHO World Report; Organisation for Economic Co-operation and Development (2010). *Sickness, Disability and Work: Breaking the Barriers: a Synthesis of Findings Across OECD countries*. Paris, France: OECD.

6. Benshoff, J., Kroeger, S.A., & Scalia, V. (1990). Career Maturity and Academic Achievement in College Students with Disabilities. *Journal of Rehabilitation 56*(2), 40–45.

7. Enright, M.S. (1996). Career and Career-Related Educational Concerns of College Students with Disabilities. *Journal of Counseling & Development 75*(2), 103–14; Lindstrom, L., Benz, M., & Doren, B. (2004). Expanding Career Options for Young Women with Learning Disabilities. *Career Development for Exceptional Individuals 27*(1), 43–63.

8. Lee, M.N., Abdullah, Y., & Mey, S.C. (2011). Employment of People with Disabilities in Malaysia: Drivers and Inhibitors. *International Journal of Special Education. 26*(1), 112–124; Paul, S. (2011). Outcomes of Students with Disabilities in a Developing Country: Tobago. *International Journal of Special Education 26*(3), 194–211; Shahnasarian, M. (2001). Career Rehabilitation: Integration of Vocational Rehabilitation and Career Development in the Twenty-First Century. *Career Development Quarterly 49*(3), 275–83.

9. United States Census Bureau (2010). *Census 2010, Detailed Tables* (Washington, D.C.: U.S. Census Bureau), Table B18120.

10. Krahn (2011), WHO World Report.

11. Barnes, C. & Mercer, G. (2005). Disability, Work, and Welfare: Challenging the Social Exclusion of Disabled People. *Work Employment and Society 19*(3), 527–546; Braddock, D.L. & Bachelder, L. (1994). *The Glass Ceiling and Persons with Disabilities*. Washington, DC: U.S. Department of Labor; Wilson-Kovacs, D., Ryan, M., Haslam, S.A., & Rabinovich, A. (2008). "Just Because You Can Get a Wheelchair in the Building Doesn't Necessarily Mean that You Can Still Participate": Barriers to the Career Advancement of Disabled Professionals. *Disability & Society 23*(7), 705–717.

12. Barnes & Mercer (2005). Disability, Work, and Welfare; Braddock and Bachelder (1994). *The Glass Ceiling*; Tororei, S.K. (2009). The Right to Work: a Strategy for Addressing the Invisibility of Persons with Disability. *Disability Studies Quarterly 29*(4), 12; Wehbi, S., & Lakkis, S. (2010). Women with Disabilities in Lebanon: from Marginalization to Resistance. *Affilia 25*(1), 56–67.

13. Gerber, P., Ginsberg, R., & Reiff, H. (1992). Identifying Alterable Patterns in Employment Success for Highly Successful Adults with Learning Disabilities. *Journal of Learning Disabilities 25*(8), 475.
14. Feldman (2004). The Role of Physical Disabilities; Osipow, S.H. (1983). *Theories of Career Development*. Englewood Cliffs, NJ: Prentice Hall.
15. Murphy, K. & Welch, F. (1990). Empirical earnings profiles. *Journal of Labor Economics 8*(2), 202–229; Topel, R., & Ward, M. (1992). Job Mobility and Careers of Young Men. *Quarterly Journal of Economics 107*(2), 439–479.
16. Paul (2011). Outcomes of Students.
17. Shandra, C.L., & Hogan, D.P. (2008). School-to-Work Program Participation and the Post-High School Employment of Young Adults with Disabilities. *Journal of Vocational Rehabilitation 29*(2), 117–130.
18. Ibid.
19. Benz, M., Lindstrom, L., & Yovanoff, P. (2000). Improving Graduation and Employment Outcomes of Students with Disabilities: Predictive Factors and Student Perspectives. *Exceptional Children 66*(4), 509–529; Fabian, E.S. (2007). Urban Youth with Disabilities: Factors Affecting Transition Employment. *Rehabilitation Counseling Bulletin 50*(3), 130–138; Fabian, E., Lent, R., & Willis, S. (1998). Predicting Work Transition Outcomes for Students with Disabilities: Implications for Counselors. *Journal of Counseling & Development* 7(3), 311–316.
20. Benz, Lindstrom & Yovanoff (2000). Improving Graduation; Fabian (2007). Urban Youth with Disabilities; Fabian, Lent & Willis (1998), Predicting Work Transition.
21. Rabren, K., Dunn, C., & Chambers, D. (2002). Predictors of Post-High School Employment Among Young Adults with Disabilities. *Career Development for Exceptional Individuals 25*(1), 25–40.
22. Fabian (2007). Urban Youth with Disabilities; Lindstrom, L., Doren, B., & Miesch, J. (2011). Waging a Living: Career Development and Long-Term Employment Outcomes for Young Adults with Disabilities. *Exceptional Children 77*(4), 423–434; Zigmond, N. (2006). Twenty-Four Months after High School: Paths Taken by Youth Diagnosed with Severe Emotional and Behavioral Disorders. *Journal of Emotional and Behavioral Disorders 14*(2), 99–107.
23. World Bank (2007). *Development and the Next Generation. World Development Report 2007*. Washington, D. C.: The World Bank.
24. Chan, F., McMahon, B.T., Cheing, G., Rosenthal, D.A., & Bezyak, J. (2005). Drivers of Workplace Discrimination Against People with Disabilities: The Utility of Attribution Theory. *Work 25*(1), 77–88; Feldman (2004). The Role of Physical Disabilities; Joly, E. (2009). Disability and Employment in Argentina: The Right to Be Exploited? *NACLA Report on the Americas 42*(2): 5–10; Wilson-Kovacs, Ryan, Haslam, & Rabinovich (2008). "Just Because."
25. Szymanski & Parker (2010). *Work and Disability*; Opini, B. (2010). A Review of the Participation of Disabled Persons in the Labour Force: the Kenyan Context. *Disability & Society 25*(3), 271–287. Wehbi & Lakkis (2010). Women with Disabilities.
26. Horvath-Rose, Stapleton, & O'Day (2004). Trends in outcomes; Krahn (2011), WHO World Report.
27. Lindstrom, L., & Benz, M. (2002). Phases of Career Development: Case Studies of Young Women with Learning Disabilities. *Exceptional Children 69*(1), 67–83.

28. Lindstrom, L., Harwick, R., Poppen, M., & Doren B. (2012). Gender Gaps: Career Development for Young Women with Disabilities. *Career Development for Exceptional Individuals 35*(2), 108–117; Parish, S., Rose, R., & Andrews, M. (2009). Income, Poverty, and Material Hardship Among US Women with Disabilities. *Social Service Review 83*(1), 33–52; Wehbi & Lakkis (2010). Women with Disabilities.

29. Gottfredson, L. (2005). Applying Gottfredson's Theory of Circumscription and Compromise in Career Guidance and Counseling. In S.D. Brown & R.W. Lent (2010), *Career Development and Counseling: Putting Theory and Research to Work* (71–100). Hoboken, N.J.: John Wiley; Lindstrom, Benz, & Doren (2004). Expanding Career Options.

30. Feldman (2004). The Role of Physical Disabilities; Hoogeveen, J. (2005). Measuring Welfare for Small but Vulnerable Groups: Poverty and Disability in Uganda. *Journal of African Economies 14*(4), 603–631; Horvath-Rose, Stapleton, & O'Day (2004). Trends in outcomes; Joly, (2009). Disability and Employment in Argentina; Singal, N., Jeffery, R., Jain, A., & Sood, N. (2011). The Enabling Role of Education in the Lives of Young People with Disabilities in India: Achieved and Desired Outcomes. *International Journal of Inclusive Education 15*(10), 1205–1218.

31. Joly, (2009). Disability and Employment in Argentina.

32. Wagner, M., Newman, L., Cameto, R., Levine, P., & Garza, N. (2006). An Overview of Findings from Wave 2 of the National Longitudinal Transition Study-2 (NLTS2). NCSER 2006-3004. Washington, D.C.: National Center for Special Education Research.

33. United States Department of Labor (2002). *Action, Independence Through Employment: New Freedom Initiative 2002*. Washington, D.C.: U.S. Dept. of Labor.

34. Anctil, T., Ishikawa, M., & Scott, A.T. (2008). Academic Identity Development Through Self-determination: Successful College Students with Learning Disabilities. *Career Development for Exceptional Individuals 31*(3), 164–174; Wagner, Newman, Cameto, Levine, & Garza (2006). An Overview of Findings.

35. Burchardt, T. (2009). *The Education and Employment of Disabled Young People: Frustrated Ambition*. Bristol, United Kingdom: Policy Press; Hasnain, R., & Balcazar, F. (2009). Predicting Community- Versus Facility-Based Employment for Transition-Aged Young Adults with Disabilities: the Role of Race, Ethnicity, and Support Systems. *Journal of Vocational Rehabilitation 31*(3), 175–188; Russell, C. (1998). *Education, Employment and Training Policies and Programmes for Youth with Disabilities in Four European countries*. Geneva, Switzerland: International Labour Organization.

36. Jones (1997). Advancement Opportunity Issues; Wilson-Kovacs, Ryan, Haslam, & Rabinovich (2008). "Just Because."

37. Magill-Evans J., Galambos, N., Darrah, J., & Nickerson, C. (2008). Predictors of employment for young adults with developmental motor disabilities. *Work 31*(4), 439.

38. Jones (1997). Advancement Opportunity Issues; Noonan et al. (2004). Challenge and Success; Wilson-Kovacs, Ryan, Haslam, & Rabinovich (2008). "Just Because."

39. Organisation for Economic Co-operation and Development (2010). *Sickness, Disability and Work*.

40. Weathers, R., & Hemmeter, J. (2011). The Impact of Changing Financial Work Incentives on the Earnings of Social Security Disability Insurance (SSDI) Beneficiaries. *Journal of Policy Analysis and Management 30*(4), 708–728.

41. Division of Labor Force Statistics (2010). *Persons with a Disability: Labor Force Characteristics*. Washington, D.C.: U.S. Department of Labor.
42. Weathers & Hemmeter (2011). The Impact of Changing Financial Work Incentives.
43. Organisation for Economic Co-operation and Development (2010). *Sickness, Disability and Work*.
44. Chan, McMahon, Cheing, Rosenthal, & Bezyak (2005). Drivers of Workplace Discrimination; Joly (2009). Disability and Employment in Argentina; Noonan et al. (2004). Challenge and Success; Wilson-Kovacs, Ryan, Haslam, & Rabinovich (2008). "Just Because."
45. Gartrell, A. (2010). "A Frog in a Well": The Exclusion of Disabled People from Work in Cambodia. *Disability and Society* 25(3), 289–301.
46. Waghorn, G., & Lloyd, C. (2005). The Employment of People with Mental Illness. *Australian E-Journal for the Advancement of Mental Health* 4(2), 129–171.
47. Shahnasarian (2001). Career Rehabilitation;
48. Jones (1997). Advancement Opportunity Issues.
49. Chan, McMahon, Cheing, Rosenthal, & Bezyak (2005). Drivers of Workplace Discrimination.
50. Ibid., 77.
51. Wilson-Kovacs, Ryan, Haslam, & Rabinovich (2008). "Just Because"; Noonan et al. (2004). Challenge and Success.
52. Noonan et al. (2004). Challenge and Success, 74.
53. Conyers, L.M., Koch, L.C., & Szymanski, E.M. (1998). Life-Span Perspectives on Disability and Work: A Qualitative Study. *Rehabilitation Counseling Bulletin* 42(1), 20.
54. Bewley, H., Dorsett, R., & Hale, G. (2007) *The impact of Pathways to Work*. London, United Kingdom: Department for Work and Pensions; Conyers, Koch, & Szymanski (1998). Life-Span Perspectives; Gottfredson (2005). Applying Gottfredson's Theory; Osipow (1983). *Theories of Career Development*.
55. Lee & Mey (2011). Employment of People with Disabilities in Malaysia; Opini (2010). A Review of the Participation of Disabled Persons; Wehbi & Lakkis (2010). Women with Disabilities.
56. Krahn (2011), WHO World Report.
57. Doren, B., Lindstrom, L., Zane, C., & Johnson, P. (2007). The Role of Program and Alterable Personal Factors in Post school Employment Outcomes. *Career Development for Exceptional Individuals* 30(3), 171–183; Gerber, Ginsberg, & Reiff (1992). Identifying Alterable Patterns; Lindstrom, Doren, & Miesch (2011). Waging a Living; Noonan et al. (2004). Challenge and Success.
58. Doren, Lindstrom, Zane, & Johnson (2007). The Role of Program; Gerber, Ginsberg, and Reiff (1992). Identifying Alterable Patterns; Roessler, R.T. (2002). Improving Job Tenure Outcomes for People with Disabilities: The 3M Model. *Rehabilitation Counseling Bulletin* 45(4), 207–12.
59. Doren, Lindstrom, Zane, & Johnson (2007). The Role of Program.
60. Gerber, Ginsberg, & Reiff (1992). Identifying Alterable Patterns.
61. Ibid., 479.
62. Gerber, Ginsberg, & Reiff (1992). Identifying Alterable Patterns; Lee, Abdullah, & Mey (2011). Employment of People with Disabilities in Malaysia; Lindstrom, Doren, & Miesch (2011). Waging a Living.
63. Lindstrom, Doren, & Miesch (2011). Waging a Living.
64. Noonan et al. (2004). Challenge and Success.

65. Hutchinson N.L., Versnel, J., Chin, P., & Munby, H. (2009). Negotiating Accommodations so that Work-Based Education Facilitates Career Development for Youth with Disabilities. *Work 30*(2), 123–36; Madaus, J.W. (2007). Employment Outcomes of University Graduates with Learning Disabilities. *Learning Disability Quarterly 29*(1): 19–31; Roessler (2002). Improving Job Tenure Outcomes.
66. Conyers, Koch, & Szymanski (1998). Life-Span Perspectives; Roessler (2002). Improving Job Tenure Outcomes.
67. Doren, Lindstrom, Zane, & Johnson (2007). The Role of Program; Hutchinson, Versnel, Chin, & Munby (2009). Negotiating Accommodations.
68. Lindstrom, Harwick, Poppen, & Doren (2012). Gender Gaps.
69. Adelman, P., & Vogel, S. (1993). Issues in the Employment of Adults with Learning Disabilities. *Learning Disability Quarterly 16*(3), 219–232; Beveridge, Craddock, Liesener, Stapleton, & Hershenson (2002). Income: A Framework for Conceptualizing; Doren, Lindstrom, Zane, & Johnson (2007). The Role of Program; Hutchinson, Versnel, Chin, & Munby (2009). Negotiating Accommodations.
70. Roulstone, A. (2003). *Thriving and Surviving at Work: Disabled People's Employment Strategies*. Bristol, United Kingdom: Policy Press, 9.
71. Doren, B., Lombardi, A., Gau, J., & Lindstrom, L. (2012). *Development and Evaluation of a Curriculum to Improve Educational and Career Outcomes for Girls with Disabilities*. Poster session, Pacific Coast Research Conference, San Diego, CA.
72. Lindstrom, L., & Post, C. (2012). *Building Career PATHS for Young Women With Disabilities*. Paper presentation, Pacific Rim International Conference on Diversity and Disability, Honolulu, HI, 26–27 March.
73. Jones (1997). Advancement Opportunity Issues; Lindstrom and Post (2012). *Building Career PATHS*; Noonan et al. (2004). Challenge and Success; Roessler (2002). Improving Job Tenure Outcomes.
74. Gerber, Ginsberg, & Reiff (1992). Identifying Alterable Patterns.
75. Ibid.; Roulstone, Alan (2003). *Thriving and Surviving at Work*.
76. Lindstrom, Doren, & Miesch (2011). Waging a Living; Noonan et al. (2004). Challenge and Success.
77. Roessler (2002). Improving Job Tenure Outcomes.
78. Gerber, Ginsberg, & Reiff (1992). Identifying Alterable Patterns.
79. Jones (1997). Advancement Opportunity Issues; Roessler (2002). Improving Job Tenure Outcomes.
80. Dix, J.E., & Savickas, M.L. (1995). Establishing a Career: Developmental Tasks and Coping Responses. *Journal of Vocational Behavior 47*(1), 93–107.
81. Bewley, Dorsett, & Hale. (2007) The Impact of Pathways to Work.
82. Fabian (2007). Urban Youth with Disabilities.
83. Jones (1997). Advancement Opportunity Issues, 56.
84. Gartrell (2010). "A Frog in a Well"; Horvath-Rose, Stapleton, & O'Day (2004). Trends in outcomes; Krahn (2011), WHO World Report; Lee, Abdullah, & Mey (2011). Employment of People with Disabilities in Malaysia; Wagner, Newman, Cameto, Levine, & Garza (2006). An Overview of Findings.
85. Parish, Rose, & Andrews (2009). Income, Poverty, and Material Hardship.
86. Wolffe, K. (2000). Critical Skills in Career Advancement for People with Visual Impairments. *Journal of Visual Impairment & Blindness 94*(8), 532–534.

87. Lindstrom, L., Doren, B., Flannery, B., & Benz, M. (2012). Structured Work Experiences. In Michael Wehmeyer and Kristine Webb (Eds.), *Handbook of Adolescent Transition Education for Youth with Disabilities*. New York: Routledge; Roessler (2002). Improving Job Tenure Outcomes.
88. Izzo, M.V., & Lamb, P. (2003). Developing Self-Determination through Career Development Activities: Implications for Vocational Rehabilitation Counselors. *Journal of Vocational Rehabilitation 19*(2), 71–78; Wolffe (2000). Critical Skills in Career Advancement.
89. Lindstrom, Doren, Flannery, & Benz (2012). Structured Work Experiences.
90. Fabian (2007). Urban Youth with Disabilities.
91. Lindstrom, Doren, Flannery, & Benz (2012). Structured Work Experiences.
92. Fabian (2007). Urban Youth with Disabilities; Lindstrom, Benz, and Doren (2004). Expanding Career Options.
93. Ibid.; Fabian, Lent, & Willis (1998). Predicting Work Transition Outcomes.
94. Fabian (2007). Urban Youth with Disabilities.
95. Ibid.
96. Lindstrom, L., & Poppen, M. (2010). *Twenty Years of the Youth Transition Program: Transition. Impact. Collaboration*. Eugene, OR: University of Oregon.
97. Ibid.
98. Benz, Lindstrom, & Yovanoff (2009). Improving Graduation; Benz, M., Lindstrom, L., & Latta, T. (1999). Improving collaboration between schools and vocational rehabilitation: The youth transition program model. *Journal of Vocational Rehabilitation 13*(1), 55–63.
99. McDonough, J., & Revell, G. (2010). Accessing Employment Supports in the Adult System for Transitioning Youth with Autism Spectrum Disorders. *Journal of Vocational Rehabilitation 32*(2), 89–100.
100. Ibid.; Olsheski, J. (2006). Career Counseling in Vocational Rehabilitation Settings. In D. Capuzzi and M.D. Stauffer (Eds.), *Career Counseling: Foundations, Perspectives, and Applications*. Boston, MA: Pearson/Allyn & Bacon, 341–470.
101. Beveridge, Craddock, Liesener, Stapleton, & Hershenson (2002). Income: A Framework for Conceptualizing; Roessler (2002). Improving Job Tenure Outcomes.
102. McDonough & Revell (2010). Accessing Employment Supports.
103. Pineda, V.S., & Cuk, V. (2007). *Young People with Disabilities in the Europe and Central Asia Region (ECA)*. Background Paper for the World Bank Conference.
104. Beveridge, Craddock, Liesener, Stapleton, & Hershenson (2002). Income: A Framework for Conceptualizing; Roessler (2002). Improving Job Tenure Outcomes.
105. Beveridge, Craddock, Liesener, Stapleton, & Hershenson (2002). Income: A Framework for Conceptualizing, 202.
106. Doren, Lindstrom, Zane, & Johnson (2007). The Role of Program; Gerber, Ginsberg, & Reiff (1992). Identifying Alterable Patterns; Izzo and Lamb (2003). Developing Self-Determination.
107. Roessler (2002). Improving Job Tenure Outcomes.; Rogers, C., Lavin, D., Tran, T., Gantenbein, T., & Sharpe, M. (2008). Customized Employment: Changing What it Means to Be Qualified in the Workforce for Transition-Aged Youth and Young Adults. *Journal of Vocational Rehabilitation 28*(3), 191–207.
108. McDonough & Revell (2010). Accessing Employment Supports.
109. Schultz, C., & Seith, D. (2011). *Career Advancement and Work Support Services on the Job: Implementing the Fort Worth Work Advancement and Support Center Program*. New York: MDRC.

110. Ibid.
111. Rudney, S. (n.d) Disability Affinity Groups. New York: Jennifer Brown Consulting. Retrieved January 23, 2013, from http://jenniferbrownconsulting.com/site/wp-content/uploads/2010/11/Disability-Affinity-Groups-Rudney_JBC.pdf.
112. Beveridge, Craddock, Liesener, Stapleton, & Hershenson (2002). Income: A Framework for Conceptualizing; Jones (1997). Advancement Opportunity Issues.
113. Noonan et al. (2004). Challenge and Success; Rousso, H. (2008). Role Models, Mentors and Muses for Women with Disabilities. Impact: Feature Issue on Employment and Women with Disabilities 21(1), 8-9; Timmons, J. (2006). *Paving the Way to Work: a Guide to Career-Focused Mentoring for Youth with Disabilities*. Washington, D.C.: National Collaborative on Workforce and Disability for Youth, Institute for Educational Leadership; Wilson-Kovacs, Ryan, Haslam, & Rabinovich (2008). "Just Because."
114. Timmons (2006). Paving the Way to Work.
115. Jones (1997). Advancement Opportunity Issues.
116. Rousso (2008). Role Models, Mentors and Muses; Wilson-Kovacs, Ryan, Haslam, & Rabinovich (2008). "Just Because."
117. Carnevale, A. (2007). Access to Opportunity. *Education Week 26*(40), 34.
118. Flannery, K.B., Yovanoff, P., Benz, M., & Kato, M. (2008). Improving Employment Outcomes of Individuals With Disabilities Through Short-Term Postsecondary Training. *Career Development for Exceptional Individuals 31*(1), 26–36; National Council on Disability (2003). *People with Disabilities and Postsecondary Education Position Paper*. Washington, D.C.: National Council on Disability.
119. Taylor, B.J., McGilloway, S., & Donnelly, M. (2004). Preparing Young Adults with Disability for Employment. *Health & Social Care in the Community 12*(2), 93–101.
120. Gilmore, D.S.& Bose, J. (2005). Trends in Postsecondary Education: Participation within the Vocational Rehabilitation System. *Journal of Vocational Rehabilitation 22*(1), 33–40.
121. Ibid.; Wagner, Newman, Cameto, Levine, & Garza (2006). An Overview of Findings.
122. Izzo & Lamb (2003). Developing Self-Determination; Lindstrom, L., Flannery, B., Benz, M., Olszewksi, B., & Slovic, R. (2009). Building Employment Training Partnerships Between Vocational Rehabilitation and Community Colleges. *Rehabilitation Counseling Bulletin 52*(3), 189–201.
123. Madaus (2007). Employment Outcomes of University Graduates.
124. Lindstrom, Doren & Miesch (2011). Waging a Living.
125. Krahn (2011), WHO World Report; Lindstrom, Flannery, Benz, Olszewksi & Slovic (2009). Building Employment Training Partnerships.
126. Flynn, W.J. (2002). More Than a Matter of Degree—Credentialing, Certification and Community Colleges. *Catalyst 30*(3), 3–12.
127. Flannery, Yovanoff, Benz, & Kato (2008). Improving Employment Outcomes.
128. de Klerk, T. (2008). Funding for Self-Employment of People with Disabilities. Grants, Loans, Revolving Funds or Linkage with Microfinance Programmes. *Leprosy Review 79*(1), 92–109; Krahn (2011), WHO World Report.
129. Barnes & Mercer (2005). Disability, Work, and Welfare.
130. Green, J.H., & Brooke, V. (2001). Recruiting and Retaining the Best from America's Largest Untapped Talent Pool. *Journal of Vocational Rehabilitation*

16(2), 83–88; Hutchinson, Versnel, Chin, & Munby (2009). Negotiating Accommodations; Jones (1997). Advancement Opportunity Issues.

131. Hutchinson, Versnel, Chin, & Munby (2009). Negotiating Accommodations; Tøssebro, J. (2007). *Report on the Employment of Disabled People in European Countries.* Utrecht, the Netherlands, and Leeds, United Kingdom: Human European Consultancy and Academic Network of European Disability Experts.

132. Jones (1997). Advancement Opportunity Issues, 68.

133. *Americans with Disabilities Act of 1990.* Federal Register 1513-91, 56 no. 144 (1990); Jones (1997). Advancement Opportunity Issues; Olsheski (2006). Career Counseling in Vocational Rehabilitation.

134. Olsheski (2006). Career Counseling in Vocational Rehabilitation.

135. Job Accommodation Network (2011). *Workplace accommodations: Low cost, high impact.* Retrieved May 17, 2012 from http://AskJAN.org/media/LowCostHighImpact.doc

136. Olsheski (2006). Career Counseling in Vocational Rehabilitation.

137. Grech, S. (2011). Recolonising Debates or Perpetuated Coloniality? Decentring the Spaces of Disability, Development and Community in the Global South. *International Journal of Inclusive Education 15*(1), 87–100; Tororei (2009). The Right to Work; Wehbi and Lakkis (2010). Women with Disabilities.

138. Chan, McMahon, Cheing, Rosenthal, & Bezyak (2005). Drivers of Workplace Discrimination; Jones (1997). Advancement Opportunity Issues; Shahnasarian (2001). Career Rehabilitation.

139. Green & Brooke (2001). Recruiting and Retaining the Best.

140. Ibid.; Jones (1997). Advancement Opportunity Issues; Rogers, Lavin, Tran, Gantenbein, & Sharpe (2008). Customized Employment.

141. Krahn (2011), WHO World Report; Seed, M. (2003). Employers' Forum on Disability. http://www.employers-forum.co.uk. *Occupational Medicine 53*(2): 152–153.

142. Employers' Forum on Disability (2012). Employer's Forum on Disability. Retreived May 5, 2012, from http://www.efd.org.uk/; Krahn (2011), WHO World Report.

143. Barnes & Mercer (2005). Disability, Work, and Welfare; Krahn (2011), WHO World Report.

144. Waldschmidt A., & Lingnau, K. (2007). *Report on the Employment of Disabled People in European Countries: Germany.* Utrecht, the Netherlands, and Leeds, United Kingdom: Human European Consultancy and Academic Network of European Disability Experts.

145. Commission for Employment Equity. *Annual report 2007–2008* (2008). Pretoria, South Africa: South Africa Department of Labour.

146. United Nations (2007). Convention on the Rights of Persons with Disabilities. *European Journal of Health Law 14*(3), 281–98.

147. Americans with Disabilities Act of 1990.

148. Barnes & Mercer (2005). Disability, Work, and Welfare.

149. Ashtiany, S. (2011). The Equality Act 2010: Main Concepts. *International Journal of Discrimination and the Law 11*(1): 29–42.

150. Opini (2010). A Review of the Participation of Disabled Persons.

151. Ibid.; Krahn (2011), WHO World Report.

152. Barnes & Mercer (2005). Disability, Work, and Welfare, 541.

153. Job Accommodation Network (2011). *Workplace accommodations*; Olsheski (2006). Career Counseling in Vocational Rehabilitation.

154. Fabian (2007). Urban Youth with Disabilities; Rabren, Dunn, & Chambers (2002). Predictors of Post-High School Employment; Zigmond (2006). Twenty-Four Months after High School.
155. Beveridge, Craddock, Liesener, Stapleton, & Hershenson (2002). Income: A Framework for Conceptualizing; Roessler (2002). Improving Job Tenure Outcomes.
156. Employers' Forum on Disability (2012). Employer's Forum on Disability.
157. Adelman & Vogel (1993). Issues in the Employment of Adults; Green & Brooke (2001). Recruiting and Retaining the Best; Timmons (2006). *Paving the Way to Work*.
158. Pineda & Cuk (2007). *Young People with Disabilities*; Roggero, P., Tarricone, R., Nicoli, M., & Mangiaterra, V. (2006). What Do People Think about Disabled Youth and Employment in Developed and Developing Countries? Results from an E-Discussion Hosted by the World Bank. *Disability & Society 21*(6), 645–650.
159. Pineda & Cuk (2007). *Young People with Disabilities*.
160. Grech (2011). Recolonising Debates or Perpetuated Coloniality?; Krahn (2011), WHO World Report.

CHAPTER 10

Preventing Job Abandonment and Facilitating Work Reintegration in High-Income Countries

RIENK PRINS

1. INTRODUCTION

This chapter focuses on disability and employment for workers who are already part of the workforce and acquire their disability during their earning years; this often happens later in their careers, when they have acquired considerable skill and experience that can become compromised by the onset of disability. To do this, the chapter explores the scope of late-onset disability among the employed population in industrialized countries, mainly Organisation for Economic Development and Co-operation (OECD) and European Union (EU) countries. The chapter begins by describing figures and trends through indicators that are available for many countries, namely sickness absence rates and disability benefit dependency rates resulting from leaving the work force because of new-onset disability. Although these indicators are not perfect and may omit important information, they are a useful way of comparing trends and outcomes across related countries.

The chapter then delves into the relationship between short-term sickness absence and uptake of long-term disability insurance, including the pathway that can lead a worker with a nascent disability to abandon the workforce and become exclusively reliant on disability benefits instead of reintegrating into employment. This section also presents the argument that labor market integration policies for workers with disabilities that have left the workforce—either short- or long-term—are socially and financially beneficial to companies, governments, and the workers themselves. The key in disability and employment is therefore to design and implement policies and programs that provide a sufficient safety net to those whose work capacity is indeed reduced and at the same time create a system of checks and incentives at the government, business, and individual levels so that workers who have acquired a disability can more easily enter, remain in, or return to the workforce.

The chapter then discusses some major findings from the OECD project *Sickness, Disability and Work*.[1] This cross-national investigation identified three types of disability policies in the ways industrialized countries deal with sickness, disability, and employment. For each type of policy an example or insights from cross-national studies will be demonstrated, focusing on what type of policies can reduce "passive" recipiency of benefits in favor of activation and integration measures.

The final section is devoted to specific measures taken in several countries to prevent the outflow from the work force into disability benefit schemes and encourage its reversal. Examples in the United Kingdom, Sweden, and the Netherlands will serve to explore how measures ranging from awareness programs to integrated service provision to increasing employer obligations are incentivizing employers and workers to remain in the workforce.

At the end of the chapter a few major challenges as to rehabilitation and labor reintegration will be discussed, including their role in adapting disability policies to changing conditions in the economy, demography, and public expectations—for example, aging populations, economic crises, and increasing expectations as to quality and accountability.

2. DISABILITY RATES IN A COMPARATIVE PERSPECTIVE

Various sources of long-term disability rates have become available over the past two decades. For a cross national insight into the scope and features of disability in persons at working age, two types of sources can be used:

1   Surveys measuring self-reported health and disability, such as household panels, living conditions surveys, health surveys
2   Comparative data derived from social security administrations (on disability benefit/pension recipients, and benefit expenditures) and employment and unemployment statistics

Mont shows that these sources do not give the same information on the same populations. There is no single definition of disability applied across countries, and different methods of data collection also affect outcomes of national studies. This heterogeneity of concepts and sources also leads to variation within countries: for example the reported disability prevalence rate (2001) for Canada ranged from 13.7% to 31.3%, depending on the type of questions used in surveys.[2]

Health surveys usually sample the entire population and not only persons in employment. The prevalence of disabilities is based on the assessment by the person interviewed, in the context of diagnosable conditions, activities of daily living, and participation. Moreover, cultural differences as to public awareness and attitudes toward persons with disabilities, including stigma, may also affect responses.

Administrative sources from social security only regard persons with disabilities who are insured (i.e., they are employed, usually in the formal sector) and who fulfilled the administrative and medical eligibility criteria for benefit receipt or rehabilitation measures.[3] Further, for compensation purposes, a minimum loss of earning capacity has to be assessed by medical and/or vocational experts.

For this category of benefit recipients, and for the population that is insured or in employment, there is comparatively more information available at the national level (including diagnoses, costs, employment, trends, rehabilitation measures, and return to work results), despite the fact that institutional criteria, which affect inflow into schemes, differ considerably across countries. This makes assessing disability benefits policies comparatively easier, although one has to bear in mind that there are groups of persons of working age who may not be covered by these schemes, either because they have not been employed the requisite amount of time to receive benefits, or because their type of employment (for example, informal work) may fall outside the scheme.

3. DISABILITY AND EMPLOYMENT: SOME CROSS-NATIONAL FIGURES

Recent UK data show that long-term sickness absence (lasting over 4 weeks) accounts for 40% of working time lost. These absences tend to be caused by musculoskeletal disorders, common mental health problems, and medical conditions like cancer, diabetes, heart disease, or stroke. About four out of five of these absences are followed by work resumption.[4]

Early intervention is one of the current leading actions for further improving these work resumption rates.[5] Work-focused health care and accommodating work places are particularly relevant here. The category of mental health disorders has proved to be less well understood by employers and therapists, particularly when dealing with the employment aspect. Not surprisingly, in many countries employees with this category of health conditions show high exit rates and increasing dependency on benefits as their only source of income, making it unlikely they will rejoin the workforce (see Figure 10.1).

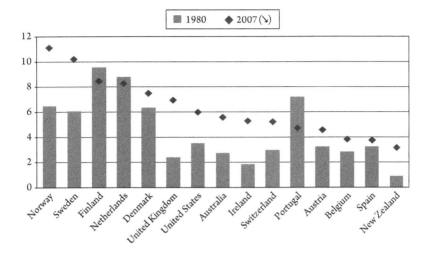

Figure 10.1
Disability benefit recipients in percent of the population aged 20 to 64 in 15 OECD countries, early 1980s and 2007/2008.[6]

The measures regarding helping persons with serious or lasting health-related problems can be classified into two groups:

1 Support to remain in the job, which may include suitable adjustments (which in many countries are supported by financial incentives to the employer, like subsidies or tax reductions) or transferring to another job within the firm
2 Change to a different employer with more suitable tasks and work place; this may be good for the employee's health and wellbeing, because continued employment has been proven to be beneficial in several aspects beyond the merely financial. It is also a source of potential savings for the employer, who is responsible for sick pay amounts, and for social security schemes.

In most countries the latter strategy of helping persons with disabilities remain in employment, albeit with a different employer, still meets many obstacles: Job brokering services are often designed so they are not available if the worker still has a labor contract or until sickness benefits have been exhausted, therefore delaying work resumption and making permanence in the workforce harder. In both the United Kingdom and the Netherlands, measures have been taken to speed up this transfer process. The United Kingdom is introducing a new job-brokering service, whereas in the Netherlands the employer is incentivized to find an adequate job for a long-term sick-listed employee who is not able to return to her or his old job and employer. If such efforts are successful, this is rewarded with a reduction of social security contributions.

Disability benefit dependency reflects the outflow from the labor market due to disabilities that reduce earning capacity. Figure 10.1 shows disability benefit dependency rates: the number of disability benefit recipients as a percentage of the population aged 20 to 64.

The data show large international variations. In 2007, the Scandinavian countries (except Norway) and the Netherlands had the highest prevalence rates for persons of working age relying on disability benefits. Despite growing evidence on the kind of interventions that can help persons with disabilities remain in the workforce, most OECD countries have been unsuccessful in containing growth in dependency rates between 1980 and 2007; only three countries (Finland, Netherlands, and Portugal) managed to reduce disability benefit dependency.

Apart from the growth in disability benefit dependency, the pattern of causes of disability for those entering benefit schemes is also shifting (Figure 10.2). In many OECD countries musculoskeletal disorders no longer comprise the largest cause of inflow; instead, it is disabilities related to mental health problems. The growth of the proportion of mental health problems in new recipients of disability benefits is particularly visible in five countries (Denmark, Sweden, Switzerland, Germany, and Austria).

This growth of mental health diagnoses is associated with changes in the health conditions of workers, as well as in the organization and conditions of their employment. But shifting cultural factors may also affect reporting, including reduced stigma and greater public awareness of mental health issues.[7] The trend is still rising; EU member states in Central and East Europe

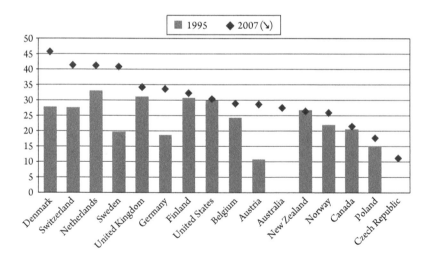

Figure 10.2
Proportion of inflows into disability benefit due to mental health conditions in 16 OECD countries, mid-1990s and 2007/08.[8]

note that this shift in morbidity patterns is now taking place in their disability benefit statistics as well.

Finally, a common feature in most developed countries is the role of aging: the older the age groups, the higher the proportion of disability benefit recipients.[9] Moreover, in most countries generally only the youngest age groups of persons with disabilities leave the schemes back into full or partial employment. The vast majority of recipients, however, leave disability benefit schemes only due to demographic reasons, namely statutory pension age or death. This speaks to failures of program design and implementation, and to the need for new approaches that can reverse this trend.

4. DISABILITY AND EMPLOYMENT: AN UNDERLYING PROCESS AND REMEDY

In many EU and OECD countries, disability policy is in a process of reconsideration and reform. Until 20 years ago, disability policies were synonymous with adequate, sometimes generous, and easily accessible disability benefits that were provided with little regard to whether the recipient could or wanted to work. However, for reasons of both fiscal prudence and integration of workers with disabilities, in more and more countries attention has shifted from a focus on the provision of "passive" benefits to activation and reintegration policies.

On a societal level there are three major policy goals for implementing this policy shift:

1. Reducing public expenditures, in order to keep health care and social security systems sustainable
2. Preventing deficits in labor market supply and using competencies in current workers for current vacancies. This argument is especially relevant in countries with comparatively low unemployment rates.
3. At the level of the individual and his or her network, ensuring continued participation in employment, which has many advantages. The generally accepted framework about work and well-being states that, when possible, sick and disabled people should be encouraged and supported to remain in or reenter work as soon as possible because it:
   - Is therapeutic, helps to promote recovery and rehabilitation, and leads to better health outcomes
   - Minimizes harmful physical, mental, and social effects of long-term sickness absence
   - Reduces the risk of long-term incapacity
   - Promotes full participation in society, independence, and human rights
   - Reduces poverty and improves quality of life and well-being[10]

5. SICKNESS, DISABILITY, AND EMPLOYMENT: CONCEPTS AND INDICATORS

This tendency toward individual benefit recipiency over social integration stands in contrast to changing attitudes toward disability. Whereas for a long time disability was mainly considered as an individual medical condition, the *social model of disability* has by now been predominant for years. This model makes a distinction between impairments and disabilities, the latter being the consequence of societal failures to recognize and accommodate differences in people. Disabilities are related to attitudinal, environmental, and institutional barriers in society.

This change in paradigm is more slowly but increasingly reflected in changes in policy focus: shifting the weight from compensation for the economic consequences of disability to increasing activation and work resumption. Sickness and disability policies try to integrate in increasingly new ways two potentially contradictory objectives: providing income support in periods of short- and long-term work incapacity, and helping persons with reduced work capacity stay in the labor force or return to work as soon as possible.[11]

Before discussing these two policies, a demarcation of some disability and employment issues is needed. Our main focus, disability in the context of work and employment, implies that our interest mainly lies in the prevalence, background, developments, and interventions that focus on persons who *acquire disabilities during their working life* (in general, age 16–65), as well as their employment or income setting, and on how to ensure that the persons that do acquire disabilities can, where possible, remain in the workforce. The period of working life plays an important role in the background of disabilities. As Mont describes, disability is not a static concept: Only 4% of people are born with disabilities, whereas 55% acquire disabilities during their lives; moreover there is a strong increase in disability prevalence after the age of 50,[12] during peak earning years for many workers.

Ill health often leads to people falling out of work. Yet many causes of absence due to ill health are relatively mild conditions that often are compatible with work or—after a few days of absence –improve or disappear. In the case of long-standing health conditions, including disability, some people continue to work whereas others with similar conditions report sick and eventually claim long-term disability benefits, often never returning to the workforce. Whether a worker with a disability falls under the former or the latter category depends on a myriad of factors, including the individual nature of the disability but also the system of incentives, policies, and programs that is in place to support the worker, and, hopefully, contribute to his or her staying in the workforce. As disability acquired during one's working life is often preceded by spells of sickness absence, adequate employer policies, including sickness management, support, adaptations at work, and occupational health interventions, also affect the incidence of disability benefit claims.

For the population of working age, two concepts can be used that, in some way, reflect the prevalence of persons in employment with health- or impairment-related restrictions:

1 Sickness absence
2 Long-term work disability

When focusing on persons in employment, both the sickness absence and the disability measure show considerable variations across countries. In most European countries, sickness absence refers to spells of work incapacity covered under public sickness benefit schemes or under employer wage payment arrangements. In many countries, these income replacement arrangements last up to a maximum of 12 months, with some exceptions where compensation is provided for longer periods such as 18 months in Germany or 24 months in the Netherlands.

When after a long period of sickness absence the underlying condition is still problematic, the worker may subsequently apply for a disability benefit or pension, under different conditions depending on the country. The timing of transfer to the disability benefit scheme affects both national sickness absence levels and the number of persons with disabilities in employment. Job protection regulations, antidiscrimination laws, and employer dismissal practices—for example, dismissal after or due to sickness—also cause considerable cross-national differences in definitions and rates. Moreover, as the overwhelming majority of sickness absences have a short duration, sickness absence rates are less valid to measure longer lasting disability in the work force.

As is the case with sickness absence, there is also no single, widely accepted, applicable, measurable definition of disability that can be used across cultures and jurisdictions. Definitions depend on the policy domain in which they are used (e.g., health and long-term care, housing, monetary benefits); related to employment, the factors affecting sickness absence also determine the content, scope, and availability of statistics on disability and employment. Consequently, comparative statistics on sickness and disability during working age years face several restrictions.

5.1 Short-Term Work Incapacity: A Relevant Risk Factor Preceding Long-Term Use of Disability Benefits

National sickness absence rates reflect the features of employment regulations, employers' obligations, and compensation systems in each country, which are often reflective of the approach particular countries take to work reintegration in the longer term. Despite the relatively short length of most cases of sickness absence, sickness benefits and long-term disability benefits are shown to be strongly linked. No less than 50%—and up to 90%—of persons entering disability benefit schemes do so after a period spent on sickness benefits. The OECD argues that "reducing sickness absence from the workplace can reduce inflow into long term disability benefits."[13] The "journey" from work to reliance on disability benefit has—in general—similar stages in most countries:

- The individual at work develops a health condition.
- This may lead to short-term absence, during which the employer is required to pay the worker's wage, fully or in part.
- If recovery is unsuccessful, the spell may turn into longer-term absence and sickness benefits will be paid from the country's social security fund.
- If there is no improvement or sick pay has been exhausted, the person will become reliant on disability benefits as the only source of income, be it temporary or permanent, or—when not meeting the eligibility criteria—unemployment benefits.[14]

This process of moving through the system is affected by decisions made by the worker, health professionals, employers, and social security. If the end result is full dependency on benefits, this is often not an unavoidable outcome but rather a function of decisions taken at every level and of the policies and programs that incentivize them. To prevent increased entry into disability benefits, interventions should be made at an early stage: "the longer someone is off sick, the higher the risk for that person never to return to work."[15]

National differences in the institutional contexts of sickness absence, such as benefit levels, job protection arrangements, and certification procedures, also affect the levels of sickness absence recorded. In order to create a common basis for comparisons, the European Union regularly carries out surveys in employed persons, which can also include some elementary features of sickness absence. Most recently published EU data from this source, 2010 figures from the Working Conditions Observatory, are featured in Figure 10.3 for a selection of West European countries (Norway, Finland, Germany, France, Belgium, the Netherlands, Sweden, Denmark, the United Kingdom, and Ireland).

The diagram indicates that—measured as self-reported absence from work due to health conditions—some countries have high rates for both short- and long-term sickness (Norway, Finland), whereas in other countries short term-absences in particular are comparatively more frequent. When focusing on indicators of long-term health conditions and disability during working life, the figures for Norway and Finland show to be twice as high as those of, for example, Denmark and Germany.

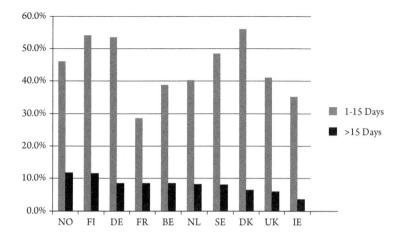

Figure 10.3
Average percent of workers absent 1 to 15 days or more than 15 days (in past 12 months) for reasons of health problems[16]

Disregarding measurement biases, these differences are also related to the characteristics of each country's social protection schemes, including amount and duration of benefits payment and degree of job protection for those who are ill frequently or long term. Also, other sources, such as a recent study based on the European Labour Force Survey, confirm the pattern in this diagram.[17]

Despite these differences, there are also many cross-national similarities regarding levels and trends in sickness absence:

1 Sickness absence increases with age of the work force, which may be explained partly by the positive correlation between age and prevalence of illness.
2 Female workers on average show higher sickness absence rates than men, which is attributed to their overall workload, including on average higher household and childrearing responsibilities.
3 Sickness absence rates vary across economic sectors.

6. DISABILITY AND EMPLOYMENT: VARIATIONS IN POLICY ANSWERS

In response to the needs of workers with disabilities, according to OECD three different disability policy models have been implemented in recent years.[18]

The "social-democratic disability policy model" shows relatively generous and accessible compensation arrangements and a broad and equally accessible labor integration program. The latter in particular focuses on vocational rehabilitation services. It is a potentially expensive model that does not necessarily result in the highest possible labor market participation. This type of policy can be found in the Nordic countries as well as in Germany and the Netherlands.

The "liberal disability policy" has a much less generous compensation goal, with lower benefit levels and a much higher threshold in the qualification for benefit receipt. It is less expensive overall, but the stronger inbuilt employment incentives due to less generous benefits are combined with average level integration policy goals. Policies applied in Australia, New Zealand, United Kingdom, Canada, and the United States fall into this category.

The "corporatist disability policy model" can be seen as an intermediate model, located between the other two. This model, which is found in European countries, includes some examples (e.g., Austria, Belgium) that stress well-developed rehabilitation systems and moderate benefit levels, and others with less well-developed employment and rehabilitation policies (e.g., Czech Republic, Italy). Benefits are relatively accessible and generous and employment programs are quite developed but not as extended as in the first model.

The OECD study used two dimensions to compare disability policies across countries and over time: the benefit system, or compensation measures, and the employment and integration measures. Applying these two dimensions, three types of policy reforms could be discerned across OECD countries for the past two decades.

The first one regards an *expansion of employment integration measures*. Disability policies of most OECD countries have shifted their focus from income replacement toward a more employment-oriented approach. Measures are aimed at helping people with disability to stay in, return to, or find work. These policies often include a combination of measures to support both workers and employers.

A measure introduced in many countries is antidiscrimination legislation. It aims to ensure equal treatment of people with disability in several areas, including employment, often covering job promotion, hiring, and dismissal procedures. When considering disability and equal treatment at work, a recent study by the Academic Network of European Disability Experts noted that several countries have introduced new laws or adapted existing regulations. Information on the impact of these rules on the job retention of persons with disabilities is very restricted or sometimes fully absent. Weaknesses reported from several countries are: poor attention to implementation and, consequently, low utilization by persons with disabilities, lack of awareness in employers, and lack of action confronting the stigma attached to people with disabilities.[19] Notwithstanding, the Trades Union Congress (a British labor union) noted that as a result of awareness of the Disability Discrimination Act, "it has become more unusual for disabled workers to face dismissal for the simple reason of being disabled, especially among larger employers.[20] The

OECD notes that antidiscrimination legislation is particularly useful for persons with new-onset disabilities who are already in employment, which is the object of this chapter.[21]

Employment quota regulations are another tool used in several countries to stimulate employers to retain or hire people with a disability. The OECD and other sources note, however, that quota obligations only apply to larger employers and in many countries are only partially fulfilled by employers; in addition, enforcement is crucial but often weak or fully missing.[22] As with antidiscrimination legislation, the quota scheme is more useful to keep workers with acquired health restrictions in the work force than to take on new workers with disabilities.

More countries apply other obligations for employers, namely providing sick pay or reasonable workplace accommodation in order to strengthen their sickness management responsibilities. Furthermore, supported employment and modernization of sheltered employment programs, which now aim at increased transfer to the open labor market, have been introduced by countries. All of these integration measures can help ensure that workers with disabilities remain in the workforce, either by making their dismissal more difficult or by facilitating adaptation to their new circumstances.

The second type of reforms focuses on *better coordination of agencies and service provision*. This may, for example, take place through the introduction of a one-stop-shop for benefits and service provision for persons with disabilities and other clients. Improved cooperation or integration of public employment services and social insurance institutions is also going forward in some countries (e.g., Norway, the Netherlands), with the goal of better sharing information and cross-funding interventions. In some countries, improvement of the institutional setup is reached by giving better incentives for benefit authorities. For instance by raising reimbursement rates for active intervention, municipalities are motivated to avoid benefit payments, as happens in Denmark. A more recent development in some countries regards outcome-based funding and payment of service providers, such as milestone payment and employment placement-related funding. In a few countries, voucher systems have been introduced to give clients more freedom of choice in selecting a provider and the services they need.

The third category of reforms mainly comprises a *tightening of benefit schemes*. Regarding sickness absence, this includes reducing benefit levels and intensifying the monitoring of absences. As for disability insurance, this may include more stringent assessment criteria and evaluation methodologies, such as making medical criteria for disability benefit entitlement more consistent. Several countries are also using more stringent vocational criteria to determine eligibility for disability benefits, for example by assessing loss of work capacity in the light of a general labor market criterion as opposed to the criterion of the applicant's employer. In some countries, reforms also include reforms in benefit payment arrangements, such as duration of payment, or in the minimum threshold for disability benefit entitlement. Although the tightening of benefit schemes is not necessarily beneficial to workers with disabilities, this category of reforms also includes stronger work incentives such as allowing the combination of disability benefits with employment income.

7. EXAMPLES OF REFORMS IN EMPLOYMENT AND DISABILITY BENEFIT DEPENDENCY

In this section, some examples of promising reforms are presented. They illustrate how some countries tackled the growth in disability benefit dependency and tried to increase return-to-work rates. They include: experiences with training and other measures (various countries), changing the service provision model (Sweden), or restricting the inflow to benefit dependency by increasing employers' responsibilities during employee sickness periods (the Netherlands).

Sources in the OECD confirm the experiences many evaluators of reforms in the disability-employment area have made before: Rigorous evaluations are lacking, implementation of reforms often lags behind the decision, and the statistical associations between innovations and outcomes are weak. Evaluations of implementation processes are more frequent than impact evaluations. Consequently, conclusions on the outcomes or impact of reforms should be interpreted with care.

7.1 Overview: Reviewing Measures on Employment of Persons with Disabilities

A review of various projects and studies in the United Kingdom showed that a robust answer to the question "what works?" in terms of employment measures for persons with disabilities and other vulnerable groups is quite problematic, due to various circumstances:

1 The *nature of the provision*: The interventions that focus on employment promotion are very heterogeneous; moreover, over time they often change as to content and form.
2 The *nature of the customer groups*: A category of clients discerned in the administration, like persons with disabilities, is shown to include persons with differing circumstances (e.g., educational levels) and needs (care, accessibility) as well as varying attitudes and motivations. One "label," based on eligibility criteria or duration of benefit receipt, simplifies the picture of measures needed.

3 The *nature of the evidence base itself*: Employment measures are not provided in an isolated way, but often are part of a package, comprising various services and provisions. Moreover, the scientific basis of success often
is weak; evaluation studies almost always lack control groups.[23]

Key findings, which were also noted to apply to other vulnerable groups, focus
on the diversity of the clients, the nature of programs and their delivery, the
role of the personal advisor in the employment office, and the relationships
with employers. Further, the study demonstrated that the timing of interventions has impact on the effectiveness of the intervention: The "ideal" timing is
dependent on the context. Besides, there is little evidence that the nature of
the provider—public employment versus private provider—has any systematic impact on effectiveness; the quality, enthusiasm, motivation, and commitment of the staff that provides the services is a far more important factor.

   In 2007, based on documentation and experts interviews in 10 countries,
we collected experiences on selected measures to keep workers with disabilities in the workforce. As to measures related to job retention, a few conclusions can be summarized.[24]

7.1.1 Education and Training

Vocational training is considered a key element for increased employability
and, consequently, is very common for specific categories of persons with
disabilities such as persons with visual, hearing, or learning disabilities
who apply for a job. For other categories, especially persons with nonspe-
cific disabilities, there seem to be fewer specific training programs applied.
In several countries, training is part of multi-stakeholder programs.
Experience (e.g., in Finland, Germany, and Norway) indicates that the close
cooperation of employers, public employment services, and training institutes stimulates employers to provide training and employment for persons with disabilities.

7.1.2 Alterations to the Premises, Adaptations to the Workplace

Adaptations to the workplace were reported to be applied quite often; in fact,
the majority of employers tend to adapt the workplace, if necessary. In many
countries, adaptations at the work site are fully or partially subsidized by
funds provided by public employment services or social insurance agencies.
However, employers often associate obtaining these subsidies with application procedures that require a lot of paperwork. On the other hand it has also
been noted that employers increasingly realize that the costs of adaptations

in general are low. The ergonomic adaptations needed (such as accessibility of venue, work site, or equipment) in general do not need to be very expensive, and adaptations in working hours or working time do not increase costs substantially either. Most common are adaptations of the working hours, followed by ergonomic adaptations. Less popular are measures in the area of organization of labor, because they require a change in working processes or attitudes and may have a larger impact on the organization. Although this impact may be positive for all, the extent of change required often incurs resistance.

7.1.3 Raising Disability Awareness in Organizations

There are considerable differences across countries as to the scope of awareness-raising activities. In Canada, the United Kingdom, and the United States disability awareness training programs for employers are quite common and are considered effective in changing employers' attitudes. In many countries, non-governmental organizations (NGOs) for disabled persons take the initiative and provide courses or seminars. In countries where NGOs have less power, this may be initiated by the government, trade unions, public employment offices, and some employers themselves. Experiences from the Netherlands and the United Kingdom indicate that awareness campaigns should not only focus on the employer but also on supervisors, who have to cooperate with and integrate employees with disabilities in working life. The effectiveness of awareness-raising activities is known to be very difficult to evaluate. However, there is some general experience that this intervention has promising results in changing employers' attitudes toward employees or job applicants with disabilities.

Finally, some facilitating and complicating factors for successful interventions for job retention of persons with disabilities can be sketched:

1 Labor shortage problems appear to make employers more willing or interested in disability management policies. This particularly was reported for the services sector (for example, hotels and retail in Germany) or information technology (for example, in Canada and the UK).
2 Three factors are particularly associated with having employed disabled staff at the workplace level: overall awareness of antidiscrimination legislation, having a policy for disabled applicants and employees, and workplace size. Promoting the application of the interventions could be improved by a better focus on and support for small employers (including information on subsidies for job adaptations and awareness campaigns).
3 Financial incentives, such as wage subsidies, seem to have no strong stimulating influence on the employer's willingness to adapt work sites or recruit persons with disabilities. A similar practical observation often heard was

that positive experiences by employers themselves have a strong impact on future disability policies in the firm.

7.2 Sweden: Integrated Service Provision in Rehabilitation

The Swedish reform in service provision started with the basic observation that persons with disabilities, and other socially excluded individuals, may suffer from a range of varied problems, such as underemployment, poor health, and reduced educational qualifications. The independence of various administrators and service providers, with their own budgets, criteria, and target groups may create fragmented services and lack of continuity in support to the client. Moreover, bureaucracy may increase as clients are being passed from one body to another or neglected altogether.

The Swedish government launched a number of projects to promote an integrated, multidimensional approach to social inclusion, thereby aiming to offer better services to individuals in need. The policy introduced allows for financial coordination at the municipality level between actors who usually operate with substantial financial and organizational independence. The public organizations involved are the social insurance offices, primary health care services, municipal social services, and the employment board.[25]

Persons with health restrictions were helped by a one-stop shop, with a pooled budget, which is administered by an independent coordinating body. In the initial pilot projects, clients' major underlying problems were related to mental health problems, musculoskeletal disorders, complex social problems, or other causes of long-term work reduction. They now could rely on one front office for intake and service delivery. The latter may include:

1 *Preventive and promotional activities*: interventions to prevent absence due to illness and combat social exclusion. Working methods include interviews and discussions, theme-based sessions, group activities, dissemination of information, and education.
2 *Socio-medical activities*, to reduce waiting times and shorten patient treatment as well as to speed up the return to work or rehabilitation. Services are provided by inter-professional teams at six primary health care centers.
3 *Occupational activities*, which have as their objective to get people back into work more quickly, or into the right rehabilitation program, with less delay. Interventions also aim to reduce passivity and increase the self-confidence and self-awareness of participants.

Evaluation studies conducted by Göteborg University showed that the model managed to create a common responsibility and ensured more structure and continuity in activities for clients. Moreover, the new collaborative structures and procedures increased the knowledge and skills of project participants. A new way of working had been introduced, in which decisions based on a common approach emerged via new communication pathways. The resulting collaborations led to new ideas about ways to meet users' needs and implement rehabilitation or treatment interventions. Also, clients indicated that they had had positive experiences with the model, compared with the traditional procedures.

On the other hand, additional research—which only focused on clients with musculoskeletal disorders—found no evidence that the model resulted in better health or a reduction in sickness absence. Despite the new working methods and procedures, clients in need of medical care received the same kind of treatment and rehabilitation as patients at control health care centers. The results showed no difference in change of health status between the groups.

Finally, an analysis of the new organizational model's effect on cost trends in the benefit systems showed a tendency toward lower costs. The national evaluation (period 1997 until 2004) showed that coordinated interventions had been strengthened, with favorable results in terms of sickness benefit costs, disability benefits, and trend changes in long-term sickness absence.

7.3 The Netherlands: More Incentives and Responsibilities for Employers

The Netherlands has a long tradition in attempting to reduce the high levels of sickness absence and the growing numbers of persons on disability benefits.[26] After various changes in the benefits system, measures showed to have impact if they included incentives and obligations for the employer. From January 1994, a compulsory wage payment period was introduced: Small employers had to pay wage during sickness for a maximum of two weeks per episode, whereas large employers had to pay for an initial 6 weeks. Subsequently, social security took over the payment of benefits.

Due to its success—sickness absence dropped by almost 20% within a year—from March 1996 onwards the wage payment period was extended to one year; sickness absence rates, however, did not decline further. In 2002 the Improved Gatekeeper Law came into force; this law aimed to affect long-term sickness absence and prevent exclusive reliance on the disability benefit scheme. The law required regular contact between employer and the sick-listed employee, as well as the use of a work resumption plan agreed upon by employer and employee. If the worker was not capable of returning to his own or to another job in the firm, the employer also faced increased responsibility to find alternative work for the worker.

Employers were further stimulated to do more on integration and prevention of disability benefit claims when—from 2004—compulsory wage payment for sick employees was extended to two years. The employer may insure that risk with private insurance, but he is also free to bear the costs. Monitoring of sickness absence, check of work incapacity, and advice on work resumption or temporary job adaptations were laid in the hands of the occupational health services. Employers are obliged by law to contract such a service, which can be either in-company, or external. In addition, in 2006 a major reform was introduced in the disability benefit system by tightening criteria and reducing benefit levels.

Several evaluative studies were held to assess the implementation and impact of the changes in the fields of sickness absence and disability policy. The combined results of increased employer tasks on sickness absence management and less attractive disability benefits reduced the level of sickness absence by 20%. Moreover, the annual inflow into the disability benefit scheme had become 40,000 by 2007–2008, down from 70,000 to 100,000 per year in the preceding decade.[27]

More importantly, beyond the reduced numbers, the innovations also affected the attitudes and behavior of various stakeholders. Employers had become more aware of the costs of failed return to work and the need for adequate personnel policy and appropriate working conditions. They also had first-hand experience of the possibilities and tools that relate to sickness absence and disability. On the other hand the new procedures also evoked complaints about the paperwork and time required.

Employee surveys showed increased workers' awareness of their own responsibilities during sickness absence, such as taking on an active role in recovery and work resumption. Workers also learned that long-term sickness and disability would imply serious income reductions. As a negative consequence, a substantial minority reported fear of pressure from their employer or occupational physician to resume work too early.

Apart from the occupational physicians, health care professionals needed the most time to adapt and initially had the most objections. They also doubted the viewpoint that—in many cases—work resumption should start before full recovery and—when feasible—early partial work resumption should be aimed at. Finally some health care professionals criticized the "de-medicalization" included in the new policies.

8. CROSS-NATIONAL EXPERIENCES AND CHALLENGES

Disability policies for workers who are already in the workforce are in a process of change, developing in various directions and with varying intensities and results. After many decades of focusing on benefit schemes that showed few pathways to the labor force, with poor or moderate results, some countries have been introducing substantial reforms, which differ as to domains, actors involved, and impact. Although cross-national differences in social security arrangements, labor relationships, or attitudes of relevant stakeholders—including social partners, NGOs, and medical professionals—can restrict the direct transfer of "foreign models," the huge amount of available information allows a much more deliberate assessment of alternative policies than one decade ago. It also allows insight into measures that seem to work well, or are considered promising.

When focusing on the situation of persons in employment who acquire disabilities during working life, lessons on several provisions or measures can be noted. In various stages—from mild health problems and temporary work incapacity up to dependency on disability benefits—a range of measures are available to keep workers with disabilities in the work force and to facilitate return to work:

1 *Sickness benefits*, which adequately replace a certain percentage of income. With a few exceptions (for example, the United States) the large majority of countries provides such a basic arrangement.[28]
2 *Early intervention* and—where possible—"intertwining" of recovery and return to work. In this way, sickness absence can be prevented from becoming permanent. Moreover, in an early stage workers with partial disabilities can be activated, as opposed to simply put onto the pathway of claiming disability benefits.
3 *Larger employer involvement*, supported by positive and negative financial incentives. It is implemented—or proposed—in a growing number of countries, aiming to manage absence instead of passively relying on medical certification and social security evaluations. Furthermore, health promotion and provision of temporary or permanent accommodation of work should be included.[29]
4 *Job protection and restriction of other exit routes*, like dismissal of workers due to sickness or disabilities. This may be facilitated further by employment quotas or antidiscrimination legislation.
5 For persons with disabilities leaving employment and becoming dependent on *disability benefits or pensions*, their benefit status should have a *nonpermanent character* (at least for younger recipients), in order to oppose the beliefs that disability is a stable situation and the end of working life. Regular assessments by social security as to capacities and needs and supporting rehabilitation measures may be helpful for leaving the disability benefit rolls after some years.

The need for applying these measures is growing because several trends may affect the scope of the health problems emerging in the working age population.

First, the global growth of *chronic diseases* not only challenges health care and health care expenditures but also employers. The lives of an increasing number of people in low- and high-income countries are being affected by heart disease, stroke, cancer, chronic respiratory diseases, and diabetes.[30] As the likelihood of developing a disabling chronic condition increases with age, the number of persons with chronic diseases will increase due to the aging of work forces and also the implementation of higher age limits to claim old-age pensions.

Second, for about a decade an additional age-related pattern becomes visible in many European countries: *Increasing numbers of younger persons with health problems* are entering disability benefit schemes. Some young persons with disabilities are meeting barriers in the transition from education to employment; others had a job and faced loss of employment due to health factors; or they had to move to sheltered employment. As the phenomenon is quite recent and more prevalent in some countries than in others, the OECD suggests an increase in awareness-raising activities among other measures.

Finally we already noted the shift in morbidity patterns in new recipients of disability benefits: *Disabilities related to mental health problems* now predominate and their proportion is on the increase (except in Australia, the United States, and Canada). Sources at the OECD indicate that depression is the leading cause of disability in high-income countries.[31] Moreover, most of the costs related to mental health problems are not in health care, but in reduced productivity at work, temporary absences, early retirement, and receipt of disability benefits with virtually no outflow back into the workforce. In various countries, new approaches and measures in areas such as public health and human resources management are being developed and tested to counteract this trend.

These trends make it increasingly important to get disability and employment schemes right. Whereas in the past, governments have relied on providing benefits based on a somewhat arbitrary "work capacity" definition of disability, it is becoming clear that the outcomes created by this approach are not socially or financially sustainable for countries, businesses, and workers themselves. For workers that acquire disabilities well into their working lives, which are a group that is only going to grow in number in the coming decades, there is an urgency to ensure that their attachment to the labor force, if it is ever interrupted, resumes whenever possible. In those cases in which disability results in a real and permanent loss of some significant degree of work capacity, an adequate safety net is necessary. However, the examples in this chapter have demonstrated that, in many others, policy and program approaches by both government and employers can lead to remaining in or (re)entering the workforce with minimal cost and tangible benefits. Although these approaches are in need of more stringent evaluations and better knowledge on transferability to different environments, sufficient evidence on what works already exists to begin to take effective action.

NOTES

1. Organization for Economic Co-Operation and Development (2010). *Sickness, disability and work: breaking the barriers. A synthesis of findings across OECD countries.* Paris, France: OECD.
2. See Mont, D. (2007). Measuring Disability Prevalence Measurement. Social Protection Discussion Paper 0706. Washington, D.C: World Bank.
3. Ibid.; also, Scheil-Adlung, X., & Sandner, L. (2010). The Case for Paid Sick Leave. World Health Report (2010) Background Paper, No 9. Geneva, Switzerland: World Health Organization.
4. Black, C., & Frost, D. (2011) *Health at work—an independent review of sickness absence.* London, United Kingdom: Secretary of State for Work and Pensions.
5. Waddell, G., Burton, A.K., & Kendall, N.A.S. (2008) *Vocational rehabilitation: what works for whom, and when?* London, United Kingdom: Department for Work and Pensions.
6. Organization for Economic Co-Operation and Development (2010). *Sickness, disability and work.*
7. Organization for Economic Co-Operation and Development (2011). *Sick on the job? Myths and realities about mental health at work.* Paris, France: OECD.
8. Organization for Economic Co-Operation and Development (2010). *Sickness, disability and work.*
9. Ibid.
10. Waddell, Burton, & Kendall (2008) *Vocational rehabilitation.*
11. Organization for Economic Co-Operation and Development (2010). *Sickness, disability and work.*
12. Mont (2007). Measuring Disability Prevalence.
13. Organization for Economic Co-Operation and Development (2009). *Sickness, Disability and Work, keeping track in the economic downturn.* High-Level Forum, Stockholm, Sweden 14-15 May.
14. Black & Frost (2011) *Health at work.*
15. Cited in Lindahl, B. (2010). *The constant hunt for ways to limit sick leave.* Nordic Labour Journal. Retrieved March 31, 2013, from http://www.nordiclabourjour-nal. org/i-fokus/in-focus-2010/theme-nordic-region-tightens-sick-leave-rules/the-constant-hunt-for-ways-to-limit-sick-leave
16. European Foundation for the Improvement of Living and Working Conditions (2010). *Absence from work.* Dublin, Ireland: Eurofound.
17. Livanos, I., & Zangelidis, A. (2010) *Sickness Absence: a Pan European study.* Munich, Germany: MPRA.
18. Organization for Economic Co-Operation and Development (2010). *Sickness, disability and work.*
19. Shima, I., & Rodrigues, R. (2009). *The implementation of EU social inclusion and social protections strategies in European countries with reference to disabled people.* Leeds, United Kingdom: Academic Network of European Disability Experts.

20. Trades Union Congress (2010). *Sickness absence and disability discrimination.* Retrieved March 31, 2013, from http://www.tuc.org.uk/tucfiles/526/Sickness_Absence_and_Disability_Discrimination_Feb2013.pdf
21. Organization for Economic Co-Operation and Development (2010). *Sickness, disability and work.*
22. See also Cheretis, J. (2008) *Onderzoek Bonus-Malus binnen de Rijksoverheid.* Leiden, The Netherlands: Instituut Bestuurskunde, Universiteit Leiden.
23. Hasluck, C., & Green, A.E. (2007) *What works for whom? A review of evidence and meta-analysis for the Department for Work and Pensions.* Research Report No. 407. London, United Kingdom: Department for Work and Pensions.
24. Prins, R. & Reijenga, F. (2007). *International exploration into specific HR measures for the employment of Persons with Disabilities: insights and lessons from selected countries.* Dublin, Ireland and Leiden, The Netherlands: Horwath/Astri.
25. Prins, R. (2007). *Sweden 2006: Integrated Services in Rehabilitation—on coordination of organisation and financing.* Synthesis report. European Commission. Retrieved March 31, 2013, from http://ec.europa.eu/employment_social/social_inclusion/docs/2006/pr_sw_en.pdf
26. Anema, H., Prinz, C., & Prins, R. (2013). Sickness and disability policy interventions. In P. Loisel & H. Anema (Eds.) *Handbook of Work Disability: Prevention and Management.* New York: Springer.
27. See e.g. De Jong, P., Veerman, T.J., van der Burg, C., & Schrijvershof, C. (2010). *Nederland is niet ziek meer Van WAO-debakel naar WIA-mirakel.* Research report. Leiden, The Netherlands: Astri.
28. Scheil-Adlung & Sandner (2010). The Case for Paid Sick Leave.
29. European Foundation for the Improvement of Living and Working Conditions (2010) *Absence from work.*
30. Van Eijndhoven, M.A.J., & Prins, R. (2010) *Adapting social security health care systems to trends in chronic diseases; Overview of policies and experiences in some ISSA member states.* Geneva, Switzerland: ISSA/CVZ/Astri.
31. Organization for Economic Co-Operation and Development (2011). *Sick on the job?*

SECTION THREE

The Role of Government

CHAPTER 11

Employment Challenges and Successes in Low- and Middle-Income Countries

SOPHIE MITRA

1. INTRODUCTION

How disability affects employment outcomes is an empirical question. The direction and magnitude of the effect is expected to vary depending on the types and severity of prevailing disabilities, how they match with available jobs and their required tasks, the accessibility of the general environment (both physical and social), schools, workplaces, the existence and success of labor market programs, and the presence of discrimination. The relevance and intensity of some of these pathways depends on cultural contexts insofar as negative attitudes toward the employment potential of persons with disabilities on the part of employers, within the household, or in society at large, might limit access to work. The policy context is also relevant; for instance, are there vocational rehabilitation programs available? Are there disability insurance or assistance programs? Such programs, depending on how they are designed and put into practice, could facilitate, constrain, or not affect access to employment for persons with disabilities. One should of course keep in mind that low- and middle-income countries are a very heterogeneous group of countries in their levels of human development and in their environments. For example, in terms of urbanization, 55% of people live in rural areas in low- and middle-income countries,[1] but this share varies greatly from country to country. For instance, in Africa, it ranges from a low of 14% in Gabon to a high of 89% in Burundi.[2]

How disability is conceptualized influences how policies and programs to improve the employment of persons with disabilities are framed. One should therefore note that, in this chapter, disability is defined within the conceptual framework of the capability approach.[3] The capability approach framework is compatible with the International Classification of Disability, Functioning and Health.[4] Disability is a deprivation in terms of functioning (i.e., what people actually do [achievements]) or capability (i.e., practical opportunities). Disability may result from four types of factors and their interaction: (1) the nature of impairment; (2) personal characteristics (e.g., age, gender, race); (3) the environment, in its physical, economic, social, political, and cultural aspects; and (4) the resources available to the individual. These factors are thus at the levels of both the individual and the environment, and policies aimed to improve employment outcomes and opportunities will therefore take place at these two levels and at their interface.

In exploring how to improve labor market outcomes for persons with disabilities in low- and middle-income countries, this chapter first reviews several labor market outcomes across disability status in low- and middle-income countries, followed by a discussion of the constraints on the employment of persons with disabilities. The third section focuses on the development of disability and employment policy and proposes a framework to guide the selection of disability and employment interventions. A review of possible interventions and available evidence for the general population and persons with disabilities follows, concluding with a discussion of next steps.

2. A SITUATIONAL ANALYSIS OF EMPLOYMENT IN LOW- AND MIDDLE-INCOME COUNTRIES

Data are available for three broad labor market outcomes in several low- and middle-income countries: employment rates, employment in the informal sector, and wages. There are of course many outcomes that are relevant in understanding the status of employment for persons with disabilities in low- and middle-income countries, including job opportunities, occupations, work hours, working conditions, type of work (in the open labor market or in sheltered workshops),and job duration (weeks or months worked on the same job). However, given that the literature on many of these is very limited, this chapter focuses on employment rates, employment in the informal sector, and wages, as these data are available in low- and middle-income countries across disability status.

2.1 Employment Rates

The employment rate (or employment-population ratio) is the number of employed persons as a percentage of the working age population.[5] Employment rate estimates for persons with disabilities in low-income countries stand at 58.6% for males and 20.1% for females, compared with 71.2% and 31.5% for males and females without disabilities, respectively.[6] In low- and middle-income countries, there are a few country case studies published in peer-reviewed journals. Studies from Uganda,[7] South Africa,[8] India,[9] Mexico,[10] Vietnam,[11] the Philippines,[12] Rwanda,[13] and Zambia[14] all find lower employment rates for persons with disabilities. Expanding to other studies, similar findings are also found in Namibia and Mozambique,[15] Lesotho,[16] Malawi,[17] and Peru,[18] but not in Zimbabwe.[19] Drawing any general conclusion from this literature is problematic given that such studies use different measures of disability. Table 11.1 gives the employment rates for persons with and without disabilities for 15 low-income countries using the same disability measure and the same data collection instrument across countries. In 13 of the 15 countries, the employment rate of persons with disabilities is consistently lower than that of persons without disabilities. In nine out of 15 countries, there is a statistically significant disability gap showing lower employment rates for persons with disabilities. There are six countries in which the difference is not statistically significant: Ghana, Kenya, Malawi, Zambia, Zimbabwe, and the Dominican Republic.[20] In Zimbabwe, Eide and coworkers find a similar result and explain that this might be due to an extensive system of specialized services for persons with disabilities, including opportunities in sheltered workshops.[21] Table 11.1 also shows employment rates for persons with single and multiple disabilities compared with persons without disabilities in 12 countries.[22] Persons with single or multiple disabilities have lower employment rates compared with persons without disabilities in eight and nine countries, respectively. Persons with multiple disabilities have even lower employment rates than persons with single disabilities. Overall, the evidence suggests that there is a disability gap in employment rates in most low- and middle-income countries and that policies that promote access to employment may be particularly important for the economic well-being of persons and households with disabilities in many low- and middle-income countries.

Table 11.1 also shows that in countries with a significant difference across disability status, there is much variation in the employment gap, from a low of eight percentage points in Lao to a high of 22 percentage points in Burkina Faso. Overall, although employment rates are lower for persons with disabilities in most low-income countries, the extent of the difference is highly variable from country to country. This heterogeneity has important implications for policy and program design because one employment disability policy may not fit all. A more in-depth analysis would be needed for each of the countries with a disability gap to develop specific and contextualized policy recommendations with respect to employment. An in-depth analysis would also be needed in countries with no significant gap in the number working, in order to determine if there may be differences in other labor market outcomes. Finally, few studies break down employment rates by disability type or run models

Table 11.1 EMPLOYMENT RATES BY DISABILITY STATUS[23]

	Persons Without Disability	Persons with Disability	Gap	Persons with Single Disability	Gap	Persons with Multiple Disabilities	Gap
sub-Saharan Africa							
Burkina Faso	0.59 (0.01)	0.00 (0.00)	0.59 ***	0.35 (0.04)	0.25 ***	0.33 (0.07)	0.26 ***
Ghana	0.77 (0.01)	0.00 (0.00)	0.77 ***	NA		NA	
Kenya	0.63 (0.02)	0.00 (0.00)	0.63 ***	0.62 (0.07)	0.01	0.41 (0.10)	0.22 *
Malawi	0.52 (0.01)	0.00 (0.00)	0.52 ***	0.53 (0.03)	-0.01	0.44 (0.06)	0.07
Mauritius	0.67 (0.01)	0.00 (0.00)	0.67 ***	0.52 (0.03)	0.15 ***	0.29 (0.05)	0.38 ***
Zambia	0.60 (0.01)	0.00 (0.00)	0.60 ***	NA		NA	
Zimbabwe	0.33 (0.01)	0.00 (0.00)	0.33 ***	0.36 (0.04)	-0.03	0.31 (0.06)	0.01
Asia							
Bangladesh	0.54 (0.01)	0.00 (0.00)	0.54 ***	0.40 (0.03)	0.13 ***	0.25 (0.03)	0.29 ***
Lao	0.81 (0.01)	0.00 (0.00)	0.81 ***	NA		NA	

Pakistan	0.52	0.00	0.52 ***	0.31	0.21 ***	0.27	0.25 ***
	(0.01)	(0.00)		(0.04)		(0.08)	
Philippines	0.55	0.00	0.55 ***	0.49	0.05 *	0.44	0.10 *
	(0.01)	(0.00)		(0.02)		(0.05)	
Latin America							
Brazil	0.61	0.00	0.61 ***	0.51	0.10 **	0.40	0.21 ***
	(0.01)	(0.00)		(0.03)		(0.06)	
Dominican Republic	0.64	0.00	0.64 ***	0.57	0.07	0.58	0.06
	(0.01)	(0.00)		(0.04)		(0.08)	
Mexico	0.56	0.00	0.56 ***	0.42	0.14 ***	0.37	0.20 ***
	(0.00)	(0.00)		(0.02)		(0.04)	
Paraguay	0.65	0.00	0.65 ***	0.53	0.12 ***	0.41	0.25 ***
	(0.01)	(0.00)		(0.04)		(0.08)	

Results by single/multiple disability status are not presented for Ghana, Zambia, and Lao due to a low number of observations of individuals with multiple disabilities. The sample size of persons with single or multiple disabilities was too small in most countries for it to be broken down by gender.

of the determinants of employment among persons with disabilities using disability types as explanatory variables. Those that do also show variation in employment across disability types.[24] This may also have implications for policy, as one policy or intervention may not affect people with different disability types in a similar manner.

In country-level studies, Eide and coworkers, Loeb and Eide, and Mitra and Sambamoorthi show that persons with disabilities in different countries have a higher propensity to be self-employed.[25] Table 11.2 shows that in a cross-country study, in nine out of 15 low-income countries, there is a significantly higher proportion of workers who are self-employed for persons with disabilities.[26] Further research is needed on informal/formal employment across disability status in low- and middle-income countries. If, in a given country, persons with disabilities are found to be disproportionately in the informal sector, then it becomes important to find the extent to which they are constrained to the informal sector due to barriers to the formal sector or the extent to which they may choose to be in the informal sector.

In most low- and middle-income countries, a large majority of persons with and without disabilities are employed in the informal sector.[27] Exceptions include a few countries in which the informal sector provides less employment than the formal sector (e.g., South Africa). Table 11.2 shows that in most of the countries studied, a majority of workers, with or without disabilities, are self-employed. Given that in low- and middle-income countries, employment is found in the informal sector most of the time, interventions to improve labor market outcomes in general and for persons with disabilities in particular, need to take place in the informal sector.

2.2 Wages

It is often reported that, once employed, persons with disabilities commonly earn less than their counterparts without disabilities. Equally important as the disparities in the employment rate is therefore the wage gap between persons with and without disabilities. There is a large empirical literature on the wage gap between persons with and without disability in high-income countries.[27] Studies in low- and middle-income countries are rare, and given the different characteristics of labor markets with large informal sectors, it is unclear whether the wage gap also affects these countries. Recent results for southern Africa and India are mixed. In southern Africa, a wage gap was found in Namibia and Malawi, but not in Zambia and Zimbabwe.[29] In India, a wage gap was found in Uttar Pradesh but not in Tamil Nadu for males in rural labor markets.[30] Further research is needed in low- and middle-income countries based on nationally representative data, especially in countries with primarily

	Persons without Disability	Persons with Disability	Difference	Persons with Single Disability	Difference	Persons with Multiple Disabilities	Difference
sub-Saharan Africa							
Burkina Faso	0.91	0.94	0.02	0.92	0.01	0.96	0.05 ***
	(0.01)	(0.02)		(0.00)		(0.00)	
Ghana	0.82	0.83	0.01	NA		NA	
	(0.01)	(0.03)		(0.00)		(0.00)	
Kenya	0.62	0.75	0.13	0.60	-0.01	0.83	0.22 ***
	(0.02)	(0.05)		(0.00)		(0.00)	
Malawi	0.74	0.84	0.10 **	0.80	0.06 ***	0.91	0.17 ***
	(0.01)	(0.03)		(0.00)		(0.00)	
Mauritius	0.20	0.29	0.09 *	0.36	0.16 ***	0.20	0.00
	(0.01)	(0.04)		(0.00)		(0.00)	
Zambia	0.81	0.89	0.07 *	NA	-0.01	NA	
	(0.01)	(0.03)		(0.00)		(0.00)	
Zimbabwe	0.45	0.68	0.23 ***	0.58	***	0.78	0.33 ***
	(0.02)	(0.05)		(0.00)		(0.00)	
Asia							
Bangladesh	0.81	0.87	0.06 *	0.88	***	0.85	0.03 ***
	(0.01)	(0.02)		(0.00)			
Lao PDR	0.83	0.84	0.01	NA	-0.01	NA	

(continued)

Table 11.2 (CONTINUED)

	Persons without Disability	Persons with Disability	Difference	Persons with Single Disability	Difference	Persons with Multiple Disabilities	Difference
	(0.01)	(0.03)		(0.00)		(0.00)	
Pakistan	0.68	0.67	-0.01	0.75	0.06 ***	0.46	-0.23
	(0.01)	(0.07)		(0.00)		(0.00)	
Philippines	0.50	0.60	0.10 ***	0.56	0.06 ***	0.66	0.17 ***
	(0.01)	(0.03)		(0.00)		(0.00)	
Latin America							
Brazil	0.41	0.55	0.14 ***	0.55	0.14 ***	0.55	0.14 ***
	(0.01)	(0.04)		(0.00)		(0.00)	
Dominican Republic	0.47	0.52	0.06	0.61	0.15 ***	0.43	-0.03
	(0.02)	(0.06)		(0.00)		(0.00)	
Mexico	0.45	0.53	0.08 **	0.58	0.12 ***	0.46	0.00
	(0.01)	(0.03)		(0.00)		(0.00)	
Paraguay	0.52	0.67	0.15 ***	0.72	0.20 ***	0.63	0.11 ***
	(0.01)	(0.04)		(0.00)		(0.00)	

Results by single/multiple disability status are not presented for Ghana, Zambia, and Lao due to a low number of observations.
The sample size of persons with single or multiple disabilities was too small in most countries for it to be broken down by gender.
The self-employment rate is the percentage of the employed who are self-employed.

wage employment and small informal labor markets such as South Africa or Ethiopia.

3. CONSTRAINTS TO EMPLOYMENT

There are many constraints on the employment of persons with disabilities in low- and middle-income countries. Understanding these constraints is essential to informing policymaking. In a country with a low employment rate of persons with disabilities compared with that for persons without disabilities, before developing a policy or program to enhance employment among persons with disabilities, one needs to find out why the employment rate is low. It could be due to several factors, including a lack of access to assistive devices or personal assistance, or contextual factors, such as a physically inaccessible work environment or negative attitudes with respect to the work capabilities of persons with disabilities. Once the main causes for the low employment rates for persons with disabilities in a particular country are better understood, it becomes feasible to develop evidence-based programs and policies to promote employment among persons with disabilities. These constraints are categorized into constraints outside the labor market and constraints inside the labor market.

3.1 Constraints Outside the Labor Market

Outside the labor market, two main types of constraints may hinder persons with disabilities' access to the labor market: limited access to education and environmental barriers.

3.1.1 Limited Access to Education

Education is a pathway toward improving employment outcomes. Research has indeed established that every year of schooling increases individual wages for both men and women by a worldwide average of about 10%. In poor countries, the gains can be even greater for persons with disabilities. One study using data for Nepal shows higher wage returns than for persons without disabilities: The estimated rate of return to education for persons with disabilities is very high, ranging from 30.4% to 33.2%.[32] Despite this high rate of return to education for persons with disabilities in Nepal, educational attainment is low compared with persons without disabilities. There is similar evidence that persons with disabilities have lower educational attainment in many low- and middle-income countries: Uganda,[33] South Africa,[34]

Eastern Europe,[35] 15 countries in Africa, Asia, and Latin America,[36] Vietnam,[37] Rwanda,[38] Afghanistan and Zambia,[39] and India.[40] There is also evidence that children with disabilities have lower school attendance rates.[41]

3.1.2 Environmental Barriers

In addition, persons with disabilities experience an array of environmental barriers on a daily basis that compound difficulties in making employment possible.[42] If persons with disabilities cannot access public transport, they will not look for work, knowing that they have no means to get to the workplace. If health care facilities are not accessible, persons with disabilities may not receive the services they need to be able to work.

Although the literature on disparities in access to health care in low- and middle-income countries is very limited, studies in India and urban Sierra Leone show that individuals with disabilities have a reduced access to health care.[43] Table 11.3 gives the percentage of persons with disabilities in seven countries in southern Africa who report that different facilities are accessible. Table 11.3 shows that in these countries, health care clinics are the most accessible, followed by hospitals and public transportation. It should be noted that figures in Table 11.3 overestimate accessibility, given that persons who have never used the facilities, including persons who never go to a hospital because of extreme accessibility issues, are not included in the sample.

The impact on environmental barriers is further compounded by limited access to assistive devices and personal assistance. Table 11.4 shows that in southern African countries, one fourth or less of persons with disabilities use assistive devices.

3.2 Labor Market Constraints

In addition to constraints outside the labor market, persons with disabilities may face constraints in the labor market. These constraints are listed in Table 11.4 and are explained in the following.

3.2.1 Limited Access to the Workplace

Barriers in the environment may include physical barriers to the actual workplace. Little information is available on the accessibility of workplaces in low- and middle-income countries. Table 11.3 provides the percentage of workers with disabilities in five countries in southern Africa that report that their workplaces are accessible. It varies from a low of 20% in Zimbabwe to a high of

Table 11.3 ACCESSIBILITY OF THE ENVIRONMENT IN SELECTED COUNTRIES
IN AFRICA AS PER THE ASSESSMENT OF PERSONS WITH DISABILITIES[44]

	Percent of Persons with Disabilities Reporting That			Workplaces Are Accessible
	Primary Health Care Clinics Are Accessible	Hospitals Are Accessible	Public Transportation Is Accessible	
Lesotho	67	59	69	88
Malawi	71	69	68	26
Mozambique	78	81	71	56
Swaziland	83	75	64	64
Zambia	85	60	65	68
Zimbabwe	87	82	79	20

Note: This question was only answered by persons with disabilities who had used the facilities (e.g., school) or where these places or facilities were available in their area.

88% in Lesotho. More than half of workers with disabilities report that their workplaces are accessible in four out of six countries. However, this result does not imply that workplace accessibility is satisfactory for most persons with disabilities in these countries, given that these numbers do not take into account the nonemployed, including people who may not have accessed jobs due to the lack of accessibility of the workplace.

3.2.2 Skills Constraints

Persons with disabilities often do not have access to formal educational or skill development opportunities. This may apply to youth with disabilities as well as to persons with adult-onset disabilities. For the latter, skill development may be particularly important if the person is returning to the labor force after a break due to disability onset. Table 11.5 gives the share of persons with disabilities who receive training services among those who report that they need vocational training in six southern African countries. Again, the range is wide across countries, from a low of 7% in Lesotho to a high of 59% in Zambia. In most countries though, a majority of those who report that they need training do receive training.

3.2.3 Lack of Labor Demand

Negative attitudes about the ability of persons with disabilities to be employed have been shown to be a major reason for their lack of access to employment,

Table 11.4 CONSTRAINTS TO EMPLOYMENT FOR PERSONS WITH DISABILITIES AND POSSIBLE INTERVENTIONS[45]

Constraint in the Labor Market		Possible Intervention	
		Evidence-Based Intervention	Mixed or No Evidence, but Theoretically Sound
Lack of access to the workplace		*Supported employment**	CBR
Skills constraint	Insufficient basic skills		Second chance programs
			CBR
	Insufficient or mis-match in technical skills	Comprehensive training programs	*Peer training*
			CBR
	Type of job—type of disability mismatch	Information on returns to technical specialties	
		*Supported employment**	
Lack of labor demand	Slow job growth economy		Public service programs
			Labor-intensive public works
	Employer discrimination	Affirmative action programs*	Antidiscrimination laws
			Quotas
		*Supported employment**	*Awareness campaigns*
			CBR
Lack of labor supply	Negative attitudes in the household		*Awareness campaigns*
	or low self expectations among persons with disabilities		*Empowerment programs*
			CBR
Job search constraints	Job matching	Employment services*	Technology-based information sharing
			CBR
Firm start-up constraint	Lack of access to financial or social capital	Comprehensive entrepreneurship programs	Microfinance
			CBR

*For this intervention, very little or no evidence is available in developing countries, but there is evidence in developed countries.
Interventions written in italics are targeted at persons with disabilities. Other interventions can be implemented as mainstream interventions (for the general population), for different target groups, including persons with disabilities, or as targeted programs only for persons with disabilities.
CBR stands for community-based rehabilitation.

Table 11.5 ACCESS TO ASSISTIVE DEVICES AND TRAINING[46]

	Percent of Persons with Disabilities	
	Who Use Assistive Devices	Who Received Training among Those in Need
Lesotho	14	7
Malawi	17	41
Mozambique	19	16
Namibia	18	19
Swaziland	22	15
Zambia	13	59
Zimbabwe	26	25

For the percentage of people who received training among those in need, the denominator includes people who self-reported if they needed vocational training services.

and, if employed, from career advancement opportunities. Negative attitudes may come from the belief that persons with disabilities are less productive than their nondisabled counterparts or from general bias.

3.2.4 Lack of Labor Supply

Negative attitudes and discrimination may not be limited to employers. They also take place on the labor supply side: Through negative attitudes and low expectations, household members may provide an environment that is not conducive to a person with disability's entry into the labor force.[47] In India, it was recently found that negative attitudes are pervasive not only among nondisabled employers, but also among family members and disabled people themselves. Persons with disabilities may have very low self-expectations about their ability to be successfully employed and therefore often do not even try to find employment. Persons who live in a household with a head who has negative attitudes were less likely to be employed than those living in a household in which the head has a positive or neutral attitude on employment and disability.[48] These negative attitudes in the household have received very little attention in the literature on employment and disability. In connection to attitudes within the household, several studies on microfinance in low- and middle-income countries have found that low self-esteem is the main barrier to microfinance.[49]

3.2.5 Job Search Constraints

Social networks, especially friends and family, are known to be good resources during the job search process. In high-income countries, evidence indicates that most of the employed and unemployed turn to friends and relatives for assistance when looking for work.[50] In addition, it has long been recognized that the informal channel of friends and relatives is the most effective way to find jobs.[51] These results apply to the short-term unemployed in general, but studies have shown that they also apply to persons with disabilities.[52] Although no such evidence on the effectiveness of different search methods could be found in low- and middle-income countries, this may be a constraint for persons with disabilities given their tendency to have more limited social networks as a result of negative attitudes toward disability.[53]

3.2.6 Firm Start-up Constraint

As noted earlier, in low- and middle-income countries self-employment is often the main form of employment (see Table 11.2). Limited access to financial and social capital (including relationships to other businesses) is what prevents many individuals in low- and middle-income countries, and persons with disabilities in particular, from starting their own firms. Although the academic literature on microfinance and disability is extremely limited, the lack of access to financial capital was documented in Uganda[54] and reported by several organizations working in low- and middle-income countries.[55]

4. DEVELOPING POLICIES AND INTERVENTIONS TO PROMOTE EMPLOYMENT FOR PERSONS WITH DISABILITIES

Promoting better employment opportunities and outcomes among persons with disabilities in the long-run requires a multidimensional approach that addresses constraints outside and inside the labor market. Any policy or intervention to promote the employment of persons with disabilities needs to start with an assessment of the employment situation of persons with disabilities.

4.1 A Situational Assessment of Disability and Employment

Efforts to improve the employment situation of persons with disabilities at a country, district, or community level need to start with an assessment of the labor market opportunities and outcomes of persons with disabilities and the constraints they face. The objective of such an assessment is first to identify the labor market outcomes that are most in need of improvement. For instance, it could be accessing jobs, retaining jobs, or the types of jobs available to them. Such an assessment needs to start with a broad general profile of disability in the country, including data on disability prevalence overall, type of disability, severity, age at onset (birth or youth, adult, older adult), and cause. It can be followed by a general labor market analysis that focuses on employment rates and the types of jobs available (formal/informal sector, by industry, main occupations, or median earnings/income). Ideally, such data on disability and the labor market need to be broken down by gender and by rural/urban areas. The study should then move onto labor market outcomes for persons with disabilities compared with persons without disabilities, and by disability type among persons with disabilities compared with persons without disabilities.

As explained earlier, there could be a variety of constraints on access to employment, both outside and inside the labor market. This assessment is broad and would also cover the constraints to the employment of persons with disabilities in general and for different subgroups. Persons with different types of disability, different severity levels, males/females, and people in urban versus rural areas may face their own constraints to employment. For this exercise, it is therefore essential to identify first the different groups of interest and second the main constraints to employment for each group.

Of course, the assessment described in the preceding requires a lot of data on disability and on employment. This data may not be available in all cases. For instance, this was found to be the case in a study on disability in 36 countries in Asia.[56] In fact, some low-income countries do not have nationally representative data on the labor market, let alone on disability. However, policy cannot wait for excellent and comprehensive data on disability and employment. In that case, research, even on a small scale, could prove useful. Small-scale participatory research involving multiple stakeholders may go a long way in developing an understanding of the employment situation of persons with disabilities and of the constraints to employment, an exercise that can inform employment and disability policy and interventions.

Stakeholders would include, of course, persons with disabilities who can contribute their expertise from lived experience. They could also include employers, service providers (e.g., social workers), and policymakers and advocates. Although new at the intersection of disability and development studies,[57] participatory research in poverty assessments has become widespread.[58] There are a variety of participatory methods that can be used flexibly, depending on the local resources and constraints.[59]

4.2 Employment and Disability Policy

Many low- and middle-income countries do not have disability policies, let alone employment policies for persons with disabilities. Disability and employment policies are expected to have different priorities across low- and middle-income countries given how different the challenges are in both nature and scope. Therefore, this chapter does not provide blanket recommendations on what a disability and employment policy should include in a low- or middle-income country context. Instead, this section makes one point regarding disability and employment policy: Progress cannot happen in a vacuum, it is linked to progress in other disability policy areas, such as accessibility, education, and rehabilitation. The level of priority of each of these areas with respect the rest is likely to vary depending on local resources and constraints. These areas are intertwined. Progress in the area of accessibility would influence education and employment. Progress in education would help youth with disabilities after they transition to the labor market.

4.3 Framework to Guide Disability and Employment Interventions

This section proposes a guiding framework for disability and employment policy and identifies relevant interventions to improve labor market outcomes for persons with disabilities[60] in low- and middle-income countries. A representation of this framework is given in Figure 11.1. At the outset, it is important to note that the framework proposed in the following can only be implemented effectively if a variety of stakeholders are involved, including persons with disabilities themselves, employers, disabled people's organizations (DPOs), policymakers, and researchers.

4.3.1 Step 1: A Situational Assessment of Disability and Employment

What this assessment needs to include and suggestions on how to conduct it were covered in Section 4.1.

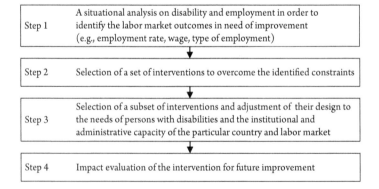

Figure 11.1
Proposed Steps toward Improving Labor Market Outcomes

4.3.2 Step 2: Intervention Selection: What Intervention(s) Can Address Identified Constraints?

After the main employment constraints have been identified, interventions to help the target groups can be identified using prior evidence if any exists. Table 11.5 and Section 5 give a summary of evidence-based labor market interventions. If the main constraints are outside the labor market, one would need to review evidence on interventions to address such constraints, which could be related to lack of access to education and the general environment, among others. The objective of this step is to develop a short list of evidence-based interventions that address the main constraints for relevant groups.

4.3.3 Step 3: Intervention Selection and Design Adjustment according to Country and Group Factors

All the interventions identified in Step 2 may not be feasible in a given country, depending on the institutional, administrative, and socioeconomic context. This is particularly relevant in low- or middle-income country contexts. This step requires assessing the realities of the labor market and the conditions for success of the intervention under consideration. For instance, an employment services intervention would be expected to have limited impact if the labor market suffers from high unemployment and limited or negative job growth. A large-scale public works program would not be feasible in a country with limited administrative capacity.

Another adjustment would need to be made to select interventions that are appropriate and expected to positively affect the relevant target groups. If for example the target group is persons with disabilities in rural areas where there is no formal employment, quotas will not be an appropriate strategy to promote employment access. This step is expected to end with a short list of interventions that are appropriate and feasible in the context and for the target groups under consideration.

4.3.4 Step 4: Program Impact Evaluation

There is a need for impact evaluations to help policymakers in government and other organizations (nongovernmental organizations, including DPOs) decide whether programs are generating the intended effects on the labor market outcomes of persons with disabilities. The impact is the difference between what actually happened as a result of the implementation of the intervention and the counterfactual; that is, what would have happened if the intervention had not taken place at all. For instance, do community-based rehabilitation (CBR) programs produce long-lasting impacts on employment outcomes for persons with disabilities? Ideally, one also needs to conduct a cost–benefit analysis to assess if the intervention was efficiently implemented.

The development field (researchers and some donors) has recently increasingly embraced impact evaluations and is moving toward assessing changes at the micro level in the lives of program participants. This move toward more impact evaluations in part contributed the evidence described in the following on labor market programs. Despite calls for program evaluations in the field of disability in low- and middle-income countries,[61] such evaluations remain rare, but they are acutely needed to assess the impact of interventions that are tailored at persons with disabilities. How do we assess impact? There are more and more resources on how to conduct rigorous evaluations[62] and sources to fund evaluations, including from donors. Evaluation needs to be incorporated at the planning stage of a program to affect design and to include a budget for evaluation activities. Impact evaluations are needed to inform stakeholders and potential program participants on the effectiveness and efficiency of interventions and to guide future policies.

5. A REVIEW OF THE EVIDENCE ON SELECTED ACTIVE MARKET INTERVENTIONS

Evidence on the impact of several labor market interventions is reviewed in the following. Interventions include laws and regulations as well as labor market programs. They may be mainstream (for the general population) or targeted (at persons with disabilities).

5.1 Interventions on Workplace Accessibility

In the formal sector of high-income countries and also some low- and middle-income countries like South Africa, there are reasonable accommodation requirements that are central to nondiscrimination legislation for persons with disabilities. As per the United Nations Convention on the Rights of Persons with Disabilities:

> Reasonable accommodation means necessary and appropriate modification and adjustments not imposing a disproportionate or undue burden, where needed in a particular case, to ensure to persons with disabilities the enjoyment or exercise on an equal basis with others of all human rights and fundamental freedoms.

Requirements for employers to make reasonable accommodations necessary for a disabled worker to fully perform his or her duties can be voluntary (e.g., Denmark) or mandatory (e.g., United States).

5.2 Interventions to Address Skills Constraints

5.2.1 Basic Skills Training

Basic skills training programs are a potential solution to address the lack of skills of individuals who have already left the schooling system. Mainstream second chance programs teach basic skills to youth who did not acquire them by the time they left the schooling system. They teach literacy and numeracy skills, sometimes in combination with technical and life skills, and may provide equivalency degrees. The *Chilecalifa* post-schooling program in Chile is designed to provide basic education and/or technical and vocational training. This program is indistinguishable from an ordinary diploma program. Although the evidence on the impact of such programs is still developing, preliminary results from evaluations or monitoring data from low- and middle-income countries are encouraging. The *Chilecalifa* program has been particularly effective in increasing wages and post-program schooling for women. Another example of such programs is the *Biruh Tesfa* program in Ethiopia that "creates safe spaces in which [program participants] are taught literacy and other skills, [which] seem to have increased literacy among participants."[63]

5.2.2 Technical Skills Training

5.2.2.1 Traditional Institution-Based Training

There is little reliable evidence on the impact of training on improving the labor market standing of the poor in high-income countries and even less in the context of low- and middle-income countries. In the latter, traditional institution-based vocational training programs have seldom been rigorously evaluated, and the evidence that is available points toward mixed results, whether the programs are mainstream[64] or targeted at persons with disabilities. Targeted programs provided in segregated centers were not shown to be effective in getting persons with disabilities jobs because they provide training in a limited range of specialized trades (e.g., carpentry, shoemaking) that do not match the labor market and lead to jobs in few occupations.[65] These training centers are typically located in a few urban areas, far from the communities where most persons with disabilities live and would need to be reintegrated at the end of training. The Government of India provides vocational services to persons with disabilities through Vocational Rehabilitation Centres (VRCs).[66] There are 17 VRCs located in state capitals, and some VRCs have rural rehabilitation extension centers whereby mobile rehabilitation counselors may organize periodic community-based rehabilitation in partnership with nongovernmental organizations. There are 11 rural rehabilitation extension centers. Training is unstructured or semistructured, and entry is allowed at any time of the year. Training is imparted in various trades, including metal, carpentry, radio and electronic equipment services, tailoring, appliance repair, tricycle assembly, and commercial education. In 2004, persons with locomotor disabilities accounted for more than 80% of the persons admitted into VRCs. Persons with visual, hearing, leprosy, and mild mental retardation represented only 7%, 10%, 0.2%, and 2%, respectively, of admitted persons, and persons with mental illness were not eligible. Of the 29,124 clients who were accepted into VRCs in 2004, following VRC only 10,490 were rehabilitated; they had found a job, begun self-employment, or been admitted to a formal training program. To the author's knowledge, there is no impact evaluation on VRC training.

5.2.2.2 Community-Based Vocational Rehabilitation

Community-based vocational rehabilitation programs provide another alternative to traditional training centers. Training takes place at a community level: Trainers are local artisans and the aim is to provide trainees the skills that are needed to become self-reliant in the community. An example of such community-based programs is presented in detail in Alade in the case of Nigeria. Over the period 1990–2002, 155 participants were provided specialized training as well as loans to become self-employed following their completion of the program. Vocations varied from community to community depending on local viability. The loan scheme was to help trainees buy equipment and materials for their new trade. In one region of Nigeria, there is evidence that this program succeeded in integrating persons with disabilities in their communities, as measured by working in the community and increased perceptions of self-worth.[67]

5.2.2.3 Information Sharing on Returns to Technical Specialties

Individuals may not know which skills are best rewarded in the labor market, especially if they have no or limited prior work experience. By providing this information, individuals may be able to increase their earnings. This is what has been shown as part of the initial results from the mainstream Jua Kali voucher program in Kenya. The Jua Kali voucher program was part of the training funds component of the Kenya Micro and Small Enterprise Training and Technology Project (MSETTP), approaching US $12 million. The Jua Kali program provided small-scale entrepreneurs with a voucher to purchase training and skills upgrading services. The program targeted mainly established entrepreneurs, and at least 20% of the vouchers had to go to women regardless of experience in the small- and medium-enterprise sector. Piloted in September

1996, 37% of the voucher recipients were women. More than 10% of the women who received the information about wages in various occupations decided to pursue more lucrative jobs (e.g., metal working, auto mechanics, and woodworking). It is important to note that although there are utilization data for the voucher program, there are limited data on its impact on earnings. However, the advantage of programs like the MSETTP voucher program is their low cost, which is estimated at about US $309 per voucher.[68]

5.2.3 Comprehensive Training Programs

A recent and increasingly common feature of training programs is to cover a broad range of skills, including behavioral skills (e.g., self-confidence, optimism, and ability to work with others) in addition to traditional technical skills, and sometimes combining them with internships and other services, such as employment services. This comprehensive form of training has been used in various contexts, including both informal and formal sectors, and in mainstream and targeted programs. A review of seven mainstream comprehensive training programs for youth in Latin America has shown that comprehensive training can increase employment rates for certain groups, specially women and younger workers, by as much as 30%, although the same program may have negligible effects in the employment rate of the general population.[69] These programs often focus on urban at-risk youths and offer short-term, demand-driven courses that are complemented by internships. In Soweto, South Africa, training in a broad range of entrepreneurial skills, such as goal setting, planning and monitoring, and networking, has been used in a targeted training program named MODE. The majority of the businesses created by MODE trainees have turnovers that are double the local disability benefit, and the survival rate of businesses started under the program are high.[70]

5.3 Interventions to Address the Lack of Labor Demand

5.3.1 Job-Creation Programs

Public works programs are construction projects financed by public funds to develop infrastructure, such as roads for the benefit of the general public. In low- and middle-income countries, mainstream public works programs have been widely used to boost labor demand during economic downturns or to alleviate poverty on an ongoing basis. Although they have been an effective short-term safety net, the evidence on their impact on future labor market outcomes beyond the program duration is inconclusive.[71] In order to improve the impact of the programs, a new model is tested in several countries but results are not available yet; this new model adds basic and behavioral skills and employment services to the program.[72] It should be noted that public works programs are likely to be inaccessible to a large portion of persons with physical disabilities due to the very nature of the work, often heavy manual labor. In order to increase the participation of persons with physical disabilities, it may be possible (depending on the nature of the program) to adjust its design to expand the scope of public works to include tasks that are less physically demanding, and to give priority to persons with physical disabilities for the realization of these tasks.[73] In India, the National Rural Employment Guarantee Act (NREGA) is one of the country's flagship programs that promises 100 days of employment in a year to rural households in all villages. The NREGA is designed to provide employment when people do not have alternate work. One state, Andhra Pradesh, made a special provision to provide 150 days of employment for persons with disabilities and an NGO, Ashagram Trust, Barwani identified parts of the work that persons with disabilities can do.[74]

5.3.2 Addressing Employer Discrimination: Nondiscrimination Laws and Quotas

Antidiscrimination laws are expected to reduce employment discrimination, increase access to the workplace, and change perceptions about the ability of persons with disabilities to be productive workers. Laws and regulations affecting employment for persons with disabilities can be found in many low- and middle-income countries (e.g., Bangladesh, Tanzania). The degree of implementation and the scope of these tools, however, vary greatly. Typically, in low- and middle-income countries, such laws and regulations are poorly enforced and at times are not well-known within their countries. Some antidiscrimination legislation requires affirmative action or the proactive recruitment and hiring of persons with disabilities. With respect to persons with disabilities in particular, some laws or regulations establish quotas or reservations on the employment of persons with disabilities in the public and/or the private sector. A quota or reservation obliges employers to set a number or percentage for persons belonging to a particular group. The implicit assumption is that without quotas, employers are turning away disabled workers because of discrimination, the perception that they are not as productive as disabled workers, or the unwillingness to bear the costs needed to accommodate disabled workers.[75] Although quotas have not been subject to thorough evaluations, evidence from several low- and middle-income countries suggests that they may not play a significant role in integrating persons with disabilities in the labor market. For instance, India has a policy of 3% reservation in government employment for those with vision, hearing, and locomotor disabilities, each allowed 1% under the 1995 Persons with

Disabilities Act. Reservation applies only to vacancies in jobs that can be performed without loss of productivity, that is, jobs that are identified as being suitable to each type of disability. The list of posts identified for persons with disabilities is very limited, accounting for only 10.2% of all posts in ministries and public establishments. The proportion of persons with disabilities in the identified posts is estimated to be 4.4%.[76] This finding suggests that reservation for persons with disabilities is followed per the letter of the law. However, the list of identified jobs is so restrictive that persons with disabilities continue to be underrepresented in government employment, with the percentage of persons with disabilities in all posts standing at 0.44%. The list of identified jobs also seems arbitrary. It is based on the assumption that the characteristics of impairment are the exclusive determinants of an individual's ability to hold a position at a particular skill level and thus ignores the potential influences of individual characteristics (motivation, age at disability onset), access to employment services, and the characteristics of the workplace and labor market. For instance, in the list of identified jobs, the job of an agricultural scientist who specializes in econometric analysis is identified as being suitable for an individual who is blind or has an orthopedic disability, but not for someone with a hearing disability.

Reducing discrimination may take place in interventions beyond the law, in particular when it comes to encouraging positive attitudes toward the employment of persons with disabilities. Some disabled people organizations already work at the community level changing attitudes toward disability. For instance, Action on Disability and Development works closely with persons with disabilities themselves and their families to encourage persons with disabilities to work and participate in society.[77] Governments and donors could bring more support to awareness campaigns that promote positive attitudes toward persons with disabilities. Lessons can be learned from past awareness campaigns targeted at specific conditions. For instance, a large-scale awareness campaign was recently conducted in India by the BBC World Service Trust to dismantle misconceptions on leprosy through a variety of channels (radio, live theater performances in villages, posters, videos, TV, film, and the media). This campaign was shown to have significantly reduced stigma against persons with leprosy.[78] Evidence is needed to improve our understanding of how interventions can shift embedded attitudes on disability.

5.3.3 Interventions to Address the Lack of Labor Supply

Large-scale awareness campaigns, as described earlier, are expected to also affect persons with disabilities: by increasing self-expectations, they may encourage them to search for work. Martinelli and Mersland provide, in the context of microfinance, some ideas on what might work to improve the self-esteem of persons with disabilities, in particular:

- Providing the opportunity for learning by doing
- Starting something small and manageable where a person can experience success
- Integrating groups of both fellow disabled persons as well as participation in mixed groups with both disabled and non-disabled members.[79]

Dedicated empowerment programs may also facilitate the development of the capacity of individuals to exert control over and direct their lives, including their decision to search for work or the choice of an occupation. Such programs could be for adults or youths with disabilities, and offered in many contexts including a school or self-help groups. Skills may include goal setting, problem solving, decision making, and self-advocacy. This is an area in which partnerships among persons with disabilities, researchers, and DPOs/NGOs seem essential in uncovering the complexities of changing attitudes, and in which further research is needed to find what approaches are most effective.

5.3.4 Interventions to Address Job Search Constraints

Employment service centers provide information about job openings and can offer other job search–related services including career counseling and training. They may also match job seekers to jobs in the formal or informal sector, and can be mainstream or targeted agencies. For example, China has 3,000 employment service agencies for persons with disabilities.[80] There is evidence that employment services have positive impacts on participants' employment and earnings,[81] especially with respect to disadvantaged workers with little access to informal search channels (e.g., family and friends). This is particularly relevant for persons with disabilities, who may have restricted social networks. An advantage of employment services programs is that their costs are relatively low. It should be noted though that employment services alone cannot be expected to improve labor market outcomes in a context with high unemployment or underemployment.

Recently, there have been several mainstream initiatives to use technology-based information sharing of job openings, that is, the use of cell phone text messaging, radio broadcasts, or Internet advertisements to share employment offers across larger geographic areas. Although there have been no evaluations of such initiatives yet, their growth is encouraging.[82] An example of technology-based information sharing is *SoukTel*, which allows firms and potential employers to contact job seekers via text messaging.[83]

5.3.5 *Interventions to Address Firm Start-up Constraints*

As noted, employment is often in the informal sector in low- and middle-income countries, in self-employment or microenterprises. The microfinance movement that has spread through many low- and middle-income countries, is based on the assumption that lack of access to credit is the sole constraint the poor face to start their businesses. Microfinance programs reduce the finance constraints by providing small loans to small businesses. According to microfinance researchers Karlan and Zinman, "despite strong claims about the effects of microcredit on borrowers and their businesses (e.g., the 2006 Nobel Peace Prize to Muhammad Yunus and the Grameen Bank), there is relatively little rigorous evidence about these programs."[84] So far, as a stand-alone program, the small but expanding empirical evidence on the impact of microfinance has been mixed, for both mainstream[85] and targeted programs.[86]

At the same time, there is very scarce but encouraging evidence in low- and middle-income countries that comprehensive entrepreneurship programs can successfully assist businesses. Comprehensive entrepreneurship programs provide a combination of financial literacy, micro-credit and/or insurance schemes, market analysis and business development training, counseling, and marketing assistance.[87] Such programs can be mainstream or targeted at persons with disabilities. When targeted, they may then include support services that meet the needs of persons with disabilities, such as medical support or rehabilitation.[88]

Another recent and novel approach related to firm start-up constraint is to provide entrepreneurship *peer training*. Peer training is community based and consists of having village entrepreneurs provide persons with disabilities with technical and business skills. This approach was implemented successfully in rural Cambodia. The International Labor Organization's Alleviating Poverty through Peer Training (APPT) project adapted the Success Case Replication (SCR) steps that were originally used by the Food and Agriculture Organization and the Economic and Social Commission for Asia and the Pacific in their poverty alleviation work in Cambodia. The eleven SCR steps are as follows:

> 1) locating successful entrepreneurs; 2) evaluating profitability and market viability; 3) assessing the willingness of the entrepreneur to be a trainer; 4) identifying trainees; 5) matching trainer to the trainees; 6) establishing a practical hands-on training programme; 7) supervising training; 8) planing the business with the trainee; 9) arranging for access to credit or providing a grant; 10) providing follow-up; and 11) arranging secondary replication (that is, for successful trainees to become trainers, if possible).[89]

Specifically, the APPT project in Cambodia has serviced a total of 958 clients between 2002 and 2007. Of these, 51% were either disabled women or women affected by disability in the family. Village-based training was imparted by 200 trainers, of whom 70% were women and 26 were former APPT clients. Of the 958 clients, 609 started their own businesses (60% of these new business owners were women). The percentage of people still in business one year or more after having received help through the APPT project has progressed from 76% in 2002 to more than 90% in 2007. Specific examples of the APPT project's success include: Mey Nith, an ice pop vendor, who, with a US $25 start-up grant and one week of training learned how to calculate the net profit of her business and how to manage it despite being blind in one eye and unable to read or write; and Choen Reuoy, a former cake seller, who, with a start-up grant, new bicycle, and some retraining, has become a mobile clothes seller and now makes US $30 per month. The one-on-one nature of peer training allows the APPT project to be adapted to the different needs of persons with disabilities within their communities. The success of the APPT project in Cambodia seems to be replicable elsewhere if peers are available to become trainers.[90]

5.3.6 Tailored Interventions to Address Multiple Constraints to Employment

Supported employment programs are designed to help integrate persons with disabilities in the competitive labor market. Supported employment provides a variety of support services that are tailored to the individual's needs, including job coaches, transportation, assistive technology, specialized job training, and individually tailored supervision. Supported employment was developed in the formal sector in high-income countries as part of government-funded programs. Supported employment has been shown to be successful in high-income countries for persons with severe disabilities (i.e., psychiatric, mental retardation, learning disabilities, traumatic brain injury).[91] For instance, an empirical review of 11 randomized controlled trials of supported employment programs serving individuals with severe mental illness concluded that employment outcomes were consistently higher than the control group programs six to 24 months after the intervention.[92] Despite an extensive body of evidence showing the positive impact of supported employment, it is not widely implemented, in part due to difficulties in financing these services.

Supported employment has been implemented in low- and middle-income countries on a smaller scale, and examples of such programs in Africa, South America, and Asia are presented in Parmenter. Supported employment can take place in both the formal and the informal sectors in a low- or middle-income country. For instance, Parmenter gives details about a program in Zambia in which more than 100 persons with development disabilities were placed in the formal sector (e.g., office workers, agricultural workers) or the informal sector (as housemaids, gardeners, or poultry workers). As in high-income countries, funding is a major obstacle to the implementation of supported employment. The project in Zambia was funded through international aid, which may not be sustainable.[93]

Community-based rehabilitation was developed over 30 years ago as a strategy to improve access to rehabilitation services for persons with disabilities in low- and middle-income countries. Community-based rehabilitation programs utilize community resources, have the community involved in planning, decision making and evaluation, and transfer knowledge on disability to communities. Since the late 1970s, CBR has considerably broadened in scope and is now multidimensional with health, education, and social empowerment as well as livelihood components.[94] Community-based rehabilitation interventions are thus very broad and may address a variety of constraints to employment, both outside and inside the labor market. For example, the key activities of Iran's CBR program include:

> training family and community members on disability.... ; providing educational assistance and facilitating inclusive education through capacity building with teaching staff and students, and improving physical access; referring persons with disabilities to specialist services.... ; providing assistive devices....; creating employment opportunities by providing access to training, job coaching and financial support for income-generation activities; providing support for social activities including for sports and recreation; providing financial assistance for living, education and home modifications.[95]

Many of the activities in the Iranian CBR program are related to employment. Other CBR activities related to labor market constraints include providing supports or adaptations to the workplace, teaching skills,[96] providing employment services (e.g., job search advice, guidance to develop relationships with employers), reducing employer discrimination, and encouraging labor supply among persons with disabilities by promoting positive attitudes with respect to their employment.

Although CBR programs can be found in many low- and middle-income countries, evidence on the impact of CBR programs in general, and on labor market outcomes in particular, is scarce and inconclusive so far. A review of published CBR evaluations by Sharma covered 21 studies published in peer-reviewed journals, with different methodologies. Most studies use a post-test design only or a pre- and posttest design, both of which are inadequate for rigorous impact evaluation. Only two studies used a randomized control trial design, six studies used a quasi-experimental design, and only one study measured the costs of the program. In addition, studies often had very small sample sizes. Employment outcomes were rarely assessed: Training was the focus of the assessment in only a few studies.[97] Of course, CBR interventions are complex to evaluate in that they include multiple components. Such evaluations are resource-intensive, which perhaps explain the dearth of evaluations in this area.

6. CONCLUSION

This chapter described, with broad strokes, the employment situation of persons with disabilities in low- and middle-income countries, their barriers to employment and policies, and interventions to address these barriers.

In most of the low- and middle-income countries in which data are available, persons with disabilities have lower employment rates and are more likely to be self-employed than their nondisabled counterparts. There are multiple barriers to employment for persons with disabilities, including lack of education and lack of accessibility of the general environment, as well as employment-specific barriers such as inaccessible workplaces and limited self-expectations about work ability.

The relative importance of these barriers is expected to vary across countries and communities. This chapter stressed the need to conduct employment and disability situational analyses before the development of policy and interventions on employment for persons with disabilities.

At the risk of generalizing for the context of low- and middle-income countries, given very limited resources and given jobs often found in the informal sector, it appears that much attention is needed toward programs that are community-based and relevant to opportunities in the informal sector. Additionally, programs that address multiple constraints to employment such as CBR are promising, whereas those that address a single constraint (e.g., technical training) may not be sufficient. However, very little evidence is available on CBR and, more generally, on employment programs, whether mainstream or targeted, that work at improving employment outcomes in low- and middle-income countries. Evidence-building is much needed to determine the impact of specific interventions and determine their relative effectiveness and costs. This chapter also offered suggestions on how to conduct an employment and disability situational analysis and on how to select programs to test. In particular, this chapter recommended the use of a participatory framework with persons with disabilities, employers, policymakers, and researchers working together to identify major constraints to employment and to develop and test solutions. Given the scarcity of resources for research and evaluations in low- and middle-income countries in general, and on employment and disability in particular, international development agencies can play an important role in low- and middle-income countries by funding and promoting the conduct of employment and disability situational analyses and program evaluations. Given the sweeping societal changes that are often required to improve the employment situation of persons with disabilities, disability policy needs to be multipronged with at least education and accessibility as core areas in addition to employment.

ACKNOWLEDGMENTS

Sophie Mitra thanks the editors for insightful comments on an earlier version and Navena Chaitoo for excellent research assistance.

NOTES

1. World Health Organization & World Bank (2011). *World Report on Disability*. Geneva, Switzerland: World Health Organization.
2. United Nations (2011). *Rural Population, Development and the Environment*. New York: Department of Economic and Social Affairs. Retrieved May 1, 2012, from http://www.un.org/esa/population/publications/2011RuralPopDevEnv_Chart/ruralpopdevenv2011wallchart.html
3. Burchardt, T. (2004). Capabilities and Disability: the Capabilities Framework and the Social Model of Disability. *Disability & Society 19*(7), 735–751; Mitra, S. (2006). The Capability Approach and Disability. *Journal of Disability Policy Studies 16*(4), 236–247.
4. Mitra (2006). The Capability Approach and Disability.
5. The unemployment rate is the number of unemployed persons as a percentage of the labor force. Because many non-working persons with disabilities do not look for jobs and are thus out of the labor force, the unemployment rate is not an adequate measure of their integration in the labor market. Instead, the employment rate is typically used as an indicator.
6. World Health Organization & World Bank (2011). *World Report on Disability*, 238.
7. Hoogeveen, J.G. (2005). Measuring Welfare for Small but Vulnerable Groups: Poverty and Disability in Uganda. *Journal of African Economies 14*(4), 603–631.
8. Mitra, S. (2008) The Recent Decline in the Employment of Persons with Disabilities in South Africa, 1998-2006. *South African Journal of Economics 76*(3), 480–492.
9. Mitra, S. & Sambamoorthi, U. (2008). Disability and the Rural Labor Market in India: Evidence for Males in Tamil Nadu, *World Development 36*(5), 934–952.
10. Organization for Economic Co-operation and Development (2003). *Transforming Disability into Ability: Policies to promote Work and income security for disabled people*. Paris, France: OECD.
11. Palmer, M.G., *et al.* (2012). Disability measures as an indicator of poverty: a case study from Vietnam. *Journal of International Development 24*(S1), S53–S58.
12. Reyes, C.M., Tabuga, A.D., Mina, C.D., Asis, R.A., & Datu, M.B.G. (2011). *Persons with Disability in Rural Philippines: Results from the 2010 Field Survey in Rosario, Batangas*. Discussion paper series 2011-06. Makati City, Philippines: Philippines Institute for Development Studies.

13. Rischewski, D., *et al.* (2008). Poverty and musculoskeletal impairment in Rwanda. *Transactions of the Royal Society of Tropical Medicine and Hygiene 102*(6), 608–617.
14. Trani, J.-F., & Loeb, M. (2012). Poverty and disability: A vicious circle? Evidence from Afghanistan and Zambia. *Journal of International Development 24*(S1), S19-S52.
15. Eide, A.H., van Rooy, G., & Loeb, M. (2003). *Living Conditions among People with Activity Limitations in Namibia. A National Representative Survey.* Oslo, Norway: SINTEF Health Research; Eide, Arne H., & Yusman Kamaleri (2009). *Living Conditions among Persons with disabilities in Mozambique. A National Representative Study.* Oslo, Norway: SINTEF Health Research.
16. Kamaleri, Y. & Eide, A.H. (2011). *Living Conditions among Persons with disabilities in Lesotho. A National Representative Study.* Oslo, Norway: SINTEF Health Research.
17. Loeb, M., & Eide, A.H. (2004). *Living Conditions among People with Activity Limitations in Malawi. A National Representative Study.* Oslo, Norway: SINTEF Health Research.
18. Maldonado Zambrano, S. (2006). *Trabajo y Discapacidad en el Perú: laboral, políticas públicas e inclusión social.* Lima, Peru: Fondo Editorial del Congreso del Perú.
19. Eide, A.H., Nhiwathiwa, S., Muderedzi, J., & Loeb, M. (2003). *Living Conditions among People with Activity Limitations in Zimbabwe. A Regional Representative Survey.* Oslo, Norway: SINTEF Health Research.
20. Mizunoya, S., & Mitra, S. (2013). Is there a Disability Gap in Employment Rates in Developing Countries? *World Development 42*,28–43.
21. Eide, Nhiwathiwa, Muderedzi, & Loeb (2003). *Living Conditions among People with Activity Limitations in Zimbabwe.*
22. Results for Ghana, Zambia, and Lao are not presented due to a low number of observations of individuals with multiple disabilities.
23. Mizunoya & Mitra (2013). Is there a Disability Gap?
24. Mitra, S., & Sambamoorthi, U. (2006). Employment of Persons with Disabilities: Evidence from the National Sample Survey. *Economic and Political Weekly 41*(3), 199–203; Mizunoya & Mitra. (2013). Is there a Disability Gap; Reyes, Tabuga, Mina, Asis, & Datu (2011). *Persons with Disability in Rural Philippines*; Maldonado Zambrano (2006). *Trabajo y Discapacidad en el Perú.*
25. Eide, Nhiwathiwa, Muderedzi, & Loeb (2003). *Living Conditions among People with Activity Limitations in Zimbabwe*; Eide, van Rooy, & Loeb (2003). *Living Conditions among People with Activity Limitations in Namibia*; Eide, A.H., & Loeb, M. (2006). *Living Conditions among People with Activity Limitations in Zambia. A National Representative Study.* Oslo, Norway: SINTEF Health Research; Eide & Kamaleri (2009). *Living Conditions among Persons with disabilities in Mozambique*; Eide, A.H., & Bhekie, J. (2011). *Living Conditions among Persons with disabilities in Swaziland. A National Representative Study.* Oslo, Norway: SINTEF Health Research; Loeb & Eide (2004). *Living Conditions among People with Activity Limitations in Malawi*; Mitra & Sambamoorthi (2006). Employment of Persons with Disabilities.
26. Mizunoya & Mitra. (2013). Is there a Disability Gap.
27. The formal economy is regulated by the government and includes employment in the public and private sectors where workers are hired on contracts, with a salary and benefits such as pension schemes and health insurance. The informal economy is the unregulated sector of a country's economy. It includes

small-scale agriculture, small-scale traders, home-based enterprises and small businesses employing a few workers.

28. Baldwin M.L., & Johnson, W.G. (2005). A Critical Review of Studies of Discrimination against Workers with Disabilities. In William M. Rodgers III (Ed.), *Handbook on the Economics of Discrimination.* Cheltenham, United Kingdom: Edward-Elgar Publishing, 119–160.

29. Eide, Nhiwathiwa, Muderedzi, & Loeb (2003). *Living Conditions among People with Activity Limitations in Zimbabwe*; Eide, van Rooy, & Loeb (2003). *Living Conditions among People with Activity Limitations in Namibia*; Eide, A.H., & Loeb, M. (2006). *Living Conditions among People with Activity Limitations in Zambia. A National Representative Study.* Oslo, Norway: SINTEF Health Research; Loeb & Eide (2004). *Living Conditions among People with Activity Limitations in Malawi.*

30. Mitra & Sambamoorthi (2008). Disability and the Rural Labor Market in India. Mitra, S., & Sambamoorthi, U. (2009). Wage Differential by Disability Status in an Agrarian Labor Market in India. *Applied Economics Letters 16*(14): 1393–1398.

31. Mizunoya & Mitra (2013). Is there a Disability Gap?

32. Lamicchane, K., & Sawada, Y. (2009). Disability and Returns to Education: A Case Study from Nepal. Paper presented at the Far East and South Asia Meeting of the Econometric Society. Tokyo, Japan, August 3-5.

33. Hoogeveen (2005). Measuring Welfare for Small but Vulnerable Groups.

34. Loeb, M., Eide, A.H., Jelsma, J., ka Toni, M., & Maart, S. (2008). Poverty and disability in Eastern and Western Cape Provinces, South Africa. *Disability and Society 23*(4), 311–321.

35. Mete, C. (Ed.) (2008). *Economic Implications of Chronic Illness and Disability in Eastern Europe and the Former Soviet Union.* Washington, D.C.:World Bank.

36. Mitra, S., Posarac, A., & Vick, B. (2013). Disability and Poverty in Developing Countries: a Multidimensional Study. *World Development 41*, 1–18.

37. Mont, D., & Viet Cuong, N. (2011). Disability and Poverty in Vietnam, *World Bank Economic Review 25*(2), 323–359.

38. Rischewski *et al.* (2008). Poverty and musculoskeletal impairment in Rwanda.

39. Trani & Loeb (2012). Poverty and disability: A vicious circle?

40. World Bank (2009). *Creating Alternative Pathways to Employment: An Assessment of the KPP Program.* Washington, D.C.: World Bank.

41. Filmer, D. (2008). Disability, Poverty and Schooling in Developing Countries: Results from 14 Household Surveys. *The World Bank Economic Review 22*(1), 141–163; Loeb & Eide (2004). *Living Conditions among People with Activity Limitations in Malawi*; Loeb, Eide, Jelsma, Toni, & Maart (2008). Poverty and disability in Eastern and Western Cape Provinces; Mete (2008). *Economic Implications*; Rischewski *et al.* (2008). Poverty and musculoskeletal impairment; Eide, Nhiwathiwa, Muderedzi, & Loeb (2003). *Living Conditions among People with Activity Limitations in Zimbabwe*; Eide, van Rooy, & Loeb (2003). *Living Conditions among People with Activity Limitations in Namibia*; Eide, A.H., & Loeb, M. (2006). *Living Conditions among People with Activity Limitations in Zambia. A National Representative Study.* Oslo, Norway: SINTEF Health Research; Eide & Kamaleri (2009). *Living Conditions among Persons with disabilities in Mozambique;* World Bank (2009). *Creating Alternative Pathways.*

42. World Health Organization & World Bank (2011). *World Report on Disability.*

43. World Bank (2007). *Persons with disabilities in India: From Commitments to Outcomes.* Washington, D.C.: World Bank; Trani, J.-F., et al. (2010). *Disability*

in and around Urban Areas of Sierra Leone. London, United Kingdom: Leonard Cheshire International.

44. Eide, Nhiwathiwa, Muderedzi, & Loeb (2003). *Living Conditions among People with Activity Limitations in Zimbabwe*; Eide, van Rooy, & Loeb (2003). *Living Conditions among People with Activity Limitations in Namibia*; Eide & Loeb (2006). *Living Conditions among People with Activity Limitations in Zambia*; Eide & Kamaleri (2009). *Living Conditions among Persons with disabilities in Mozambique*; Kamaleri & Eide (2011). *Living Conditions among Persons with disabilities in Lesotho;* Loeb & Eide (2004). *Living Conditions among People with Activity Limitations in Malawi.*

45. Table based on author's research and using evidence summarized in Cunningham, W. , Sanchez-Puerta, M.L., & Wuermli, A. (2010). *Active Labor Market Programs for Youth: A Framework to Guide Youth Employment Interventions.* World Bank Employment Policy Primer No. 16. Washington, D.C.: World Bank; and in Morrison, N. (2006). *Active Labor Market Programs: Evidence from Evaluations.* World Bank Employment Policy Primer, No. 7 Washington, D.C.: World Bank.

46. Eide, Nhiwathiwa, Muderedzi, & Loeb (2003). *Living Conditions among People with Activity Limitations in Zimbabwe*; Eide, van Rooy, & Loeb (2003). *Living Conditions among People with Activity Limitations in Namibia*; Eide & Loeb (2006). *Living Conditions among People with Activity Limitations in Zambia*; Eide & Kamaleri (2009). *Living Conditions among Persons with disabilities in Mozambique*; Kamaleri & Eide (2011). *Living Conditions among Persons with disabilities in Lesotho;* Loeb & Eide (2004). *Living Conditions among People with Activity Limitations in Malawi.*

47. Mitra & Sambamoorthi (2008). Disability and the Rural Labor Market in India.

48. World Bank (2007). Persons with disabilities in India.

49. Martinelli, E., & Mersland, R. (2010). Microfinance for people with disabilities. In T. Barron (Ed.), *Poverty and Disability.* London, United Kingdom: Leonard Cheshire International.

50. Holzer, H.J. (1988). Job Search by Employed and Unemployed Youth. *Industrial and Labor Relations Review 40* (4), 601–611.

51. Ibid.

52. Hotchkiss, J.L. (2003). *The Labor Market Experience of Workers with Disabilities: The ADA and Beyond.* Kalamazoo, MI: W.E. Upjohn.

53. See, for example, Gartrell, A. (2010). "A Frog in a Well": the Exclusion of Disabled People from Work in Cambodia. *Disability and Society 25*(3), 289–301.

54. Mersland, R., Nakabuye Bire, F., & Mukasa, G. (2009). Access to mainstream microfinance services for persons with disabilities—lessons learned from Uganda. *Disabilities Studies Quarterly 29*(1).

55. For example, Handicap International (2006). *Good practices for the economic inclusion of persons with disabilities in developing countries: Funding mechanisms for self-employment.* Lyon, France: Handicap International.

56. United Nations Economic and Social Commission for Asia and the Pacific (2009). *Disability at a Glance 2009: A Profile of 36 Countries and Areas in Asia and the Pacific.* Bangkok, Thailand: United Nations Economic and Social Commission for Asia and the Pacific.

57. Katsui, H., & Koistinen, M. (2008). The Participatory Research Approach in nonWestern Countries: Practical Experiences from Central Asia and Zambia. *Disability and Society 23*(7): 747–757.

58. Chambers, R.(2007). Participation and Poverty. *Development 50*(2), 20–25.

59. Ibid.
60. This framework is in part inspired by a framework proposed by Cunningham, Sanchez-Puerta, & Wuermli (2010). *Active Labor Market Programs*, with the objective of promoting youth employment.
61. Stone, E. (1999). Disability and development in the majority world In E. Stone (Ed.) *Disability and Development: Learning from action and research on disability in the majority world*. Leeds, United Kingdom: The Disability Press, 1–18.
62. See, for example, Khandker, S.R., Goolwal, G.B., & Samad, H.A. (2009). *Handbook on Impact Evaluation: Quantitative Methods and Practices*. Washington, D.C.: World Bank.
63. Cunningham, Sanchez-Puerta, & Wuermli (2010). *Active Labor Market Programs*.
64. Attanasio, O., Kugler, A., & Meghir, C. (2011). Subsidizing Vocational Training for Disadvantaged Youth in Colombia: Evidence from a Randomized Trial. *American Economic Journal: Applied Economics 3*(July), 188–122; Card, D., Ibarraran, P., Regalia, F., Rosas, D., & Soares, Y. (2007). *The Labor Market Impacts of Youth Training in the Dominican Republic: Evidence from a Randomized Evaluation*. National Bureau of Economics research, Working Paper 12883. Washington, D.C.: NBER; Betcherman, G., Olivas, K., & Dar, A. (2004). *Impacts of Active Labor Market Programs: New Evidence from Evaluations with Particular Attention to Developing and Transition Countries*. Social Protection paper No. 0402. Washington, D.C.: World Bank.
65. Alade, E.B. (2004). Community-based vocational rehabilitation (CBVR) for persons with disabilities: experiences from a pilot project in Nigeria. *British Journal of Special Education 31*(3), 143–149; Coleridge, P.(2007). Economic Empowerment. In T. Barron & P. Amerena (Eds.), *Disability and Inclusive Development*. London, United Kingdom: Leonard Cheshire International; Mitra, S., and Sambamoorthi, U. (2006). Government Programmes to Promote Employment among Persons with Disabilities in India, *Indian Journal of Social Development 2*, 195–213.
66. Mitra & Sambamoorthi (2006). Government Programmes to Promote Employment.
67. Alade (2004). Community-based vocational rehabilitation
68. Adams, A. (n.d.). Assessment of the Jua Kali Pilot Voucher Program. Retrieved on June 20,2012, from http://siteresources.worldbank.org/EDUCATION/Resources/278200-1099079877269/547664-1099079934475/ 547667-1135281552767/ Jua_Kali_Pilot_Voucher_Program.pdf; Cunningham, Sanchez-Puerta, & Wuermli (2010). *Active Labor Market Programs*.
69. Some information on each of the seven programs is given below and is taken from Ibarraran, P., & Rosas, D. (2009). Evaluating the Impact of Job Training Programs in Latin America: Evidence from IDB Funded Operations. *Journal of Development Effectiveness 1*(2), 195–216. The *Probecat* program in Mexico, which was started in 1984, seeks to increase the employability of its participants. Although the program is not focused on youth or the disadvantaged in particular, it offers short-term, demand-driven courses that are complemented by internships, which emphasize on-the-job training. The *Joven* program in Chile, which was started in 1992, caters specifically to the urban, "at risk" youth. Like the *Probecat* program, it also offers short-term, demand-driven courses that are complemented by internships. Following Chile's successful implementation of the *Joven* program, five programs were developed in other countries as replicates of the Chile program. Argentina started *Proyecto Joven* in 1994, Colombia started

Jovenes en Accion in 2002, the Dominican Republic started *Juventud y Empleo* in 1999, Panama started *ProCaJoven* in 2002, and Peru started *Projoven* in 1996. While the Dominican Republic program did not demonstrate any significant effect on youth employment rates, earnings were shown to be 17% higher for participants than nonparticipants. The Colombia program had more widespread and large effects on women than men; women participants were 14% more likely to be employed and earned 18% more than those not offered training. The Panama program also showed significant increases in employment and earning rates for women participants. Peru's program resulted in positive and statistically significant increases in formal employment rates and earnings for both males and females between the ages of 16 and 21. Argentina's program resulted in an increase in the likelihood of formal employment by 5% to 10%. Mexico's program resulted in greater rates of salaried employment and higher earnings. Finally, Chile's program resulted in about a 30% increase in income for young trainees but not for adults and a 30% increase in employability for young adults but not older adults.

70. Coleridge (2007). Economic Empowerment.
71. Betcherman, Olivas, & Dar (2004). *Impacts of Active Labor Market Programs.*
72. Cunningham, Sanchez-Puerta, & Wuermli (2010). *Active Labor Market Programs.*
73. Mitra, S.(2006). Disability and Social Safety Nets in Developing Countries. *International Journal of Disability Studies 2*(1), 43–88.
74. Cordaid (2012). Network of persons with disability organisations India. Retrieved June 15, 2012, from http://www.cordaid.nl/nl/Projects/Network-of-persons-with-disability-organisations-India.html
75. Mont, D. (2004). *Disability Employment Policy.* Social Protection Discussion Paper No. 0412. Washington, D.C.: World Bank.
76. Mitra & Sambamoorthi (2006). Government Programmes to Promote Employment.
77. Action on Disability and Development (2006). *A Report on our Activities 2005-06.* Bangalore, India: Action on Disability and Development.
78. World Bank (2007). Persons with disabilities in India
79. Martinelli & Mersland (2010). Microfinance for people with disabilities.
80. World Health Organization & World Bank (2011). *World Report on Disability.*
81. World Bank (2009). Creating Alternative Pathways.
82. Cunningham, Sanchez-Puerta, & Wuermli (2010). *Active Labor Market Programs.*
83. *Souktel* is a Palestinian-Canadian NGO that has created an application, which uses short SMS surveys to help job-seekers build a short CV and employee-seekers a job description (see Houssian, A., Kilany, M., & Korenblum, J. (2009). Mobile Phone Job Services: Linking Developing-Country Youth with Employers via SMS. *3rd International Conference On Information and Communication Technologies and Development 2009 Proceedings.* Carnegie Mellon University in Doha, Qatar, 491). *Souktel* matches job seekers to jobs based on the CV that they have entered into *Souktel*'s database. These job matches are sent directly to the job-seekers via SMS. Between 2006 and 2009, *Souktel* has helped 2,000 youth find work and internships through their SMS-based job search and matching application. See Cunningham, Sanchez-Puerta, & Wuermli (2010). *Active Labor Market Programs.*
84. Karlan, D. & Zinman, J. (2011). Microcredit in Theory and Practice: Using Randomized Credit Scoring for Impact Evaluation. *Science 332*(6035),1278–1284.

85. Ibid.
86. See for example Dyer, S. (2003). Credit is a Need and a Right: Inclusive Policy and Practice in Micro Finance. In K. Heinicke-Motsch & S. Sygal (Eds.), *Building an Inclusive Development Community: A Manual on Including Persons with disabilities in International Development Programs.* Eugene, OR: Mobility International.
87. Cunningham, Sanchez-Puerta, & Wuermli (2010). *Active Labor Market Programs*; Karlan, D., & Valdivia, M. (2011). Teaching Entrepreneurship: Impact Of Business Training On Microfinance Clients and Institutions. *Review of Economics and Statistics 93*(2), 510–527.
88. Muñoz, W., Last, U., & Kimsean, T. (2010). *Good Practices from the Project: Towards Sustainable Income Generating Activities for Mine Victim and Other Persons with Disabilities in Cambodia.* Phnom Penh, Cambodia: Handicap International.
89. International Labour Organization (2007). *Replicating Success: A Handbook and Manual on Alleviating Poverty through Peer Training.* Geneva, Switzerland: International Labour Organization, 9–10.
90. International Labour Organization (2007). *Replicating Success.*
91. See, for example, Wehman, P., Revell, G., & Kregel, J. (1998). Supported employment: A decade of rapid growth and impact. *American Rehabilitation 24*(1), 31–43.
92. Bond, G.R., Drake, R.E., & Becker, D.R. (2008). An update on randomized controlled trials of evidence-based supported employment. *Psychiatric Rehabilitation Journal 31*(4), 280–290.
93. Parmenter, T.R. (2011). *Promoting training and employment opportunities for people with intellectual disabilities: International experience.* Employment Working Paper No. 103 2011. Geneva, Switzerland: International Labour Organisation.
94. World Health Organization (2010). *Guidelines on Community Based Rehabilitation:.* Geneva, Switzerland: World Health Organization.
95. Ibid., 16.
96. International Labour Organisation (2008). *Skills Training through Community Based Rehabilitation (CBR): A Good Practice Guide.* Geneva, Switzerland: International Labour Organisation.
97. Sharma, M. (2007). Evaluation in Community Based Rehabilitation Programmes: A Strengths, Weaknesses, Opportunities and Threats Analysis. *Asia Pacific Disability Rehabilitation Journal 18*(1), 46–62.

CHAPTER 12

Government Policy and Employment of Persons with Disabilities in Peru

STANISLAO MALDONADO

1. INTRODUCTION

The employment conditions in Peru are extremely precarious, as is the case in many low- and middle-income countries. Despite the impressive process of economic growth experienced by the country over the past 10 years, for most Peruvians it is increasingly difficult to find decent jobs with adequate levels of income to meet their basic needs. In the last 20 years the country has experienced an expansion in the number of workers in informality and under-employment, with low wages and no access to social security.

The employment numbers of people with disabilities in Peru are proportionally even lower. According to statistical evidence, the unemployment rate of persons with disabilities is almost double the overall unemployment rate, reaching 18.1% in Lima, the capital city.[1] However, this indicator misses the high proportion of persons with disabilities who are not in the labor force. According to the information available for Lima, 76% of working-age persons with disabilities are economically inactive. Moreover, even those employed are usually overrepresented in low-productivity jobs in the informal sector, which implies that most of them are facing poor labor conditions and lack of, or inadequate access to, basic social rights.

As a consequence of this situation, in recent years persons with disabilities and their families have been attracting, through their organizations, the attention of the state and the rest of Peruvian society due to the acute conditions of economic and social exclusion that they face every day. This effort led to the enactment of law 27050 in 1998, known as the Law of People with Disabilities, during Alberto Fujimori's government (1990–2000). This law establishes—for the first time in the country—a legal regime for the protection, health care, work, education, rehabilitation, and social security of persons with disabilities, with the aim of improving their economic and social integration.[2]

This legal progress, although important, has not been accompanied with significant changes in human development prospects for this population. The shared view among activists, public officials, policymakers, and politicians is that the State could do more in practice to enforce and monitor compliance with the law. This is a consequence of the disability policy-making processes in the country, which are markedly characterized by lack of coordination, instability, weak technical capacity, low quality of implementation, and weak political will. Following some recent scholarship in political economy, what seems to matter in this case is more the quality of the disability policymaking rather than its orientation.[3]

This chapter studies the employment policies for persons with disabilities in Peru and their results in terms of improving labor market conditions. After providing some basic institutional details, we briefly characterize the Peruvian labor market as one in which underemployment and informality are prevalent despite the high economic growth rates experienced by the Peruvian economy during the past decade. We also describe the Peruvian population with disabilities in terms of their stock of human capital and gender differences, showing that important differences arise when these factors are taken into account. Particularly, we show that women with low levels of education are more exposed to labor market exclusion and, even when employed, suffer from unfavorable labor market inclusion conditions in terms of access to social benefits and other rights recognized by law.

We then discuss the most important policy instruments employed by the Peruvian state to reach that goal and analyze, exploiting the available information, their effectiveness. These policy instruments include employment services, training and other labor programs, financial supports, quota systems, and antidiscrimination measures. Although the lack of information was the most important barrier in the development of this study, we do find some areas of progress but even more areas in which adjustments are needed.

We have identified two policies that seem to be relatively effective in terms of improving labor market conditions for persons with disabilities: participation in general workfare programs such as "Construyendo Perú" and the preferential treatment of promotional enterprises that provide good and services to the state. In both cases, the employment opportunities that were created are basically in the informal sector, specifically in construction. These results are consistent with the low levels of human capital that characterize this group. Whereas only 2% of the population without disability has no level of education, about 21% of persons with disabilities are in the same situation; 13% of persons with disabilities have some level of tertiary education, compared with

24% for those without disability. Given the lower levels of formal education, it should not be surprising that precisely those instruments that are targeted to unskilled groups are the most promising ones in terms of improving the labor market conditions for persons with disabilities.

Although the lessons from this chapter are only valid for Peru, they may be useful for understanding the case of societies with similar levels of economic and political development in Latin America, such as Ecuador and Bolivia in the Andean region, which possess similar social structure and economic and political institutions. However, a more careful analysis of these comparisons is an area of future research.

The rest of the chapter is organized as follows. Section 2 provides basic institutional details as well as basic labor market information about persons with disabilities. Section 3 studies the set of policies contained in the current legal framework. Section 4 concludes.

2. CONTEXT AND BACKGROUND

2.1 Basic Statistics about Persons with Disabilities in Peru

When providing a general overview about the characteristics of persons with disabilities in the country, the first task is to estimate the size of their population in Peru. This depends mainly on the definition of disability employed, with current estimates ranging from 1.3% to 31.28%. The first figure is obtained by the Ninth National Population Census carried out in 1993 and the second was developed by the National Institute of Rehabilitation (INR) in its study, *Prevalence of Impairments, Disabilities and Handicaps in Peru, 1993*.[4]

In the first case, the estimates are based on a bounded and exclusionary definition, which considers only the total loss of a function or capacity, whereas in the second case, the definition is broad and inclusive, although heavily grounded on a medical approach to disability. Alternative numbers from other surveys and censuses fall between these two extremes and are based on more modern definitions of disability.[5] For instance, the Encuesta Continua (ENCO) of 2006 estimated that 8.4% of the total population had a disability,[6] whereas the census of 2007 put this number at 11.86%.[7] This last number means that more than 3 million Peruvians have at least one disability. Differences in terms of the wording of the question regarding disability status may explain this difference.

Using the census of 2007,[8] it is possible to characterize the composition of the population with disabilities in the country according to type of disability. About 46% have visual limitations, 20% physical disabilities, 20% have hearing or speech limitations, and 14% have other type of disabilities.[9]

Additional information for the case of Lima, the capital city, was collected by the Encuesta de Hogares con Discapacidad (EHODIS) for 2005.[10] This instrument estimated that the prevalence of disability was 5.7%, significantly lower than the ENCO estimate of 11.7% for Lima.[11]

2.2 Labor Market Conditions of Persons with Disabilities

Like most low- and middle-income countries, the labor market in Peru is characterized by high levels of informality and low-quality employment. According to statistics produced by the Ministry of Labor, about 60% of employed workers are in the informal sector.[12] Wages are low and they grew very modestly (6.8%) between 2000 and 2009, despite the high economic growth rates experienced over the period (about 8%).[13] These high growth rates were led by the mining sector, in a context of high prices of mineral products, as well as by the construction sector due to the expansion of public investment by the central and regional governments, also linked to the increase in mineral rents. Therefore, although employment levels experienced an important increase because of the mineral boom, the quality of employment and wages did not change in a significant way.

Unfortunately, there are no current statistics on the working conditions of persons with disabilities in Peru.[14] The latest figures correspond to those in the surveys and censuses already discussed, but none of these cover in detail the labor market characteristics of this sector. For this reason, this chapter focuses on the statistics provided by the National Household Survey (ENAHO) carried out by the Ministry of Labor and Employment in 2002 and 2003.[15] These numbers are complemented by more recent estimates from EHODIS 2005 and the census of 2007. One limitation of this source is its limited coverage, but it still can provide a good starting point to frame the employment policies to be discussed in the following.

The labor market outcomes for persons with disabilities in Peru can be characterized in the following way:

1 Labor market participation rates for persons with disabilities are low compared with nondisabled people, and are especially low for women with disabilities.

According to survey data for 2002 and 2003 from ENAHO, the gap in participation rates among people with and without disabilities was about 40% (63.8% vs. 23.6%, respectively). This implies that almost eight out of 10 disabled persons in the country were not working or looking actively for jobs, which is extremely high if we consider that less than four out of 10 persons with no disabilities are in the same situation. These numbers graphically show the magnitude of the economic exclusion of persons with disabilities in the Peruvian labor market.

There are important gender differences to take into account in our analysis. The gaps of participation rates were 45% for men and 38% for women (Table 12.1). Using the survey, we have estimated that for each 10 men with disability, three were active, whereas for each 10 disabled women, fewer than two were actively looking for jobs in the market. This calls for employment policies with a gender perspective. Unfortunately, this aspect has been neglected so far in disability policymaking.

2 Unemployment is not the basic mechanism to explain the labor market exclusion of persons with disabilities.

As discussed, most persons with disabilities in Peru simply do not look for employment opportunities. This significantly reduces the scope of disability and employment policies in the country. For this reason, unemployment, which only measures those looking for work, does not seem to be the most relevant indicator. Evidence from the ENAHO survey for 2003 shows that the unemployment rate for persons with disabilities was 18.4%, certainly higher than the 8.2% experienced by nondisabled people, but this is not comparable to unemployment gap rates in developed countries. Although this result seems initially better than international evidence which suggests that unemployment rate of persons with disabilities is about three times higher than the rates faced by people without disabilities,[16] it is largely due to the large number who are too discouraged to seek work.

Gender differences are also important. Whereas the unemployment rate gaps between people with and without disabilities for men is 5.6%, the gap for the case of women it is 16%. Hence, although labor market exclusion for men with disabilities is mostly explained by low participation rates, high unemployment levels seem to be important in the case of women also.

3 Employment opportunities available to persons with disabilities are basically in the informal and low productivity sectors.

Table 12.1 LABOR MARKET INDICATORS BY GENDER AND DISABILITY STATUS

Labor Market Indicators	Participation Rate			Unemployment Rate		
	Male Population	Female Population	Total	Male Population	Female Population	Total
People with Disabilities	28.8%	16.7%	23.8%	14.6%	27.9%	18.4%
People without Disabilities	74.0%	54.8%	64.1%	8.9%	11.8%	10.2%
Total Population	**72.9%**	**54.2%**	**63.2%**	**9.0%**	**11.9%**	10.3%

Figure 12.1 shows the distribution of employed persons with disabilities by type of occupation. The most salient characteristic is the fact that about 46% of those employed work as independent workers: 23% are blue collar workers in the private sector and 6% are white collar workers in the public sector. This indicates that this population not only faces constraints in their access to the labor market, but also that their inclusion is usually linked to occupations characterized by low levels of pay and benefits.

Important gender differences are also present here. Whereas on average 46% of persons with disabilities work as independent workers, this percentage grows to 75% for women. This is about 40 percentage points higher than for men with disabilities, suggesting that a significant part of the gaps observed between workers with and without disability is mainly driven by the magnitude of the labor exclusion of disabled women.

This information can be complemented with information regarding the occupational groups in which persons with disabilities tend to work. Figure 12.2 shows that persons with disabilities tend to work, in most cases, as sellers (39%), services providers (15%), and craftspeople (11%). These contrast with the 23%, 14%, and 16% for nondisabled workers, respectively. Only 9% work as professionals or technicians (vs. 18% for nondisabled workers).

4 Low levels of human capital are linked to low labor market participation and employment for persons with disabilities.

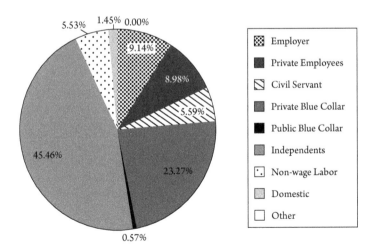

Figure 12.1
Distribution of Employed Persons with Disabilities by Type of Occupation

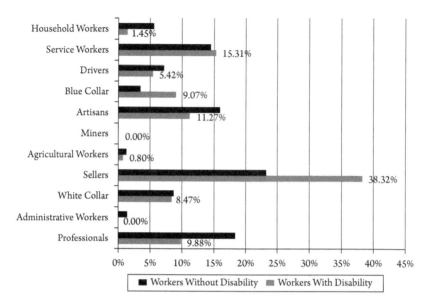

Figure 12.2
Distribution of Employed Persons with and without Disabilities by Occupational Group

The evidence suggests that human capital accumulation by persons with disabilities is linked to participation in the labor market. Figure 12.3 shows that those individuals with disabilities with low levels of education are less likely to actively participate in the labor market. For instance, those persons with disabilities with no education have an inactivity rate of 90%, whereas those with college degrees have an inactivity rate of 50%. Interestingly, even for those with high level of education, the levels of labor market participation are relatively low, suggesting that, although education matters, it is a necessary but not sufficient condition to improve the levels of labor market inclusion for this group.

This element is critical because the fraction of persons with disabilities with low levels of education is significant. Recent evidence from the 2003 ENAHO survey indicate that whereas only 2% of the population without disability has no level of education, about 21% of persons with disabilities are in the same situation. On the other hand, only 13% of persons with disabilities have some level of tertiary education, versus 24% for those without disability. Despite the progress, the gap among those with and without disability is still significant.

However, this does not mean that those persons with disabilities with higher levels of education are necessarily as well off as their educational peers who have no disabilities. Figure 12.4 shows that the probability of being employed for those persons with disabilities with the highest level of

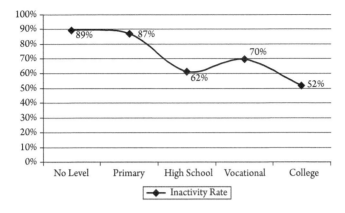

Figure 12.3
Labor Market Participation of Persons with Disabilities by Educational Level

education is still lower than the probability of employment of those nondisabled with the lowest level of education, using data for 2003. This result is critical and requires public policies to address the barriers that remain.

5 Lower wages and employment chances for persons with disabilities are not fully explained by differences in education and other observable characteristics.

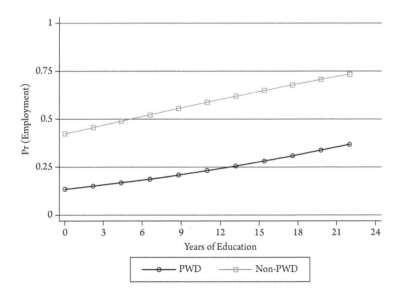

Figure 12.4
Probability of Being Employed by Educational Level and Disability Status
PWD stands for persons with disabilities

The gaps observed in terms of probability of employment and wages between persons with and without disabilities cannot be fully explained by differences in endowments of education and other valuable economic assets. Maldonado (2007) uses a set of econometric techniques to address this issue, and finds that, in the case of gaps in employment, there is a gap of 21.62% that cannot be explained by differences in stock of human capital and other relevant controls.[17] This latter result is slightly higher than that found by Mitra and Sambamoorthi (2006), who estimate this number to be 18.6% in the case of India.[18] In the case of the decomposition strategy based on the matching method suggested by Ñopo,[19] the author found that 52% of the gap in probability of labor market participation is not explained by differences in observable characteristics between the groups compared or by differences in the support of the distributions of these characteristics. Results obtained from alternative matching strategies go in the same direction.

In the case of wage gaps, the author found that this difference, computed using the decomposition strategy proposed by Reimers,[20] is about 70%. Using the nonparametric technique suggested by Ñopo,[21] the unexplained component of the wage gap is estimated at 32%. According to these results, persons with disabilities not only face high levels of labor market exclusion (expressed as a low probability of employment) but also suffer from wage discrimination.

2.3 Institutional Background

Disability policymaking is relatively new in Peru. Although there have been policies targeted to this group in the past, they were mainly sectorial efforts weakly connected to each other and highly fragmented.[22] As a consequence, they had almost no impact on the human development of persons with disabilities.

Along with the development of policy instruments regarding disability (like the National Plan of Equality of Opportunities for Persons with Disabilities), and the enactment of Law 27050, a set of governmental offices were created in order to deal with the implementation and enforcement of the law, together with other instruments. This section briefly discusses those most relevant to disability and employment.

2.3.1 National Council for Integration of People with Disabilities

The most important instrument is an autonomous office—called the National Council for Integration of People with Disabilities (CONADIS)—that was created to oversee compliance with the law and to serve as the technical focal point for disability issues. The National Council for Integration of People with Disabilities also has the responsibility of developing policy initiatives, studies, and projects related to disability issues. Despite its broad set of responsibilities, CONADIS in practice lacks technical capacity and its annual budget is insufficient to fulfill the tasks entrusted to it by the state. Because its goal is very broad and somewhat ambiguous, its performance has been erratic, and successive governments have had different views regarding its role. This erratic performance has contributed to its low level of professionalization, which has been compounded by the pressure of disabled peoples' organizations toward particular agendas in a context of limited resources.[23]

2.3.2 Special Commission on Disability Studies

In recent years, different sectors of the Peruvian state have also developed specialized offices or units to address disability. In many cases, these new offices are the result of individual efforts by policymakers or politicians with special sensitivity to the disability rights agenda. For instance, in 2001 the Congress of Peru implemented the Special Commission on Disability Studies (CEEDIS) under the leadership of a congressman with a disability.[24] This is a practice that has been repeated since then under slightly different names.

Although its original goal was oriented to the development of knowledge regarding the social and economic conditions of persons with disabilities,[25] over the course of the years this commission has been reorienting its activities toward the attention of more specific demands from individuals with disabilities, neglecting its original goal of being a research commission. In a way, the magnitude of social exclusion faced by this group makes this adjustment needed because politicians are sensitive to the demands of this constituency, but at a high cost in terms of critical knowledge needed for the development of effective public policies for this group.

2.3.3 National Direction of Labor Promotion for People with Disabilities

The Ministry of Labor recently created the National Direction of Labor Promotion for People with Disabilities, and charged it with the responsibility of coordinating labor services targeted to this sector. This direction is relatively new and its activities are basically oriented toward the defense of the labor rights of people with disabilities and other legal services. Although the implementation of a unit like this is positive, there are important limitations to be addressed before this office can become an effective tool for improving labor conditions. First, the development of units like this must be accompanied by budget and other resources, which is not happening in this case.[26] Also, efforts in this direction require training for public officials and the development of knowledge regarding labor market conditions for persons with disabilities. The Ministry of Labor can support this by providing research funds or using alternative mechanisms to create incentives for researchers, particularly from academia, which is a sector that has been largely uninterested in disability issues in contexts such as Peru's.

2.3.4 Municipal and Regional Offices for People with Disabilities

As part of Law 27050, local and regional governments have also created special offices for the provision of services to persons with disabilities, called OMAPED (Oficina Municipal de Atención a la Persona con Discapacidad) and OREDIS (Oficina Regional de Atención a las Personas con Discapacidad), respectively. We know little about the workings of these offices because systematic evidence about their performance has not been collected yet. Although many provincial and local governments have created offices during the past years, the law is not precise regarding their role. In practice, most offer basic services in terms of information and counseling about disability rights. The link with employment opportunities for persons with disabilities is limited, although some organize exhibitions of products manufactured by promotional enterprises.

The problems highlighted in the preceding regarding limited budgets and weak technical capacities are more acute in this case. Only a few local governments in rich areas of Lima (like the districts of Miraflores and San Isidro) were able to build high-profile OMAPEDs. In most cases, these offices are poorly funded.

2.3.5 Policymaking on Disability Issues

Despite these developments, the perception among experts is that the state has no clarity in respect to the orientation it wants for public policies for persons with disabilities. This is the natural consequence of a political and social environment that does not favor the formulation of coherent, stable, and enforceable policies. Due to the lack of resources and technical capacity, the coordination role of CONADIS in the policymaking process is very weak, creating a vacuum that is occupied by several actors with fragmented agendas in diverse circumstances. This is reinforced by the absence of cooperative behavior among critical actors in the policymaking arena, which in turn weakens advocacy efforts and political accountability.[27] The resulting public policies tend to lack coherence and be weakly enforceable.

3. EMPLOYMENT POLICIES: POLICY INSTRUMENTS AND IMPACT

3.1 Overview

This section provides an overview of the set of policies for promoting the employment of persons with disabilities that has been implemented in Peru. Over the past years, the set of policies and instruments regularly used by governments for expanding employment opportunities for persons with disabilities have typically included: (1) employment services; (2) training for employment; (3) financial supports; (4) technical and personal support; (5) quota systems; (6) antidiscrimination legislation; (7) persuasion measures and; (8) disability management.[28] In Peru, most governments have used some combination of these practices, at least from the 1990s, although in some cases these can be traced back to the 1960s.[29] It is beyond the goal of this chapter to provide complete coverage of these instruments. Rather, it focuses on those mechanisms that are more directly connected to employment opportunities for this group.

The most important developments with regard to current labor policies for persons with disabilities happened during the late 1990s. The existing policies are contained in Law 27050 and its amendments (particularly, Law 28164). This latter law devotes two chapters (Chapter VII: Promotion and Employment, and Chapter VIII: Promotional Enterprises) to promote employment for persons with disabilities.[30]

In order to properly evaluate policies that promote the labor inclusion of persons with disabilities contained in the current legal framework, as well as in other policy instruments such as the National Plan of Equality of Opportunities for Persons with Disabilities, it is necessary to establish some basic criteria for classification. Here we follow the proposal of Hills (2002), who suggests that it is possible to classify the policies for persons with disabilities in a dynamic framework as follows:[31]

- *Prevention policies*: Policies designed to reduce the risk of a person falling in a non-desirable state.
- *Protection policies*: Policies aimed at reducing the impact of a negative shock or a similar event on the well-being of a person.
- *Promotion policies*: Policies oriented to increasing the chances of a person exiting an undesirable state.
- *Propulsion policies*: Policies designed to reinforce the benefits of leaving a non-desirable state as well as to avoid the return to this state.

A detailed discussion of the full set of employment policies for persons with disabilities in Peru is beyond the scope of this short chapter; instead, the chapter focuses mainly on protection, promotion, and propulsion policies. Because the focus of this chapter is on employment opportunities for those who already have a disability, it seems natural to focus on those policies that assume a pre-existing disability. Prevention and protection policies are designed for those without disability or who have recently acquired such condition.

In order to understand the scope and impact of the current set of policies, it is crucial to first analyze the disability certification requirement established in the Peruvian legal framework.

3.2 Certification of Disability as a Source of Exclusion

According to the Peruvian legal framework, individuals with disabilities need to certify their disability status in order to have access to the rights and benefits recognized by the law. As a consequence, the certification of disability can play an exclusionary role if the state does not provide the means to facilitate access to this document for disabled people. Using 1993 census estimates as reference, Maldonado showed that only 0.46% of the population with disability had access to this certification in 2004,[32] meaning that a very small fraction of persons with disabilities were, in practice, the target of the disability policy in the country.[33] Using the same methodology and information updated to 2011, it is possible to estimate that only 1.90% of persons with disabilities have a disability certificate, suggesting that no significant changes have happened over the past 7 years.[34] One challenge for policymakers and NGOs working in this area is to think of alternatives to facilitate and democratize access to the disability certificate.

3.3 Protection Policies

Protection policies for persons with disabilities are usually based on antidiscrimination mechanisms in access and job retention. These are also related to social protection schemes and access to services and financial assistance to mitigate the impact of a disabling event. In terms of specific protection policies, this discussion is focused on antidiscrimination laws.[35]

According to Law 27050, nobody can be discriminated against because of disability status, considering "... invalid any act based on discriminatory grounds that affect access, retention and/or employment conditions of the person with disabilities." It also states that the person with disability must "... enjoy all the benefits and rights recognized by the labor laws." The regulations of this law provide a greater detail in this regard. According to this legal instrument, any person who "... arbitrarily impedes, obstructs, restricts, or otherwise impairs the full exercise of persons with disabilities' rights, will be forced, at the request of the affected, to stop the discriminatory act."[36] In the specific case of labor rights of workers with disabilities, it establishes the role of the Ministry of Labor in order to punish acts of discrimination in relation to job offers and access to technical or vocational training.

It is important to note that, for a long time, the antidiscrimination rules discussed in the preceding did not contain mechanisms to discourage discrimination against persons with disabilities. Article 2 of the regulations of Law 27050 established no penalty for those who discriminate against a person with disability. Moreover, the welfare losses associated with an act of discrimination against a person with disability were not compensated either by the discriminating party or by the state. This contradicts antidiscrimination mechanisms existing in other countries. For example, in Brazil, in accordance with Law 7853/89, discrimination against a person based on disability is a punishable offense subject to a fine and imprisonment for up to four years.[37] Other low- and middle-income countries, such as Mauritius, have similar schemes. An additional limitation of the Peruvian regulatory framework is that it does not establish the precise set of acts that can be considered discriminatory. A significant number of countries include in their antidiscrimination legislation a detailed list of discriminatory acts liable for punishment.[38]

Very recently, this situation changed, at least formally. Law 28867, enacted in August 2006, modified article 323 of the Penal Code to include disability as a form of discrimination, making it a cause for imprisonment for up to three years. In addition, Law 29392, which establishes a set of penalties for those who do not comply with Law 27050, was enacted in August 2009. The perception among experts on disability is that the lack of enforcement is the most important barrier for these instruments to be effective.

In regard to labor rights, the law establishes equality between workers with and without disability. This is consistent with point 10 of Recommendation 168 of the International Labour Organization, and is commonplace in similar laws in other countries of the region such as Ecuador, Colombia, and Argentina. However, despite the importance of the principle of equal rights, this principle is ineffective if it is not accompanied by concrete measures to provide support to employers interested in hiring workers with disabilities. What is needed is substantially a legal framework that encourages hiring without necessarily increasing the firms' labor costs, but that in turn ensures access to benefits and social rights recognized by law to workers with disabilities. Schemes based on shared responsibility between employers and the state need to be explored in order to create incentives that promote labor inclusion of disabled workers.

3.4 Promotion Policies

Promotion policies are designed with the aim of improving opportunities to escape from an undesirable state. In our case, this is linked to creating conditions for persons with disabilities in such a way that they can develop greater autonomy and better prospects for achieving well-being through access to decent work. Among the available policy instruments, we may consider measures to encourage the hiring of disabled workers through tax incentives, wage subsidies, and training programs, just to mention some of the most common practices.[39]

Law 27050 assigns to CONADIS the role of coordinating and monitoring the implementation of training and retraining programs for persons with disabilities.[40] In addition, the law establishes that this office, in coordination with the Ministry of Labor, must support measures to promote employment and special programs for this group.[41] In order to encourage the recruitment of persons with disabilities in the public and private sectors, the law incorporates the deduction of expenses on the total wages paid at a rate set by the Ministry of Economy and Finance: 50% if the company has up to 30% of its workforce made up of persons with disabilities and 80% if this percentage exceeds 30%.[42] Additionally, the law states that CONADIS must coordinate with the Ministry of Labor to ensure that no less of 2% of total beneficiaries of services and training programs offered by the latter must have a disability.[43]

In addition, Law 28164 (enacted in December 2003) states that the executive branch, its decentralized offices, constitutionally autonomous units, state enterprises, and regional and local governments are required to employ persons with disabilities that meet the established requirements in an amount no smaller than 3% of their entire staff. Furthermore, the same instrument provides that those applicants with disabilities will get a scoring bonus of 15% in merit competitions for public sector jobs if they have received a passing score and meet the requirements for the position for which they are applying for.[44]

3.4.1 Training, Retraining, and Special Labor Programs for Persons with Disabilities

In relation to measures of training and retraining, it is important to note that little progress was made in this direction, and the efforts made by institutions responsible have been insufficient. The law assigns CONADIS a central role in that regard, but this office was able to do very little in this direction. The central reason for such modest progress is the low budget allocated to CONADIS and the Ministry of Labor to carry out these activities.

Regarding the special employment programs mentioned by the law, there is no consensus on the need to design and implement a special program. Indeed, specialized employment programs for persons with disabilities are currently subject to severe criticism because the curricula are often related to jobs traditionally thought of as appropriate for this population. The problem with schemes of this nature is that they are usually in permanent mismatch with market needs, thereby undermining the real labor market opportunities available to this group. From this perspective, it would be best to create conditions of equal access to regular labor programs, so persons with disabilities can take advantage of them rather than developing specific programs. This will be consistent with a broad goal of promoting social inclusion in society. This, however, does not mean that this alternative can be useful in all cases. For instance, persons with severe disabilities are usually excluded from these general programs.

One of the most important programs currently offered by the Ministry of Labor is a workfare program called Construyendo Perú. This program provides funds for labor-intensive and small scale projects proposed by local communities. The targeted population is usually characterized by low levels of formal education and limited formal economy participation. Given the social conditions they previously faced, some workers with disabilities have found access to temporary income via this program. Another important program is ProJoven. This program offers training services for youth (16–24 years old) in high-demanded technical skills as well as labor intermediation services. Since 1997, this program has offered its services to 50,000 youths, mostly from poorer environments. Finally, labor intermediation services are offered through Red-CIL. This program was created in 1996 with the goal of reducing the informational frictions in labor markets via intermediation services that match labor supply and demand.[45] For the past decade, these programs have been increasingly incorporating beneficiaries with disabilities, although they are still far below the goal of 2% established by the Supreme Decree 003-2006-MIMDES.[46]

Using 2005 data, Maldonado showed the poor performance of labor programs in reaching persons with disabilities. Table 12.2 summarizes this result. None of the programs were able to comply with the 2% target mentioned in the preceding. For instance, ProJoven has only managed to train 11 young people with disabilities from a total of 34,000 participants throughout its 11 calls. A Trabajar was able to reach only 96 persons with disabilities out of a total of 194,000 beneficiaries, whereas in the case of Mujeres Emprendedoras only 46 women with disabilities were able to use the services provided by the program. A similar behavior is observed in other programs, such as the Red CIL-PROEmpleo and Peru Entrepreneur.[47]

More recent data suggest that the situation did not change dramatically over the past five years. For instance, according to information provided by the Ministry of Labor for this study, ProJoven trained only 85 youths with disabilities in 2009 and 58 in 2010. In the case of RED-SIL, over five years 1996 persons with disabilities participated, and 264 found employment, a modest result.[48]

The exception to this pattern is Construyendo Perú, the successor of A Trabajar. Whereas in 2005 only 96 persons with disabilities benefited from the program, in 2009 this number was 1,118, and in 2010 1,836. This is a

Table 12.2 PARTICIPATION OF PERSONS WITH DISABILITIES IN LABOR PROGRAMS CIRCA 2005[49]

Name	PROJoven (1)	A Trabajar Urbano (2)	Perú Empren-dedor (3)	Mujeres Empren-dedoras (4)	Programa de Autoempleo y Micro-empresa (5)	Red CIL-PRO Empleo (6)
Beneficiaries with disability	11	96	39	46	42	60
Total beneficiaries	34,136	194,756	n.d.	3,628	24,308	36,909
Participation rate of PWD	**0.03%**	**0.05%**	**n.d.**	**1.27%**	**0.20%**	**0.16%**

PWD stands for persons with disabilities

remarkable result, because the kind of activities performed in projects funded by the program are typically physically intensive.

It is important to keep in mind that labor demand can be a constraint, as is illustrated by 2005 data for ProJoven.[50] If we follow the 2% rule, this implies that at least 683 youth with disabilities must be accepted to the program. However, only 282 applied to the selection of courses. That is, the number of vacancies was more than twice the number of applicants. The limited number of applicants may reflect insufficient outreach by the program to persons with disabilities or the program being perceived as inaccessible, as well as actual levels of demand. Therefore, although programs need to make adjustments to incorporate persons with disabilities more effectively, this would not work if we do not pay attention to demand.

3.4.2 Quota Systems and Public Employment

In the case of the quota mechanism established by Law 28164, information collected by CONADIS in 2010 indicates that only 0.5% of the labor force of state agencies is composed by persons with disabilities. This is far below the legal target of 3%. This poor performance raised some concerns among policymakers and civil society, and the state's response was the creation in 2011 of a special commission to analyze this situation and propose a set of policy recommendations to overcome it.[51] Unfortunately, its recommendations did not get implemented due to a lack of political will.

There is much room for improvement in this regard. Even in tasks traditionally assigned to persons with disabilities, it is frequently observed that persons without disabilities are those who take these positions. Part of this poor performance is related to a set of austerity norms enacted by the Peruvian government over the past decade by which hiring is restricted. In this scenario, most of the available vacancies of public jobs are usually offered under temporal contracts, which are not regulated by the laws that favor persons with disabilities.

A similar situation is observed for the additional points in favor of persons with disabilities in merit competitions for public sector jobs.[52] The use of this benefit is severely limited because the hiring practices of the Peruvian state are dominated by the abuse of temporal contracts such as the Administrative Services Contract (CAS). This form of contract only recognizes a limited set of social rights and can be signed only for one year. As a result, the practical consequences of this instrument are very limited.

Moreover, persons with disabilities have had difficulties when trying to assert their rights. The Ombudsman Office has received multiple complaints by persons with disabilities who have faced difficulties in achieving the recognition of the additional 15% score. Only between August 1999 and June 2003, the Ombudsman Office was informed of 23 complaints, six information requests, and seven petitions regarding compliance with Article 36 of Law 27050 on additional points. The common pattern of these complaints was the failure to recognize the bonus of 15% in the regulations issued for public sector job competitions. It was found that this was due mainly to lack of knowledge of the law on the part of public officials.

Another limitation detected in the implementation of the bonus of 15% is the uncertainty regarding the stage of the competition at which it is appropriate to apply the percentage mentioned. For example, Maldonado found that in the case of the Ministry of Education the bonus was applied during the evaluation of the curriculum vitae, whereas at the National Judicial Council, this bonus was awarded at the end of the curriculum evaluation and knowledge test.[53] These differences are mainly due to the lack of clarity of the law on this regard.

3.4.3 Tax Incentives

Although the deductions of expenses provided by law have been regulated by the Ministry of Finance through Supreme Decree 102-2004-EF for some years now, there is no information available to assess its effectiveness. Interviews with public officials and policymakers suggest that no significant progress exists in this regard. If no progress is made in the certification of disability, it is likely that additional rules would have little impact.

3.5 Propulsion Policies

In regard to propulsion policies, the law establishes a set of rules aimed at contributing to the development of business initiatives by persons with disabilities, mainly in its Chapter VII, which is dedicated to promotional enterprises. Such measures include access to credit, preferential purchase of products by the state, and the creation of a bank of projects for promotional enterprises.

One of the first issues to evaluate here is the definition of a promotional enterprise. Current law provides that the promotional enterprise category is acquired if at least 30% of workers in an economic unit are workers with disabilities.[54] The accreditation and supervision of these enterprises is the responsibility of the Ministry of Labor.

Although systematic information about the characteristics of promotional enterprises has not been collected yet, anecdotal evidence suggests that they are mainly small firms, composed of individuals with physical disabilities, they lack access to credit, and their workers' wages are low compared with the average worker in the Peruvian labor market. In many ways, this is consistent with previous evidence collected by Sicchar.[55]

It is important to mention that this law represents a significant improvement regarding previous legal instruments.[56] However, although the requirements for the creation of promotional enterprises are relatively more flexible now than they were during the previous regulatory framework, there was little progress during the first years of implementation of the law. According to information from the Ministry of Labor, only two promotional enterprises were registered in 2003. This situation has changed in the past years. For instance, in 2010, 380 promotion enterprises were incorporated to the register and by early 2013 this number had risen to almost 550.[57] The rapid growth experienced in recent years creates positive expectations regarding the potential of this mechanism to improve employment conditions of persons with disabilities.

These improvements have been made despite the existence of two important constraints for the development of such enterprises. The first is essentially structural in nature and is associated with the context of informality characteristic of most of these enterprises. According to a study conducted by the Agency for Promotion of Small and Medium Enterprises (PROMPYME) for the case of Metropolitan Lima and Callao, about 70% of micro and small businesses that hire persons with disabilities are informal.[58] The other constraint lies in the difficulties already mentioned regarding the disability certificate, a requirement for enrollment in the register.

3.5.1 Legislation Implementing Procurement Preference

A first evaluation of the law leads us to conclude that the way in which it was designed did not promote, in practice, the development of enterprises by persons with disabilities. The law was very ambiguous about the preferential treatment for promotional enterprises, which has led to the small amount of progress observed in past years.

This situation changed after the publication of the Supreme Decree 184-2008-EF in January 2009, which contains the regulations of the State Contracting Law.[59] This legal instrument established that, in the event that two proposals obtain equal scores after a competitive evaluation process, the contract must be awarded to the promotional enterprise. In a context of large increases in government budgets due to high international prices of mineral resources, contracting with the state has become a profitable business for small and medium enterprises. In turn, this has created incentives to hire persons with disabilities with the expectation of taking advantage of the benefits established by the law. The direct consequence has been the increase in the number of promotional enterprises, starting in 2009, along with an increase in employment opportunities available for persons with disabilities.

Mechanisms developed by regional and local governments to promote labor market opportunities for persons with disabilities can offer a different view. According to the law, these levels of government are responsible for the constitution of regional and municipal offices to attend to people with disabilities (OREDIS and OMAPED, respectively). In turn, these entities are called upon to coordinate and formulate regional and local policies for this sector. Among these policies, the promotion of goods produced by persons with disabilities is a critical role recognized by the law. Despite this, there has been relatively little progress, because of the low priority assigned to this activity within the set of activities normally organized by municipalities and regional governments.

In fact, local and regional governments have shown very little interest on the topic. According to information provided by the Ombudsman Office, only 350 municipalities have established offices of this type.[60] This is equivalent to 19% of all municipalities in the country. From all of these, very few have used their purchasing power to support enterprises by persons with disabilities. In fact, a study elaborated by the Ombudsman Office some years ago showed that there is no a single case in which municipalities supported products made by persons with disabilities.[61] There is definite room for improvement in this area.

3.5.2 Access to Credit

With regard to the issue of credit, according to Article 37 of Law 27050, CONADIS, in coordination with the Ministry of Economy and Finance, has the role of developing mechanisms to provide preferential loans for financing promotional enterprises. However, there has not been much effort to move in that direction, besides some experimental initiatives. For instance, the

Development Finance Corporation (COFIDE) provides resources for microfinance institutions interested in assisting persons with disabilities.[62] Whether these schemes work is a pending area of research, not only because of the lack of information, but also because these initiatives have been recently implemented and it is premature to assess their impact.

4. CONCLUSION

This chapter has studied the set of policies employed by the Peruvian state in order to improve labor conditions for persons with disabilities. It discusses policy instruments and evaluates their effectiveness, taking into account informational constraints. After characterizing the labor market for persons with disabilities as one in which participation rates are low and informality is high, it is shown that the impact of most policies is currently modest.

Some tentative lessons emerge from our analysis. Despite the weak enforcement of the law, it is possible to argue that some progress has been made. In most cases, this improvement is linked to the development of labor opportunities for persons with disabilities in small and medium enterprises. This is consistent with the labor market conditions in low- and middle-income countries, where the formal sector is relatively small. Furthermore, the low levels of formal education that characterize persons with disabilities in Peru because of previous exclusion also work as a constraint.

A set of policy recommendations can be derived from our discussion. In the first place, better information systems are needed to monitor and evaluate the policies implemented. Available information is scarce and fragmented, making any attempt to study this issue very costly. New protocols and instruments to collect information are required because the existing ones, when they exist, are outdated. Although there has been some progress in this regard, little can be achieved without political will.

A second recommendation is related to human capital accumulation. Low levels of education are related to the way in which persons with disabilities participate in the labor market. Those with little education are more likely to be inactive or workers in the informal sector; therefore, education policy has a critical role to play.

A third recommendation would be to reassess the emphasis that current policies have on formal employment. Most of these policies seem to assume a level of formality that the country does not have, putting too much weight on policy instruments that will have limited impact. Along the same lines, these policy instruments are based on the assumption that the average worker with a disability has a set of labor skills that are not consistent with their actual levels of human capital. This does not mean that these policies must be discarded because there are workers with disabilities who are taking advantage of them; it is only a matter of emphasis. Given the lack of technical capacity and resources, policymakers should allocate more effort to what is working.

Finally, it is important to explore more policy alternatives regarding the development and sustainability of promotional enterprises as well as ways to expand job market opportunities for a labor force characterized by low levels of human capital. Given the role played by the state as the most important buyer of goods and services over the past years, there is a window of opportunity to create jobs for low-skilled workers with disabilities.

There are dimensions that require but have not received much attention. Perhaps the most important is to pay special attention to differences in gender and, by extension, ethnicity. The evidence presented here suggests that the labor market exclusion faced by women with disabilities is particularly acute. Disability policies need to take these issues into account.

Although overall progress in disability and employment in Peru is slow, there is also room for optimism. Just 15 years ago the topic was invisible for the Peruvian state and the rest of society. More political will and better institutional capacities are, in our view, the key ingredients for achieving the social inclusion of persons with disabilities.

ACKNOWLEDGMENTS

This chapter was prepared for the conference Disability and Work: Global Strategies for Equity, organized by the Institute for Health and Social Policy at McGill University. The author thanks the organizers of the conference for the invitation and their patience. Comments, inputs, and suggestions by the editors, Luis Miguel del Aguila, Antonio Salazar, Javier Díez Canseco, Susana Stiglich, and Liliana Peñaherrera are highly appreciated. Usual disclaimers apply.

The author wishes to dedicate this chapter to the memory of Javier Díez Canseco, who was a tireless fighter for the rights of persons with disabilities in Peru. His courage in advancing the agenda for the rights of persons with disabilities will be deeply missed.

NOTES

1. Although information for other parts of the country is available, only in the case of Lima do we have access to better quality data in an ample set of labor indicators for persons with disabilities.
2. Before this law, there were fragmented policies targeted to different groups of persons with disabilities but not an integral approach.
3. Spiller, P. & Tommasi, M. (2007). *The Institutional Foundations of Public Policy in Argentina*. Cambridge, United Kingdom: Cambridge University Press.

4. This broad range may seem disconcerting at first. However, these are common in countries in which more than one definition of disability is used. For example, in Colombia, the Census of 1993 estimated the proportion of persons with disabilities at around 2% while, in 1997, the National Information System estimated this proportion at 23.8%. Additionally, two years later, the National Disability Plan calculated this indicator about 18%.
5. It is beyond the goal of this chapter to discuss the advantages and shortcomings of the definitions used in these sources of information. For an interesting discussion about the measurement of disability, see Loeb, M., Eide, A., & Mont, D. (2008). Approaching the measurement of disability prevalence: The case of Zambia. *ALTER, Revue européenne de recherché sur le hándicap* 2, 32–43. For a detailed discussion on the measures available for the Peruvian case, see Maldonado, S. (2006). *Trabajo y Discapacidad en el Perú: Mercado Laboral, Políticas Públicas e Inclusión Social.* Fondo Editorial del Congreso del Perú and Programa de Naciones Unidas para el Desarrollo. Lima. For a discussion about measurement issues about disability in other Latin American countries, see: Dudzik, P., Elwan, A., & Metts, R. (2002). *Disability Policies, Statistics, and Strategies in Latin America and the Caribbean: A Review.* Washington, D.C.: Inter-American Development Bank; Hernández-Licona, G. (2002) *Disability and the Labor Market: Data Gaps and Needs in Latin America and the Caribbean.* Washington, D.C.: Inter-American Development Bank; Montes, A., & Massiah, E. (2002) *Disability Data: Survey and Methods Issues in Latin America and the Caribbean.* Washington, D.C.: Inter-American Development Bank.
6. See Instituto Nacional de Estadística e Informática (2006). *Encuesta Nacional Continua.* Lima, Peru: INEI. This survey was carried out by the National Statistical Institute. It has national coverage and a sample size higher than 300,000 observations. The data collection process covered the whole year.
7. Lima, Peru: INEI. This census was collected in a single day in 2007 under the leadership of the National Statistical Institute. It was designed to replace the ENCO survey, which originally was introduced as a new methodology to collect information about the socioeconomic characteristics of the whole Peruvian population, replacing the standard census methodology.
8. This is a preferable source to ENCO 2006 because it is the official information used by the Peruvian state.
9. Instituto Nacional de Estadística e Informática (2007). *Censos Nacionales 2007.* One potential problem with this source is that it can overestimate the extent of disability in the population. This is clear from the proportion of people who declare that they have visual limitations.
10. This was a specialized survey on disability issues in the capital city, which represents about 30% of the country's population. It was a joint effort of CONADIS and INEI. From a methodological point of view, the EHODIS is the best source of information available in the country. It is based on a carefully designed instrument that measures loss of function following the recommendations of the World Health Organization. Unfortunately, this survey did not get the attention of civil society and policy-makers because it provided an estimate of the prevalence of disability lower than the commonly accepted 10%. This is important, since there is a political use of disability prevalence estimates by activist and disabled peoples' organization, who consider that the size of the population with disabilities matters in order to advocate for more resources and attention from the Peruvian state.

11. Instituto Nacional de Estadística e Informática (2005). *Encuesta Nacional de Hogares sobre Discapacidad en Lima Metropolitana y Callao*. Lima, Peru: INEI and CONADIS.
12. These numbers were computed from the Encuesta Especializada de Niveles de Empleo, carried out yearly by the Ministry of Labor and Employment. See Ministerio de Trabajo y Promoción del Empleo (2008). Informe de la Encuesta de Hogares Especializada en Niveles de Empleo, Lima Metropolitana 2008. Retrieved March 25, 2013, from: http://www.mintra.gob.pe/archivos/file/ estadisticas/peel/publicacion/ENAHO_PRELIMINAR_2008.pdf
13. The estimates of GDP growth were taken from the Central Bank of Peru. See Banco Central de Reserva del Perú (2013). Estadísticas. Retrieved March 25, 2013, from: http://www.bcrp.gob.pe/estadisticas.html
14. A recent study in this regard is CEDAL-POETA (2010). *Diagnóstico de la Situación Laboral de las Personas con Discapacidad en el Perú*. Lima, Peru: OAS. However, this work does not exploit the most recent household surveys to produce a consistent description of the labor market for persons with disabilities. For basic references for a complete description of labor market issues for persons with disabilities in the country, see Maldonado (2006). *Trabajo y Discapacidad en el Perú*, and Maldonado, S. (2007). *Exclusión y Discriminación en contra de la Población con Discapacidad en el Mercado Laboral Peruano: Un Análisis de Descomposiciones Paramétricas y no Paramétricas*. Lima, Peru: CIES and CEDEP.
15. Unless noted, all the estimates provided in the rest of this chapter were computed by the author using microdata from the ENAHO survey for 2002-2003. The data can be consulted at: Instituto Nacional de Estadística e Informática (2013). Consulta de Encuestas. Retrieved March 25, 2013, from: http://www.inei.gob.pe/srienaho/enaho197.htm
16. Metts, R. (2000). Disability Issues, Trends and Recommendations for the World Bank. *Social Protection Discussion Paper Series 0007*. Washington, D.C.: World Bank; Mont, D. (2004). Disability Employment Policy. *Social Protection Discussion Paper Series 0413*, Washington, D.C.: World Bank.
17. Maldonado (2007). *Exclusión y Discriminación*.
18. Mitra, S., & Sambamoorthi, U. (2006). Disability and the Rural Labor Market in India: Evidence for Males in Tamil Nadu. World Development 36 (5), 934–952.
19. Ñopo, H. (2004). Matching as Tool to Decompose Wage Gaps. *IZA Discussion Paper Series 981*. Bonn, Germany: IZA.
20. Reimers, C. (1983). Labor Market Discrimination against Hispanic and Black Men. *Review of Economics and Statistics* 65 (4), 570–579.
21. Ñopo (2004). Matching as Tool to Decompose Wage Gaps.
22. For an evaluation of previous attempts to develop a disability policy by the Peruvian State, see Maldonado (2006). *Trabajo y Discapacidad en el Perú*.
23. During a set of interviews with the author for this chapter, several respondents complained about the significant amount of time that public officials in CONADIS spend in responding to particular and narrow demands by groups or individuals with disabilities.
24. This commission was originally led by Javier Díez Canseco for the term 2001-2006; he was replaced by Micheal Urtecho for term 2006-2011. The commission was renamed as "Commission of Social Inclusion and Disability" for the term 2011-2016, now under the leadership of the congresswomen Rosa Mavila.
25. In 2006, this commission published several monographs regarding labor, health, and accessibility conditions for persons with disabilities. No similar effort in

terms of promoting research about disability issues in the country has been developed since then.

26. As part of the research for this chapter, I visited the Ministry of Labor to interview one of the officials working in this unit. The team (composed of about 4 officials) shared a small office in the first floor of the Ministry. Concerns regarding the lack of resources to carry out their work were expressed by officials of this unit during the interview.

27. Interestingly, this contrasts with the relative electoral success of candidates with disabilities in the last election for Congress. For the first time, Congress has 5 members with disabilities (out of 130).

28. O'Reilly, A. (2007). *El Derecho al Trabajo Decente de las Personas con Discapacidades*. Working Paper. Geneva, Switzerland: International Labour Office.

29. The most important legal instrument was Decree 24560 of July 11, 1963. This instrument required that government agencies and other units of the public sector had to provide state-paid work in vacancies for qualified disabled people for tasks that they are in a position to perform. This rule was intended to explicitly link existing rehabilitation systems (such as the Instituto Nacional del Ciego and other rehabilitation centers for persons with disabilities) with the labor market through employment in the public sector. Also, the Peruvian government agreed to create centers of industrial production in order to provide permanent employment to graduates of the centers mentioned above. For an historical overview of employment policies for persons with disabilities in the Peruvian context, see Maldonado (2006). *Trabajo y Discapacidad en el Perú*.

30. For a compilation of laws and other legal instruments related to employment opportunities for persons with disabilities, see Salazar, A. (2011). *Las Personas con Discapacidad y el Trabajo: Compendio de Normas Laborales*. Lima, Peru: Oficina Nacional de Promoción Laboral de las Personas con Discapacidad, Ministerio de Trabajo.

31. Hills, J. (2002). Does a focus on "social exclusion" change the policy response? In J. Hills, J. Le Grand and D. Piachaud (Eds.). *Understanding Social Exclusion*. Oxford, United Kingdom: Oxford University Press. 226–243.

32. Maldonado (2006). *Trabajo y Discapacidad en el Perú*.

33. CONADIS has a register for persons with disabilities. Although one person with a disability can have a disability certificate and not be registered in CONADIS, some public officials have interpreted that a registration in CONADIS is needed to have access to the benefits and rights recognized by the law. For that reason, this information is a good proxy to estimate the extent of potential beneficiaries of the current legal framework.

34. According to CONADIS, about 16,502 persons with disabilities had disability certificates in 2004. This number was 68,125 in 2011. Notice that we are using the prevalence rates computed by the INR study of 1993. Using the population numbers of the Census of 2007, this estimate will be 2.12%, still very low. Those interested in the evolution of the disability certification the past decade can visit the following link: http://www.conadisperu.gob.pe/web/documentos/registro/estadisticas/estadisticas.pdf

35. Another reason for this decision is the poor development of financial assistance for those recently affected by disability. Although these mechanisms exist, they are available only for formal workers. Moreover, many firms (76%) do not pay

insurance, so their workers are unprotected in practice. See Maldonado (2006). *Trabajo y Discapacidad en el Perú*.

36. See Ley 27050, *Ley General de la Persona con Discapacidad*. According to Degener, T. & Quinn, G. (2000). A Survey of International, Comparative and Regional Disability Law Reform. Retrieved March 25, 2013, from http://www.dredf.org/international/degener_sp.html, most countries, especially developed countries, do not use criminal law-based mechanisms against discrimination against persons with disabilities. However, there is a strong debate because a strictly civil law-based approach is found to be too weak to avoid discrimination against persons with disabilities. For a discussion of the importance of advancing the criminalization of anti-discrimination rules in the context of Netherlands, see Van Vijnen, A. (2003), El derecho a vivir y a ser tratado con respeto en este mundo: Las posibilidades del derecho penal. Retrieved March 25, 2013, from http://www.disabilityworld.org/01-03_03/spanish/gobierno/law.shtml.

37. Lei 7.853, de 24/10/1989.

38. O' Reilly (2007). *El Derecho al Trabajo Decente*.

39. This classification may be controversial for some readers. We proceed in this way since we believe these instruments are more consistent with the goal of promotion, but it is obvious that for some instruments there is not a clear line between types of policies.

40. Ley 27050, *Ley General de la Persona con Discapacidad*, Article 32.

41. Ley 27050, *Ley General de la Persona con Discapacidad*, Article 33.

42. Ley 27050, *Ley General de la Persona con Discapacidad*, Article 35.

43. Ley 27050, *Ley General de la Persona con Discapacidad*, Article 49.

44. Ley 28164, *Ley que Modifica Diversos Artículos de la Ley N° 27050, Ley general de la Persona con Discapacidad*, Article 36.

45. These programs were named "A Trabajar," "ProJoven" and "Red CIL-PROEMPLEO" respectively during Alejandro Toledo's administration. The new government of Ollanta Humala decided to change these names again, a usual practice among politicians after a change of government, but this chapter keeps the names these programs had during Alan Garcia's earlier administration because the information available comes from these years. It is important to mention that other minor programs are also offered by the Ministry of Labor, such as those targeted to specific groups like women (Mujeres Emprendedoras) and workers affected by the 2008 international crisis (Revalora Perú).

46. This 2% was established by the Ministry of Social Development as a complementary measure to expand employment opportunities for persons with disabilities in the public sector. See Decreto Supremo No.003-2006-MIMDES, *Modifican Reglamento de la Ley General de la Persona con Discapacidad, aprobado por D.S. N° 003-2000-PROMUDEH, publicado el jueves 30 de marzo del 2006 en el diario oficial El Peruano*. Due to the lack of enforcement, few governmental offices are reaching this goal.

47. It is possible that, due to the lack of good instruments for collecting information about the disability status of the participants in these programs, the number of participants with disabilities was being underestimated. However, according to local experts on the topic, it seems highly unlikely that this is the case. In any case, the bias, if it exists, must be minimal.

48. Data from this section was provided by the National Direction of Labor Promotion for People with Disabilities at the Ministry of Labor. I thank Antonio Salazar for sharing this information.

49. Maldonado (2006). *Trabajo y Discapacidad en el Perú.*
50. As most training programs, ProJoven selects its participants based on a selection process. Those selected are offered the training services for a limited period.
51. This commission was composed of representatives of the Ministry of Labor, Ministry of Production, the Presidency of Council of Ministers, CONADIS, the Congress and the Ombudsman Office. Its final report was delivered in August 2011 but its implementation is still uncertain. This issue has become shelved after a change in the direction of the Ministry of Labor. Whereas the former minister was sensitive to the agenda of labor rights for persons with disabilities, for the new administration this agenda was of secondary importance.
52. According to the current legal framework, all permanent jobs at any governmental office must be allocated after a competitive process in which previous experience and qualifications are assessed. Each job posting includes a set of rules regarding the points allocated to each part of the evaluation, which usually includes a personal interview. The law establishes that these merit competitions must provide extra points to applicants with disabilities.
53. Maldonado (2006). *Trabajo y Discapacidad en el Perú.*
54. Besides this criterion, no systematic information about the characteristics of these enterprises is available. This issue is an area for future research.
55. Sicchar, J. (2003). *Características de las pequeñas y microempresas que emplean personas discapacitadas.* Lima, Peru: Comisión de Promoción de la Pequeña y Microempresa PROMPYME.
56. During the 1980s, the category of promotional enterprises already existed but it was very modest in terms of size. One potential reason could be the fact that, to be considered as such, a promotional enterprise had to have a labor force composed of at least 65% of persons with disabilities, which is quite a steep requirement.
57. This information was provided by the National Direction of Labor Promotion for People with Disabilities of the Ministry of Labor. The interested reader can consult the quarterly reports of this direction at: http://www.trabajo.gob.pe/mostrarContenido.php?id=119&tip=9
58. Sicchar (2003). *Características de las pequeñas y microempresas.*
59. Decreto Supremo184-2008-EF, *Reglamento de Contrataciones del Estado.*
60. For more details, see Defensoría del Pueblo (2013). Grupos de especial protección. Personas con discapacidad. Retrieved March 25, 2013, from http://www.defensoria.gob.pe/grupos-eatencion.php?des=18
61. Defensoría del Pueblo (2003). *Resolución Defensorial Nº 039-2003/DP del 17 de Diciembre del 2003 que recomienda al Congreso de la República modificar el Artículo 36º de la Ley Nº 27050, Ley General de la Persona con Discapacidad.* Lima, Peru: Defensoría del Pueblo.
62. This initiative is developed under the Guarantee Fund for People with Disability (known as FOGADIS for its name in Spanish) under COFIDE. Some microfinance institutions (MFI) as well as a state-owned bank are starting to use these funds to provide credit to small entrepreneurs with disabilities. One of the first MFIs to take advantage of this fund is the Caja de Piura. A credit program, called "CrediAmigo," was developed, and 50% of the risk of no payment is covered by COFIDE, allowing for lower interest rates and transaction costs. The size of these credits are relative small (from 140 to 2000 US$).

CHAPTER 13

Restructuring Disability Policy and Improving Employment Outcomes in the United States

DAVID C. STAPLETON AND DAVID R. MANN

1. INTRODUCTION

The United States is struggling to undertake a transition to disability policies that are appropriate for the 21st century. In many ways, America's struggles with disability policy are similar to those in other democracies with advanced economies. The wealth of these nations has allowed them to build complex safety nets for people with disabilities. As measured by public expenditures, these safety nets are very large, demonstrating the high willingness of taxpayers in these countries to assist this population. Historically, such safety nets have primarily used a "caretaker" model, designed to provide for the basic needs of those assumed unable to provide for themselves. Only a tiny share of public resources has been devoted to helping those with disabilities take better advantage of their capabilities. In fact, many features of existing safety nets have the effect of discouraging work and self-sufficiency.

The central challenge for policymakers is to change these large complex systems in a manner that will empower people with disabilities to realize their full productivity while 1) preserving basic supports for those with the very limited self-sufficiency capabilities or who have become highly dependent on the existing system, and 2) slowing growth in public expenditures for their support during a time of fiscal austerity.

This chapter describes the limited progress that has been achieved in these areas thus far in the United States. It first considers why past policy initiatives have not been more successful and then presents a road map for greater success in the future.

2. CURRENT CHALLENGES

The core feature of the American support system that discourages employment is the common medical eligibility criterion for the two programs that provide most of the public income support for working-age people with disabilities and are the gateway to health benefits and many other supports.[1] Social Security Disability Insurance (SSDI) is social wage-replacement insurance for workers; benefit amounts are based on past wages, without regard for assets. Supplemental Security Income (SSI) is a means-tested welfare benefit, available only to those with extremely low assets, and provides a benefit amount that is inversely related to income from other sources. Their common medical eligibility criterion is inability to work more than a minimal amount for a period of at least 12 months or until death because of a medically determinable impairment. This criterion excludes entry into either program by individuals with disabilities earning more than a low threshold amount—US $1,010 per month for non-blind individuals in 2012.[2] In addition, individuals already receiving SSDI benefits lose their benefits completely if they earn more than the same threshold amount for more than 12 months, whereas all SSI recipients lose US $1 in monthly benefits for every $2 earned above a $65 disregard.[3]

The SSDI/SSI gateway to the disability support system is a policy structure that discourages work and perpetuates the misconception that people with disabilities cannot work. Recent research demonstrates the effect of this structure on employment. One study provides convincing evidence that at least 18% of new recipients of SSDI benefits are able to earn more than the annual equivalent of US $1,010 per month within two years after program entry, but only 5% choose to do so.[4] Other strong evidence is consistent with this finding.[5]

The first *World Report on Disability (WRD)*, issued by the World Health Organization (WHO) and the World Bank, provides a framework for evaluating American disability policy.[6] The *WRD* identifies legislation and policies considered central to improving employment outcomes of people with disabilities, including, among others, antidiscrimination laws, affirmative action, quotas, support for employment, and vocational rehabilitation and training. Of those identified, antidiscrimination legislation is the only policy that is firmly in place in the United States; the Americans with Disabilities Act (ADA) was enacted into law more than two decades ago, and has been emulated in many respects by disability rights legislation in other countries and the United Nations Conventions of the Rights of Persons with Disabilities.[7] The United States also has a somewhat impressive record of expanding employment services to people with disabilities. But the United States has, at best, only weakly addressed other aspects of the *WRD* recommendations, and, at worst, ignored some entirely.[8]

The key to reversing past trends might well be to bring policy more in line with the *WRD* recommendations, most notably: moving away from benefits that are predicated on "inability to work" toward benefits that enhance the capabilities of individuals and their value to employers; harmonizing employment incentives with the ADA's objectives; and ensuring social protection while supporting employment. Addressing these recommendations requires fundamental restructuring of America's disability programs.

However, there are three major barriers to structural reform. The first is inadequate evidence on how to best support successful structural changes. Although some countries are implementing elements of the *WRD* recommendations, the body of evidence on specific approaches is weak. Further, differences between American institutions and those in the rest of the world—most notably with respect to the health care system and political institutions—limit the applicability of findings from other countries. Even with the best intentions, structural changes not firmly grounded in evidence could further undermine the economic status of people with disabilities, or accelerate growth in government expenditures for their support. Reliable evidence is also needed to forge a consensus among advocates and overcome the political polarization that confronts nearly all new social legislation in the United States.

The second barrier to structural reform is a national fiscal crisis that is likely to dominate federal and state government decision making for many years to come. Myopic focus on immediate deficit reduction in Congress makes it difficult to move forward with reforms that do not produce short-term results or savings, or that require testing via demonstrations and a long implementation period. Advocates and other stakeholders are understandably unwilling to give up the status quo in favor of new, untested programs. Hence, policymakers oppose reform legislation requiring higher short-term costs with no certainty of lower future costs, whereas stakeholders insist that structural reforms be evidence-based.

The third barrier is the fragmented nature of American disability programs. The types of reforms needed require structural changes that cut across the current responsibilities of multiple agencies at multiple levels of government. That, in turn, requires breaking down current institutions, which is often not in the interest of the many existing stakeholders. Although individual program administrators and others do have incentives to innovate within the present system, such reforms fail to take advantage of more attractive opportunities that cut across multiple programs, and sometimes improve one program's performance at the expense of another's.

In summary, an inadequate evidence base, the nation's fiscal challenges, and the fragmentation of the current disability support system all pose major challenges to improving disability policy in the United States. A concerted effort will be required to effectively address all three of these barriers.

The chapter is organized as follows. In the first section we review the disappointing trends in the employment, economic status, and reliance on public support of working-age Americans with disabilities since 1980. In the second section, we summarize the policy road traveled during the same period, and offer our diagnosis of why the results have been so unsatisfactory. We also briefly summarize the successes and failures of major structural reforms in the assistance provided to low-income families over the same period, commonly referred to as "welfare reform." The experience of welfare reform offers important lessons on how to move forward with disability policy reform—some encouraging, others cautionary. The final section provides a road map for future progress that addresses the barriers identified in the preceding ones.

3. THREE DECADES OF DISAPPOINTMENT

Our review of the recent history of disability policy in the United States highlights lessons from previous reform efforts that are applicable to policymakers worldwide and identifies the origins of the current barriers to reform. The summary begins in 1980 for two reasons. First, before 1980 data limitations make it much more difficult to assess trends in employment and economic status for people with disabilities. Second, policymakers first became alarmed about growth in the reliance of working-age people with disabilities on government support in the late 1970s, which led to a long series of policy initiatives. Although we present data for the entire period, the discussion in this section focuses on comparing 1980 data to 2010 data. We save consideration of the interim period for the following section where we review major disability policy changes and their impact on economic and government support trends.

3.1 Employment and Economic Status

The longest uninterrupted employment rate series by disability status in the United States is from the Current Population Survey (CPS). The CPS uses a "work-limitation" definition of disability: the presence of a physical or mental condition that limits the respondent's ability to work. Although there is much to criticize about the CPS disability definition, extensive analysis has shown that, over subperiods, trends in employment rates by disability status from the CPS are quite comparable to those measured in other surveys, using other measures of disability, especially when comparisons are made at comparable points in the business cycle.[9]

The CPS measure shows that since the late 1980s, the employment rate for those with work limitations has steadily declined relative to those without work limitations (Figure 13.1, bottom line). In 2010, the employment rate of those with work limitations was just 21% of the corresponding rate for those without work limitations. In 1981, the earliest year with comparable data, the corresponding figure was 34%. Over the entire period, the relative employment rate declined by 37%. To help put this change in perspective, if the relative employment rate in 2010 was the same as it was in 1981, and holding 2010 employment of those without work limitations constant, then employment for those with work limitations in 2010 would have been approximately 900,000 higher than it actually was.[10]

Statistics from the CPS also show that the mean household income of those with work limitations has steadily declined relative to the mean for other households (Figure 13.1, top line). As we shall see, household income from disability benefits increased over the same period. However, the increase in disability benefit payments for those with work limitations did not fully compensate for the decline in wage income.

3.2 Reliance on Government Support

As relative employment rates and earned income among working-age people with disabilities have declined, their reliance on government support

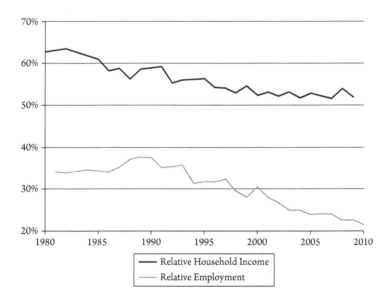

Figure 13.1
Relative Employment and Household Income of Working-Age People with Work Limitations, 1980–2010[11]

has steadily increased. This section describes the extent of these increases across several programs. We first consider caseloads and expenditures for the main program that provides benefits for workers who have left the labor force because of a long-term disability, the Social Security Disability Insurance program. We then consider expenditures for Medicare, the public health insurance program SSDI beneficiaries automatically enter after 24 months of benefit receipt. Complete data for both programs are available from 1970 to the present. Finally, we consider estimates of support expenditures from a much broader array of government programs. These estimates are available from 2002 through 2008 only. As will be seen, expenditures for all other programs combined exceed those for SSDI and Medicare alone.

3.2.1 Social Security Disability Insurance and Medicare

The SSDI caseload nearly tripled in size from 1980 to 2010, although part of this growth can be attributed to growth in the number and change in the age-sex composition of workers covered by the program. To control for the gradual increase in the age at which SSDI beneficiaries are converted to Social Security retirees after 2003, the data presented are only for beneficiaries under age 65. The (December) caseload grew from 2.9 million in 1980 to 7.9 million in 2010 (Figure 13.2, solid line).

Figure 13.2 also projects what the caseload would have been in December of each year based on 1980 participation rates for qualified workers within age-sex categories. The projected series incorporates the growth in the number and change in the age-sex composition of workers covered by SSDI on the size of the caseload. The difference between the two series represents the aggregate effects of changes in participation rates within age-sex categories between 1980 and the projection year.

It is apparent from Figure 13.2 that factors other than changes in demographics have led to an increase in the SSDI caseload. The projected series shows that the 2010 caseload would have been 2.2 million lower than the actual caseload had changes in worker demographics been the only cause of caseload growth—28% lower than the actual number.

Rapid SSDI caseload growth combined with rapid growth in the cost of health care are driving ever increasing federal expenditures to support SSDI beneficiaries. From 1980 to 2010, SSDI expenditures and Medicare expenditures for SSDI beneficiaries grew at a faster rate than gross domestic product (GDP) and all federal outlays (Figure 13.3). SSDI benefits alone grew 53% more than GDP, whereas Medicare expenditures for SSDI beneficiaries outpaced GDP growth by 153%. In 2010, the sum of these

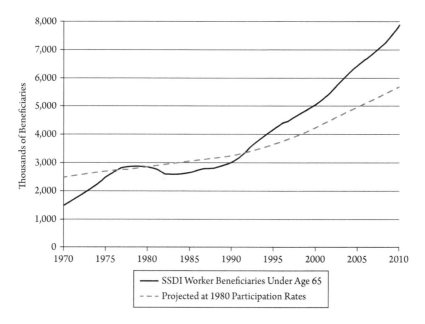

Figure 13.2
SSDI Worker Beneficiaries under Age 65, 1970–2010[12]

expenditures accounted for 1.3% of GDP and 5.0% of all federal outlays. In 1980, these expenditures accounted for just 0.7% of GDP and 3.5% of federal outlays.

The Trustees of the SSDI Trust Fund and the Congressional Budget Office both project that the fund will be exhausted in 2016.[13] If no action is taken by Congress, the program will not be able to pay all SSDI benefits on time.

3.2.2 All Programs That Support the Working-Age Population with Disabilities

Although federal expenditures for SSDI benefits and Medicare coverage for SSDI beneficiaries represent a large share of federal expenditures for the working-age population with disabilities in the United States, total federal expenditures for this population are more than twice as high. Estimated total federal expenditures for this population accounted for 12% of all federal outlays in federal fiscal year 2008, or US $358 billion.[14] In the same year, states spent an additional $71 billion for federal-state programs to support this population.

The bulk of these expenditures are for income support and health care (95%). The second-largest income support program, following SSDI, is

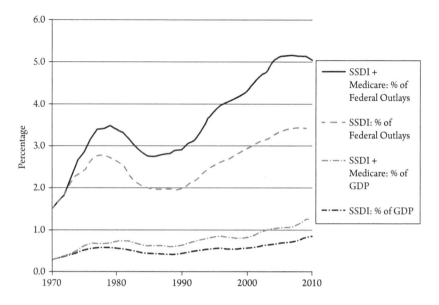

Figure 13.3
SSDI and Medicare Expenditures for People under Age 65 Relative to GDP and Federal Outlays, 1970 to 2010[15]

Supplemental Security Income (SSI), which is means tested. After Medicare, the second largest health program is Medicaid, a means-tested federal-state benefit that, unlike Medicare, pays for disability services such as personal assistance and institutional care. Other major income and health programs are those that provide support for disabled veterans. Only a very small, and shrinking, share of federal expenditures for this population are directed toward work (Table 13.1).

Since at least 2002, total expenditures for these programs have also grown faster than both all federal outlays and GDP. After adjusting for inflation, the 2008 estimate for federal expenditures is 31% higher than a comparable estimate for 2002,[16] and 28% higher when state expenditures are included. The 2002 federal figure represents 11.4% of federal outlays in that year, compared with 12.0% in 2008. Federal and state expenditures combined grew from 2.7% of GDP in 2002 to 3.0% in 2008.

Like many other high-income countries, the United States is facing a prolonged period of fiscal austerity. Politicians from both parties are looking for ways to reduce future government expenditures. The share of federal outlays devoted to the working-age population with disabilities will make it difficult for Congress to make such reductions without trimming eligibility and benefits for disability programs. The pending exhaustion of the SSDI Trust Fund

TABLE 13.1 FEDERAL EXPENDITURES FOR WORKING-AGE PEOPLE WITH DISABILITIES BY MAJOR EXPENDITURE CATEGORY, FISCAL YEARS 2002 AND 2008[17]

Category	FY 2008 Expenditures (US $ millions)	Percent Change Since FY 2002, Inflation Adjusted
Income maintenance	169,801	29.5
Health care	169,099	34.4
Housing and food assistance	11,643	17.9
Education, training, and employment	4,321	−2.6
Other services	2,492	2.3
Total	357,356	30.6

and the rapid growth of Medicare and Medicaid expenditures make these programs prime targets for budget cuts. Tightening eligibility and benefits is worrisome, however, because it will impose further hardship upon a very vulnerable population.

In summary, over the past three decades, the economic status of Americans with disabilities has fallen further and further behind that of their peers without disabilities. At the same time, growth in government outlays for their support has outpaced growth in both GDP and other government expenditures. This unsustainable growth combined with the country's fiscal problems are making it increasingly difficult for Congress to avoid tightening eligibility and reducing benefits, despite the hardship such changes would create for persons with disabilities. Equally troubling, these adverse trends have occurred despite substantial policy changes that were designed to improve economic outcomes for people with disabilities and reduce their reliance on government support.

4. THE POLICY ROAD TRAVELED

4.1 Major Policy Initiatives

The first relevant policy initiative occurred in 1980. Alarmed at the rapid growth in the number of SSDI beneficiaries in the late 1970s (see Figure 13.2) and growth in federal expenditures for their support (see Figure 13.3), Congress enacted amendments to the Social Security Act that require the Social Security Administration to conduct more systematic reviews of the medical status of existing beneficiaries. As a result of these reviews, the benefits of many beneficiaries were terminated in 1981 and 1982, which coincided with the worst recession since the Great Depression.

Negative political reaction to the large number of benefit terminations following medical reviews, including some highly publicized cases of individual hardship, led to an end of the heightened reviews in 1983 and passage of the Disability Benefits Reform Act of 1984.[18] The Act expanded the ways in which beneficiaries could meet the medical eligibility criteria for SSDI and SSI. Among other things, the 1984 amendments made it easier to obtain benefits if the functional symptoms of a chronic condition prevented work even if the medical evidence about the cause of the symptoms was ambiguous—most importantly for psychiatric disorders and lower back pain. After the new law was implemented, in the latter half of the 1980s the SSDI caseload started to grow again (see Figure 13.2), as did expenditures for their support (see Figure 13.3). The pace of caseload growth during this period was modest, but nonetheless slightly higher than what would be expected from growth in the size of the covered workforce and change in its age-sex composition, and despite the fact that the country was enjoying a vigorous economic expansion. Note also that relative employment of those with work limitations actually increased during this period (see Figure 13.1)—the only sustained increase observed over the entire three-decade period.

The passage of the ADA in 1990 was a major milestone for disability policy in the United States. The ADA established the rights of people with disabilities with respect to a wide array of social activities, including employment. Title I of the ADA prohibits employer discrimination against job applicants or employees with disabilities and also requires employers to provide reasonable accommodations for their disabilities. Provisions under other titles for accessibility of public places, commercial facilities, transportation, and telecommunications were designed to make it easier for people with disabilities to participate in all social activities, including employment.

Early research on the ADA concluded that it was responsible for the relative decline in employment for people with disabilities shortly after its passage.[19] The researchers hypothesized that the Title I provisions imposed costs on employers for hiring and retaining workers with disabilities that exceeded the benefits of avoiding potential litigation. More recently, however, others have pointed out that these early results are quite sensitive to the data used and the definition of both disability and employment. Perhaps most importantly, there is substantial evidence that the decline in employment of people with long-term disabilities predates the passage of the ADA, starting as early as 1986, and coinciding with the implementation of the Disability Benefits Reform Act.[20]

The passage of Individuals with Disabilities Education Act (IDEA) in 1990 represented a major commitment to investing in the human capital of children with disabilities. Although not explicitly focused on developing the capacity of children with disabilities to become employed as adults, presumably improvements in educational opportunities for such children would enable more to work in later years. The IDEA firmed up the rights of children with disabilities to receive education in the public school system. Under the IDEA, public schools that received federal funding were required to provide a tailored educational program to each child with a disability.

A judicial decision in 1990 concerning children with disabilities likely also had substantial implications for their employment and dependence on government support as adults. The Supreme Court's decision in the Sullivan v. Zebley case forced the Social Security Administration to make a large class of children with disabilities eligible for SSI benefits.[21] The result was a very rapid rise in the number of children receiving SSI, from just under 265,000 in 1989 to 955,000 in 1996.[22] Congress passed legislation in 1996 to reduce the number of children that became eligible following Sullivan v. Zebley and also required every child SSI recipient to undergo an age 18 redetermination as an adult. Despite the 1996 legislation, more than 1.2 million children received SSI in 2010, and nearly 60% of child SSI recipients remain on the SSI rolls after their age 18 redetermination, and approximately 10% more return to the SSI rolls within four years following a successful appeal of a denial or a new application.[23] The SSI expansion for children might have enabled the children's parents to invest more in their children's human capital, increasing the chance of employment as adults, but it likely also made them aware that might jeopardize their adult eligibility for SSI by working or even preparing themselves for work.

The 1992 amendments to the Rehabilitation Act were also designed to improve employment outcomes for people with disabilities. The Rehabilitation Act, first enacted in 1973, provides funding for state vocational rehabilitation agencies to serve people with disabilities, includes a number of affirmative action provisions related to federal employment and the use of federal funds, and also supports Independent Living Centers, which provide limited assistance to people with disabilities living independently in the community. The Department of Education is responsible for its administration. The federal government funds 80% of services provided by state vocational rehabilitation agencies, with the state required to pay for the remainder. The 1992 amendments promoted "consumer choice" with respect to career options; required vocational rehabilitation agencies to focus on competitive employment as the most desirable outcome; and also specified that SSDI and SSI beneficiaries were presumptively eligible for these services.

In an effort to coordinate and integrate employment services for people with disabilities with employment services delivered to others, Congress incorporated the Rehabilitation Act in the Workforce Investment Act in 1998. The latter governs federal-state employment programs under the jurisdiction of the Department of Labor. Under the Workforce Investment Act, state Workforce Investment Boards provide job search and training services to workers through local offices, now called American Job Service Centers (AJCs). Before the Act, local Workforce Investment Board offices often referred clients with disabilities to state vocational rehabilitation agencies, rather than providing them with services, a practice that was encouraged by limited budgets and performance-based incentives. Because AJC performance was based on the extent to which clients successfully obtained employment, and the AJCs expected less employment success for those with significant disabilities, it was in AJCs' interest to send such clients elsewhere. The Workforce Investment Act included provisions to improve the accessibility of AJCs and encourage greater cooperation with the state vocational rehabilitation agencies. It also promoted use of customized employment strategies, such as job carving, self-employment, supported employment, job restructuring, developing partnerships with local businesses, and assigning personal agents for customers.

The 1999 Ticket to Work and Work Incentive Improvement Act (Ticket Act) was designed specifically to increase employment of people with disabilities and reduce their reliance on public benefits. The Ticket Act states that "it is the policy of the United States to provide assistance to individuals with disabilities to lead productive work lives." The many provisions of the Ticket Act are focused on improving outcomes for those who are already SSDI or SSI beneficiaries. In some cases they also extend to those who meet the medical qualifications for those programs but who are working.

The Ticket Act's signature program, Ticket to Work, is in essence a performance-based voucher program, available to essentially all SSDI and SSI beneficiaries, administered by the Social Security Administration. Each beneficiary receives a "ticket" that he or she can attempt to assign to an array of prequalified public or private providers, called Employment Networks, in return for employment services. The Social Security Administration makes monthly payments to the provider when the beneficiary achieves specified earnings amounts. Most payments are made only when beneficiaries earn so much that they are no longer eligible for an SSDI or SSI payment, and are paid over many months (currently 36 for SSDI beneficiaries and 60 for SSI-only beneficiaries).

Before Ticket to Work, state vocational rehabilitation agencies were eligible for payments from the Social Security Administration under a different system that provided capped cost reimbursements if the beneficiary engaged in substantial work for a period of nine months, but these payments were not tied to exit from the rolls. Ticket to Work was designed to encourage competition between the state vocational rehabilitation agencies and other providers, offer more service options to beneficiaries, increase provider incentives to help beneficiaries exit the SSDI and SSI rolls, and reduce disability program costs. State vocational rehabilitation agencies became Employment Networks under Ticket to Work in the sense that they could accept tickets and use the new payment systems. Rehabilitation agencies were also permitted to continue use of the existing payment system on a case-by-case basis.

Initial use of Ticket to Work was low and few ticket users actually left the rolls for work. Most tickets were assigned to state vocational rehabilitation agencies under the existing payment system. Many providers that had qualified to become Employment Networks started to let their contracts with the Social Security Administration lapse because they were unable to recover their costs through ticket payments.[24] The Social Security Administration then made major changes to the Ticket to Work program in an attempt to invigorate both beneficiary and provider interest. These were implemented in 2008, so any effects of the new regulations have been confounded with the effects of the worst recession since the Great Depression. The Department of Labor has also taken significant steps to encourage AJCs to participate as Employment Networks.

Ticket to Work also expanded the Medicaid Buy-in program (initially authorized in 1997) and provided funding for improving the health infrastructure for workers with disabilities.[25] Medicaid Buy-in is an option available to states under the federal-state Medicaid program that allows qualified workers to buy-in to the federal-state Medicaid program. It was designed to provide health insurance to SSDI and SSI beneficiaries who work, or for those who would be eligible for benefits if they were not working. Such individuals are often unable to purchase private coverage from an employer (many employers do not offer employee health plans) or need services that are not covered by employer plans, such as personal assistance services. Medicaid Buy-in allows qualified workers to buy in to the federal-state Medicaid program. The premium amount is based on income. Work requirements, premium schedules, and covered services vary by state, and not all states have adopted the Medicaid Buy-in option.

The Ticket Act had a number of other provisions to make it easier for SSDI and SSI beneficiaries to work. Most notably, the Ticket Act: established grant programs to expand the availability of benefits counselors and legal advocates; extended the period during which SSDI beneficiaries continue to be eligible for Medicare after leaving SSDI because of work to from 39 months to 93 months (8.5 years); protected Ticket users from medical reviews that could lead to a finding of benefit ineligibility because of medical improvement; and instructed the Social Security Administration to create an expedited reinstatement process for SSDI beneficiaries who have already given up their benefits for work but are unable to continue working because of their disability.[26]

The Affordable Care Act (ACA), passed in 2010 and scheduled for full implementation in 2014, was primarily designed to expand health insurance coverage to all Americans and start a process of reducing growth in the cost of health care in the United States. Its implications for people with disabilities who work are potentially important but unclear. The ACA aims to improve the employer-based coverage system, but also provides coverage for those ineligible for employer-based coverage. Employees are essentially required to purchase coverage from their employer and all but small employers are penalized if they fail to cover their employees. Those individuals ineligible for employer-based coverage must purchase potentially subsidized coverage from their state's Health Insurance Exchange, unless their incomes are sufficiently low to qualify for Medicaid. The ACA also severely limits the extent to which insurers can experience-rate premiums.

The ACA's effect on employment among people with disabilities will likely depend on how its provisions affect the extent to which employers must pay for the health care of their own workers. Currently, employers who offer insurance share in the liability of all of their covered employees. Hence, workers with exceptionally high health care needs can be much more costly to employ than otherwise comparable workers.

The impact of the ACA on employer costs for workers with disabilities will likely be positive for some and negative for others. On the one hand, employers will find it more costly to avoid offering health care coverage, which by itself would diminish their willingness to hire workers with low skills, and workers with disabilities are a disproportionately large share of low-skilled workers. On the other hand, the ACA's limits on the use of experience rating might mean that the difference between an employer's liabilities for workers with high health care costs and those with low health care costs will diminish markedly.

4.2 Assessment

The three-decade record of declining economic status and growing reliance on government support is all the more disappointing because of the significant efforts undertaken to increase the employment and economic self-sufficiency of working-age people with disabilities during the same period. Why have these changes not produced the desired results? As will be seen, when key policies and programs developed between 1980 and 2010 are viewed against the employment recommendations of the World Report on Disability it is apparent that they have fallen far short in critical areas.[27]

Our assessment is summarized in Table 13.2. As evidenced by the dearth of checkmarks, only one recommendation has been substantially met: anti-discrimination legislation and enforcement. Some critics might argue that the ADA's provisions and enforcement are inadequate to prevent discrimination and need to be strengthened, but, although not perfect, the country is much closer to compliance with this recommendation than with any of the others.

Table 13.2 ASSESSMENT OF RECENT DISABILITY LEGISLATION IN THE UNITED STATES

World Report on Disability Employment Recommendations	Social Security Act Amendments	Disability Benefits Reform Act	Americans with Disabilities Act	Individuals with Disabilities Education Act	*Sullivan v. Zelbley*	Rehabilitation Act	Workforce Investment Act	Ticket to Work and Work Incentives Improvement Act	Affordable Care Act
	1980	1984	1990–2009	1990–1997–2004	1990	1973–1986–1992–1998	1998	1999	2009
Laws and Regulations									
• Antidiscrimination legislation and enforcement			√						
• Harmonize employment incentives								+	?
Public Programs									
• Accessible employment and training programs						+	+	+	
• Tailored services				+		+		+	
• Ensure social protection while supporting employment	–	–			+/–			+	+/?
• Provide services needed to support work						+	+	+	+
• Focus eligibility on capabilities, not disabilities	–	–				–		–	
• Monitor and evaluate innovations; scale up successful ones						+/–	+/–	+/–	
• Adequate and sustainable funding for training programs				+		+	+		

Key: √ substantially accomplished; + positive steps toward meeting; – negative step. Note: The recommendations are abbreviated versions of those that appear in the *World Report on Disability*.

Although no other recommendation has been substantially accomplished, multiple policy initiatives have made positive contributions to address barriers to the employment of persons with disabilities. Most of these concern improving the delivery of education, employment services and training, and include the IDEA, the Rehabilitation Act, the Workforce Investment Act, and the Ticket Act. In addition, the Ticket Act makes steps toward harmonizing employment incentives with the objectives of the ADA and ensuring social protection while supporting employment. More generally, however, the policy record on employment services is not as impressive as it might first appear because funding for these services represents a tiny share of all federal and state expenditures that support persons with disabilities. Funding limitations are illustrated by the fact that applicants for state vocational rehabilitation services often wait many months to receive assistance, especially if they are not already receiving SSDI or SSI benefits.

The Rehabiliation Act, the Ticket Act, and the Workforce Investment Act have all provided support for monitoring and evaluation. The records of these acts on monitoring and evaluation are mixed, however.[28] Although some major demonstrations have used experimental methods to produce methodologically rigorous estimates of impacts, others have not, and the non-experimental evaluation methods available have not been able to convincingly control for various confounding factors. As an example, the Ticket Act required the Social Security Administration to roll out a major new program, Ticket to Work, without a pilot or demonstration. Thus far, the evaluation of Ticket to Work has not been able to produce reliable estimates of impacts.

Both the Rehabilitation Act and the Ticket Act perform negatively with respect to determining eligibility based on capabilities, not disabilities. Both acts aim to improve employment services for those with very significant disabilities. Further, the Ticket Act gives providers incentives to serve those SSDI and SSI beneficiaries who need the fewest services to return to work. But most services under the Ticket Act are available only to SSDI or SSI beneficiaries. The Rehabilitation Act does not impose this requirement, but when funding is limited the state vocational rehabilitation agencies are required to give preference to SSDI and SSI beneficiaries. Hence, both increase the importance of inability to work in determining eligibility for services.

The 1980 Social Security Act Amendments, which tightened eligibility for SSDI and SSI, and the 1984 Disability Benefits Reform Act, which expanded eligibility, both perform poorly when evaluated based on empowering individuals to work. Neither program endeavors to "ensure social protection while supporting employment," nor do they "focus eligibility on capabilities, not disabilities" (Table 13.2); instead, both reinforce the fundamental idea that only those unable to work are worthy of support.

Existing policies also fall far short with respect to a third WRD recommendation, "harmonize employment incentives" (Table 13.2). State agencies and providers have incentives to help individuals with disabilities obtain SSDI and SSI rather than work supports because federal funding for SSDI and SSI is not limited, unlike federal and state support for state vocational rehabilitation agency services. Further, the welfare reforms of the 1990s, described in the following section, increased state incentives to help low-income parents with disabilities enter SSI or SSDI rather than provide them with family income and work supports using limited federal welfare funding. The most obvious of the employer disincentives is the way that health insurance is financed in the United States, which might or might not be moderated in the future by the ACA.

There are other significant issues with disability policy in the United States that make it difficult for policymakers to follow the WRD recommendations. The most notable of these is the substantial fragmentation of support, which makes support determinations and delivery highly inefficient. As the Government Accountability Office has documented, a plethora of federal and state disability support programs create pervasive inefficiencies, including service overlaps, service gaps, misaligned incentives, and conflicting objectives.[29] Incentives that encourage inefficient behaviors are prevalent at all levels. The previously mentioned incentives that states and providers have to encourage entry into SSDI and SSI reflect this fragmentation. Another example is that the federal agencies that provide employment supports for people with disabilities, the Departments of Education and Labor, gain nothing from helping workers with disabilities avoid entry into SSDI or SSI because the costs of the latter programs are not in their budgets. Program fragmentation is also a barrier to structural reform. Stakeholders in existing structures have incentives to oppose such reforms. Not surprisingly, program administrators limit their improvement efforts to those that increase measured performance for their own programs, often at the expense of other programs. These examples just scratch the surface of the enormous inefficiencies caused by fragmentation of support.

4.3 Lessons from Welfare Reform

The final section of this chapter offers a road map for addressing these critical issues. That road map draws on the lessons from "welfare reform"—the major structural changes in the support system for low-income families, many of which are headed by single mothers, implemented in the 1990s. Welfare reform addressed work disincentives and pervasive inefficiencies related to how welfare programs were financed. The system in place before that period—primarily income support under Aid to Families with Dependent Children (AFDC), and health insurance under Medicaid—provided benefits to low-income families with no expectation that the parents would work to support their families and no time limit other than the attainment of age 18 by the youngest child.[30] Each state had its own rules and administered its own programs, but the federal government paid a fixed share of the income and health benefits. Income benefits were low, so many families on welfare lived in poverty. Parental employment was also very low and many children who grew up in welfare families eventually received welfare benefits as adults. During this period, caseload sizes and program expenditures grew very rapidly.

Welfare reform replaced this system with a "work-first" system that features a very different financing structure. Under Temporary Assistance to Needy Families (TANF), parents are now required to work or participate in activities that will quickly lead to work. Benefits have a lifetime limit of 60 months for each family. An expanded earned income tax credit for families increases the incentive for parents in such families to work. The old federal-state cost-sharing formula with open-ended entitlements has been replaced by federal "block grants" under which the federal government makes annual grants commensurate with past federal expenditures, thereby increasing the incentive for the state to help welfare parents find work and leave the welfare rolls.

The work-first approach of welfare reform was widely regarded as successful for many years, even by those who initially opposed the reform. Employment of single mothers increased substantially. Welfare caseloads and costs plummeted. Researchers have attributed these early gains to increased incentives for parents to work and support their children, increases in the incentives for state agencies to help them work and leave the welfare caseload, and exceptionally strong economic growth.

Not all of the effects of welfare reform are considered to be positive, however. One such effect was that welfare reform pushed parents with disabilities into SSI. Moving to SSI allowed parents to avoid welfare's new work requirements and time limits. For the state, moving a parent to SSI meant moving the costs for their support from a state budget to a federal budget and avoiding the responsibility of providing child care and other services that might be necessary for the parent to work.[31] More recently, a second major problem has emerged: the inability of the block grant financing mechanism to fund benefits appropriately during all phases of the business cycle.[32]

The history of welfare reform contains several lessons. The first is that it took decades for policymakers to determine an approach that proved promising for achieving the twin goals of improved economic outcomes and less reliance on government support. Development of the evidence base was critical for both designing effective policy and building the political consensus to move forward.[33]

The second lesson from welfare reform is that major structural changes that affect a vulnerable population can have a positive and dramatic impact on employment, income, and self-sufficiency. Of course, the issues faced by people with disabilities are fundamentally different from those faced by low-income families, so the same reforms applied to people with disabilities could have different, and potentially negative, effects. For those people with disabilities who can work, however, welfare reform suggests that changing work expectations, increasing the incentive to work, and integrating work support and other services with benefit payments can lead to greater economic success and self-sufficiency.

Welfare reform also showed, however, that the reform's financing mechanism had substantial shortcomings in the long term. During the strong economic expansion of the late 1990s several states had excess welfare program funding that they spent on other programs rather than saving to fund their welfare programs during an economic downturn. This spending occurred at least in part because of the expectation that Congress would reduce future welfare funding if the excess funds were not quickly spent. As a result of this spending, states have had insufficient funds to pay for welfare benefits following the recent recession. More funds were appropriated as part of the federal government's economic stimulus expenditures, but states have run through those funds, and it seems unlikely that additional federal welfare funding will become available.[34]

The history of disability policy reform in the United States stands in sharp contrast to the history of welfare reform. The former established the right of people with disabilities to work and was accompanied by incremental changes designed to increase employment within a fragmented policy structure that continues to define disability as "inability to work." Results for employment and disability program trends have been extremely disappointing. Welfare reforms included a fundamental change in the programmatic support for low-income families combined with a complementary change in the structure of financing. Employment of unmarried mothers rose rapidly and welfare caseloads diminished. Our critique of disability policy suggests that structural reforms are required to reverse disability employment and program trends; welfare reform suggests that structural reform can achieve both goals at once. But it would be a serious mistake for disability reforms to closely follow the example of welfare reform for several reasons. The barriers to successful employment of people with disabilities are very different from those of low-income parents; the set of supports available to those with disabilities is quite different from those available to low-income families before welfare reform; and welfare reform was not an unmitigated success—most notably with respect to the adequacy of funding during all phases of the business cycle. The next section offers a strategy for disability policy reforms that reflect all of these considerations.

5. A POLICY ROAD MAP FOR POLICY REFORM IN THE UNITED STATES

In a recent working paper, we described programmatic and financial reforms that have the potential to address the structural problems of current disability policy.[35] Although many details remain to be specified and the evidence base is insufficient to implement them quickly, these reforms hold out the promise of more economic success for people with disabilities, while reducing growth in public expenditures for their support. In what follows, we first sketch the programmatic reforms, and then describe an approach to federal and state financing that would support the programmatic reforms. We conclude with a discussion of how to build the evidence base needed to inform change.

5.1 Programmatic Reforms

The programmatic reforms proposed in this section are intended to illustrate the magnitude and complexity of the structural changes that would be required to bring US disability policy in line with the recommendations of the WRD. Many other proposals have been put forth that would at least partially address some of the WRD recommendations, but we are not aware of any that do so as comprehensively as this one. Although many variations are possible within the proposal described in the following, and many of the details are yet to be specified, a comprehensive programmatic approach to reform is necessary to transform current disability policy.

Programmatic reforms should focus on consolidating support administration at the state or local level, provide important but limited federal oversight, empower people with sufficient earnings capacity to at least partly support themselves through work, protect and strengthen supports for those with insufficient earnings capacity, and increase beneficiaries' ability to control decisions that affect their lives.

Under these reforms, responsibility for all eligibility determinations and support delivery would be consolidated under Disability Support Administrators (DSAs), new entities that would operate at the state or sub-state level, but receive federal as well as state financial support. Every DSA would have the same responsibilities but potentially different organizational structures. A DSA could be run by state or local government, a private organization, or a coalition of multiple entities—whatever administrative structure is best for each service area. Regardless of the organizational structure, each DSA would be responsible for determining what supports each beneficiary needs and ensuring their delivery in a timely and coordinated fashion. To help achieve this goal, a single case manager would be responsible for each beneficiary's case and serve as the beneficiary's primary point of contact. The federal government would oversee the DSAs by establishing national eligibility criteria, adjudicating appeals, and monitoring and reporting key outcomes. Establishing a strong oversight mechanism would be critical to the acceptance of the DSA system by the disability community and their advocacy organizations. The federal government would also encourage DSAs to continually innovate and share best practices via dissemination and technical assistance activities.

The reformed system's success would depend, in part, on receiving timely feedback from the beneficiary population. To facilitate this communication and oversight, we propose the creation of consumer boards at both the national and DSA level. The national board would ensure that the federal government vigorously exercises its oversight responsibilities, whereas boards at the DSA level would share consumer feedback and monitor programmatic efforts.

The national eligibility criteria to be applied by DSAs would focus on potential work capacity rather than chronic inability to work. Each applicant's potential work capacity would be measured as part of the eligibility determination process. Inability to work would no longer be a criterion for benefit eligibility. Consequently, workers would be able to apply for benefits while remaining in the labor force. Development of the eligibility criteria and a model process for applying them are key challenges to the restructuring of disability policy.

We envision that DSAs would provide an array of supports and services that are matched to the individual's characteristics and circumstances. Table 13.3 provides examples of supports tailored to the circumstances of three hypothetical individuals. While the best approach to these three hypothetical settings can be debated, they represent our proposal as authors and are illustratives. The first individual has substantial earnings potential as well as high disability-related costs. Such an individual might receive some combination of counseling services, an income allowance designed to offset the costs of disability not conditioned on earnings, necessary training and education to reach his or her earnings potential, an earned income tax credit designed to increase both the incentive to work and income from work, services specific to employment, or subsidies that lower the cost to the individual for a variety of disability services and supports. The duration of all supports would be determined by the beneficiary's medical condition, potential work capacity, and employment effort.

In the second scenario, an individual who is close to retirement age has acquired a condition that has reduced his or her earnings capacity to a very low level, following a long work history. Consistent with the intent of the SSDI program when it was introduced in 1956, existing benefits for such workers would be preserved.[36] The rationale reflects both efficiency and equity considerations. The cost of helping a worker regain substantial earnings capacity might be high relative to the earnings generated over what would be at best a short period of work. Such an individual could be provided with the same SSDI and Medicare benefits as are available under current policy. Given greater availability of work supports outside of SSDI (such as those provided for the individual in the first example), the medical criteria for such benefits

Table 13.3 EXAMPLES OF BENEFITS MATCHED TO INDIVIDUALS

Individual Characteristics*	Benefits Available**
• Substantial earnings potential • High disability costs	• Counseling services • Disability allowance • Training and education • Earned income tax credit • Employment services • Subsidized disability services, equipment, and accommodations
• Substantial work history • Over age 50 • Very low earnings potential	• SSDI benefits • Medicare after 24 months
• Age 18 or older • Very low earnings potential	• Disability allowance • Counseling services • Subsidized disability services, equipment, and accommodations • Assistance with individual and social activities

*All beneficiaries must have a significant, long-lasting medical condition or impairment.
**Benefits for the first and third hypothetical participant would be customized to their individual needs, whereas those for second would not change relative to current law.

might be stricter than under current SSDI rules, and the complex SSDI work incentives could be eliminated.

The third illustration concerns an individual who has little or no work history and very limited earnings capacity. By limited earnings capacity we mean that cost of training, education, and services designed to build earnings capacity are excessive relative to any earnings generated. Such individuals would not be expected to contribute to their own support through work and would qualify for income and in-kind benefits that are at least as generous as those currently available. Efficiency gains resulting from support integration and coordination of care could help improve the lives of such individuals, even though they would not benefit from enhancement of their earning potential. Others might argue for increased work in all three of these hypothetical cases, both to ensure no age discrimination and because the value of work goes beyond earning capacity.

The proposed reforms would most dramatically affect those people with disabilities who have substantial work capacity, or potential capacity, including a substantial share of those who would be eligible for SSDI or SSI under current law. With appropriate supports and assistance, such individuals would be expected to contribute to their own financial support through work. Those who are not employed would need to demonstrate a good faith employment effort to continue receiving benefits. Acceptable employment efforts could include active job search; medical rehabilitation preparatory to work; and goal-oriented, time-limited (re)education and retraining.

The provision of supports to those who work will likely increase the total number of support recipients. To offset the cost of these additional beneficiaries, savings generated from more efficient delivery of supports under the restructured programs would need to be at least as large. The proposed reforms create government savings through increases in lifetime earnings and tax payments by those with work capacity, reductions in their reliance on government support, and program integration. Historical data suggest that these savings could be tens of billions on an annual basis.[37] It is important to proceed with caution, however, because it will be challenging to strike an acceptable balance between improving supports and reducing expenditure growth.

Under the reformed system, most beneficiaries would receive basic health care coverage from the same sources as other Americans. Under the Affordable Care Act, beneficiaries eligible for employer-based health insurance would be required to enroll; all others would buy coverage from their state's Health Insurance Exchange or, if household income is below 133% of the federal poverty level, enroll in Medicaid. Those over 50 who are eligible for SSDI benefits would also be eligible for Medicare.

5.2 Financial Reforms

Although the proposed programmatic reforms deal with much of the structural fragmentation and inefficiency responsible for rapid expenditure growth in the current system, financial reforms are required to ensure adequate funding and alignment of financial incentives with programmatic objectives. Most importantly, DSAs should be incentivized to make eligibility and benefit decisions that meet federal standards but are not excessive and do not unnecessarily drive up costs. Financial reforms should ensure adequate funding, encourage efficient decisions, contain federal and state expenditure growth, make federal expenditures responsive to external factors such as the business cycle, and avoid precipitous declines in support for those who depend on it.

Federal funding sources would be a mixture of revenues from payroll taxes and general revenues, as under current law. Federal funding would not be open-ended, however. Rather, federal expenditures would remain under a threshold determined by Congress that is consistent with national fiscal objectives. Each DSA's federal funding allocation would be a function of its catchment area's current funding levels, projected needs, payroll tax revenues, and ability to pay. Federal funding would also be adjusted as DSA catchment areas change demographically and beneficiaries migrate across catchment areas. Because demand for services would be sensitive to the business cycle, it will also be important for the funding mechanism to intentionally increase funding during economic downturns and decrease funding during rapid expansions.

Each DSA's share of federal funding would be allocated in two steps. The Social Security Administration and the Centers for Medicare and Medicaid Services would first directly pay all proposed income benefits and Medicare costs, respectively, for eligible beneficiaries in the DSA's catchment area. The federal funds that remain after the income benefits and Medicare costs are paid would then be granted to the DSA. The DSA would use the federal grant combined with state funding to finance all other supports, particularly the supports provided to the expanded group of workers with disabilities.

The two-step federal funding allocation has several advantages. By receiving grants that exclude all income and Medicare payments, DSAs would be incentivized to responsibly determine eligibility and award supports. The more income benefits and Medicare cases allowed, the smaller the grant amount that would come to the state to support other services, and vice versa. In addition, using a national cash payment system already in place avoids costly payment system duplication and supports federal monitoring of cash payments.

In the 2008 fiscal year, states contributed US $71 billion to joint federal-state disability programs for working-age people. Under the reformed structure, states would be required to contribute commensurate disability support funding, even if the state does not operate DSAs within its borders. Initially, each state would divert funds currently used to pay Medicaid and other state or federal/state benefits for the working-age population with disabilities. Maintenance of effort requirements would change gradually, as circumstances warrant. Each state's minimum funding requirement would eventually be a percentage of federal grants to the DSAs in the state.

This funding scheme would dramatically alter the financing of public disability programs in the United States. To illustrate, Figure 13.4 shows the distribution of disability support funding under current law and also illustrates how funding might be allocated under the proposed reforms after a transition period. Federal matching grants and block grants to states, which comprise 22% and 1% of current funding, respectively, would be eliminated in favor of grants to DSAs. About one third of federal disability program funding would also be rechanneled to DSAs. States would initially provide the same level of funding under the reformed policy as they do under current law. The collective effect of these changes would be to provide the DSAs with much more flexibility to tailor supports to individuals than any local entity has now. They would also have a strong incentive to be accountable for the well-being of their clients.

Financial reforms that create incentives for employers to retain workers with disabilities could generate additional funding and promote employment

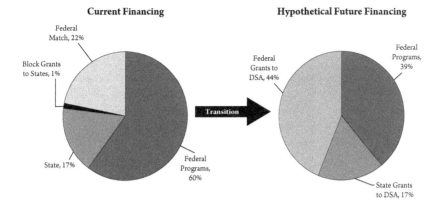

Figure 13.4
Illustration of the Financing Transition[38]

for program participants. For instance, the federal government could "experience rate" payroll taxes by levying surcharges on employers whose former employees frequently require disability supports, and vice versa.[39]

5.3 How to Move Forward

The reforms we describe require major structural changes to the nation's disability support system. These reforms can potentially benefit both Americans with disabilities and American taxpayers, but a policy transition that is too quick and not evidence-based could do more harm than good.

The first step in a successful transition to a new disability policy must be a substantial demonstration period—perhaps 10 years or longer. The purpose of this period is to build the evidence base and policy consensus needed to move forward. Following the example of the research that preceded welfare reform, numerous pilot projects would be initiated during the demonstration period by federal and state agencies, municipalities, counties, and various private organizations. Many would likely be unsuccessful, just as they were with welfare reform. But even unsuccessful demonstrations provide valuable information to policymakers. Just as under welfare reform, those interventions and policies discovered to be effective and viable would be incorporated into the new policy.[40]

Federal legislation is needed to initiate such a demonstration period. It must authorize and encourage pilot projects, define demonstration objectives and requirements, guarantee the cooperation of pertinent agencies, and create a national disability demonstration commission. The commission would encourage government agencies and other organizations to plan and conduct

Table 13.4 COMPARISON OF CURRENT AND FUTURE DISABILITY POLICY FEATURES

	Current Law	New Policy
Work	• "Disability" defined as inability to work because of medical conditions • Program rules and culture discourage work	• Focus on remaining work capacity, given physical or mental conditions • Program rules and culture encourage work
Eligibility Determinations and Support Delivery	• Fragmented among many federal, state, and local agencies • Multiple points of contact	• Fully integrated/coordinated by DSAs • Single point of contact
Income Benefits	• SSDI: all beneficiaries receive income benefit. Size of benefit based on work history • SSI: Size of benefit based on a maximum not of countable income from other sources • Some states supplement income benefit	• SSDI still available to some older workers • For others, income benefit's size and duration based on various beneficiary characteristics, including work capacity and impairment severity • Some receive other supports, but no income benefit
Work Supports	• Secondary benefit for most	• Primary benefit for many • Targeted at those with substantial potential work capacity
Federal and State Funding	• Spread around a variety of separate programs • Open-ended expenditures for major programs • Encourages cost shifting	• All funneled through DSA • Government expenditures not open-ended • Expenditures adjust to DSA-area demographic and economic factors
Innovation and Reform	• Fragmented authority stifles innovation	• Demonstration period initially promotes tests of innovations • DSAs have authority and incentives to improve continuously

demonstrations, ensure that risks to participants are minimized, and foster a spirit of innovation and learning.

The nation's long-term fiscal problems are creating an urgent need for structural reform to programs that support working-age people with disabilities. Expenditures for these programs account for a large share of the federal budget and will almost inevitably have to be reduced. As summarized in Table 13.4, we have outlined a set of structural changes that have the potential to both improve economic outcomes for those with disabilities and reduce growth in government expenditures for their support. Without structural changes, current programs will likely be forced to make cuts. The cuts might be made in ways that try to minimize harm, but will likely have severe consequences. Even though the process requires time, policymakers should instead consider instituting an evidence-based structural reform process to improve performance and reduce costs in the long term, while affording more protection to current programs in the short term than would otherwise be feasible.

5.4 Lessons for High- and Low-Income Settings

Although this proposal focuses on US disability policy, it is relevant beyond the US context. Most notably, the history of US disability policy illustrates a broader theme. Economically advanced democracies have historically tended to develop extensive safety nets for people with disabilities following a caretaker model and are consequently now struggling to incorporate economic and social supports and opportunities into these existing programs. These nations have the wealth and technology needed to be successful at reform, yet still struggle to change policies that have become entrenched in complex laws, programs, and institutions. Although the system proposed here would need to be adjusted for each country's context, it can serve as a model for aligning national policies with international recommendations.

There is a lesson here for nations that have not yet developed extensive policies and programs for people with disabilities. Although some people with disabilities have limited work capacity, many others have great work capacity. If such nations follow in the footsteps of American disability policy and build systems designed almost exclusively to meet the needs of those who cannot work, they might eventually find themselves in the same position as the United States. It might be far better to chart a different course now—a course that recognizes the significant actual and potential capabilities of many of those with very significant impairments and medical conditions, and helps them become, or continue to be, productive members of society, while providing for those whose actual and potential earnings capabilities are more limited. Finding a way to strike the right balance is challenging, but essential.

NOTES

1. A more detailed description of America's disability safety net and how it discourages people with disabilities from taking better advantage of their capabilities appears in Stapleton, D. C., O'Day, B. L., Livermore, G. A., & Imparato, A. J. (2006). Dismantling the poverty trap: disability policy for the 21st century. *The Milbank Quarterly* 84(4), 701–732.

2. For blind individuals, the monthly earnings maximum was US $1,690 in 2012. These values are adjusted annually for inflation.
3. Some additional disregards are available on an individual basis. The US $65 disregards is not adjusted for inflation annually, and has been in place since the early 1980s.
4. Maestas, N., Mullen, K., & Strand, A. (2011). *Does Disability Insurance Receipt Discourage Work? Using Examiner Assignment to Estimate Causal Effects of SSDI Receipt.* Santa Monica, CA: RAND.
5. See also Chen, S., & van der Klaauw, W. (2008). The effect of disability insurance on labor supply of older individuals in the 1990s. *Journal of Econometrics 142*(2), 757–784; French, E., & Song, J. (2011). *The Effect of Disability Insurance Receipt on Labor Supply.* WP 2009-05. Chicago: Federal Reserve Bank of Chicago.
6. World Health Organization & the World Bank (2011). *World Report on Disability.* Geneva, Switzerland: World Health Organization.
7. See Stein, M. A., & Stein, P. J. S. (2007). Beyond disability civil rights. *Hastings Law Journal 58*, 1203–1241.
8. Stein, M. A., & Stein, P. J. S. (2011). Beyond Disability Civil Rights, summarizes the status of American policy in a different, although similar fashion. The nation leads the world in establishment of the civil rights of people with disabilities, but has not yet recognized the human right of people with disabilities to utilize their capabilities and develop their individual talents, let alone established the programs and policies needed to fulfill those rights.
9. Weathers, R. R. II, & Wittenburg, D. C. (2009). Employment. In A. J. Houtenville, D. C. Stapleton, R. R. Weathers II, & R. V. Burkhauser (Eds.), *Counting Working-Age People with Disabilities: What Current Data Tell Us and Options for Improvement, 101–144.* Kalamazoo, MI: The Upjohn Institute for Employment Research.
10. The contributors to Stapleton, D. C., & Burkhauser, R. V. (Eds.) (2003). *The Decline in Employment of People with Disabilities: A Policy Puzzle.* Kalamazoo, MI: W. E. Upjohn examined various possible explanations for this decline, including measurement issues, changes in severity of disability, changes in the nature of the labor market, rapid growth in the cost of health care, and public policy. The editors conclude that there is much we do not know about the decline, but that the most compelling evidence concerns the effect of public policy on employment. Additional evidence on the role of public policy appears later in this chapter.
11. *Source:* Employment rate of persons age 18 to 64 with health-related work limitations relative to the employment rate of those without such limitations. Derived from: von Schrader, S., Erickson, W. A., & Lee, C. G. (2010). *Disability Statistics from the Current Population Survey (CPS).* (Ithaca, NY: Cornell University Rehabilitation Research and Training Center on Disability Demographics and Statistics).
12. *Source:* Statistics are for December of the year. Projected series is based on actual number of disability-insured workers by age and sex multiplied by the 1980 participation rate (beneficiaries per disability-insured worker) within the age-sex category. Beneficiaries by year, age and sex are from Social Security Administration (2011). *Annual Statistical Report of the Social Security Disability Insurance Program, 2010* (Baltimore, MD, Social Security Administration) 2011, Table 19. Beneficiaries age 65 and over are excluded starting in 2004, when some age 65 workers first became eligible for benefits because of the increase in

the Full Retirement Age. Number of disability insured workers by age and sex are from Social Security Administration, Office of the Actuary (n.d.), Statistical Tables. Retrieved February 28, 2011, from http://www.ssa.gov/oact/STATS/table4c2DI.html

13. Social Security & Medicare Boards of Trustees (2011). *A Summary of the 2011 Annual Reports: Social Security and Medicare Boards of Trustees*. Baltimore: Social Security Administration; Congressional Budget Office (2011). *The Budget and Economic Outlook: Fiscal Years 2011 to 2021*. Washington, DC: CBO.

14. Livermore, G. A., Stapleton, D. C., & O'Toole, M. (2011). Health care costs are a key driver of growth in federal and state assistance to working-age people with disabilities. *Health Affairs 30*(9), 1664–1672, Table 2.1.

15. *Sources:* For SSDI expenditures: Social Security Administration, Office of the Actuary (n.d.), Statistical Tables. Retrieved February 28, 2011 from http://www.ssa.gov/oact/STATS/table4a6.html; for under-65 Medicare Part A and B expenditures: Centers for Medicare and Medicaid Services (2012) Medicare and Medicaid Statistical Supplement, 2010 Edition, Table 3.2. Retrieved February 28, 2011, from http://www.cms.gov/MedicareMedicaidStatSupp/10_2010.asp; for GDP and Federal Outlays: Bureau of Economic Analysis (n.d.). National Income and Product Accounts, Interactive Tables. Retrieved February 28, 2011, from http://www.bea.gov/interactive.htm

16. Goodman, N. J., & Stapleton, D. C. (2007). Federal expenditures for working-age people with disabilities. *Journal of Disability Policy Studies 18*(2), 66–78.

17. *Source:* Livermore, Stapleton, & O'Toole (2011). Health care costs. FY is fiscal year. FY 2002 dollar values were adjusted for inflation using the annual Consumer Price Index for all Urban Consumers. Working age defined as ages 18 to 64.

18. Collins, K. P., & Erfle, A. (1985). Social Security Disability Benefits Reform Act of 1984: legislative history and summary of provisions. *Social Security Bulletin 48*(4), 5–32.

19. Deleire, T. (2000). The wage and employment effects of the Americans with Disabilities Act. *Journal of Human Resources 35*(4), 693–715; Acemoglu, D., & Angrist, J. (2001). Consequences of employment protection? The case of the Americans with Disabilities Act. *Journal of Political Economy 109*(5), 915–957.

20. A recent review of the mixed evidence on the ADA's impacts, along with further mixed evidence based on analysis of longitudinal data, appears in Donohue, J. J. III, Stein, M. A., Griffin, Jr., C. L., & Becker, S. (2011). Assessing post-ADA employment: some econometric evidence and policy considerations. *Journal of Empirical Legal Studies 8*(3), 477–503.

21. Sullivan v. Zebley, 493 U.S. 521 (1990).

22. See Table 7A.8 in: Social Security Administration (2013). *Annual Statistical Supplement to the Social Security Bulleton.*Baltimore, MD: Social Security Administration.

23. Hemmeter, J., & Gilby, E. (2009). The age-18 redetermination and postdetermination participation in SSI. *Social Security Bulletin 69*(4), 1–25.

24. The performance of TTW during this initial period is evaluated in Stapleton, D., et al. (2008). *Ticket to Work at the Crossroads: A Solid Foundation with an Uncertain Future*. Washington, DC: Mathematica Policy Research.

25. Kehn, M., Croake, S., & Schimmel, J. (2010). *A Government Performance and Results (GPRA) Report: The Status of the Medicaid Infrastructure Grants Program as of 12/31/09*. Washington, DC: Mathematica Policy Research.

26. The Ticket Act also mandated that SSA conduct a demonstration under which SSDI benefit rules would treat earnings more generously than under current law. Under current law, SSDI beneficiaries may essentially earn any amount they can without benefit loss for 12 months, but after that they keep 100% of their benefits if their monthly earnings (after allowable disregards) are below a maximum amount (currently US $1,010). If they earn even a dollar more than this amount, they lose 100% of their benefits. This program feature, known as the "cash cliff" is believed to discourage many beneficiaries from earning more than the maximum amount. The rules change, known as the benefit offset, would instead reduce benefits by US $1 for every $2 in earning above the same maximum amount. After conducting small pilots in four states, SSA launched a nationwide randomized test of the rules change, called the Benefit Offset National Demonstration, in 2011. See Stapleton, D., Bell, S., Wittenburg, D., Sokol, B., & McInnis, D. (2010). *BOND Implementation and Evaluation. BOND Final Design Report, submitted to the Social Security Administration, Office of Program Development & Research.* Cambridge, MA: Abt Associates, Inc. and Washington, DC: Mathematica Policy Research. Estimates of impacts from four pilot programs are provided by Weathers, R. R. II, & Hemmeter, J. (2011). The impact of changing financial work incentives on the earnings of Social Security Disability Insurance (SSDI) beneficiaries. *Journal of Public Policy Analysis and Management* 30(4), 708–728.

27. More extensive discussions of disability policy and employment can be found in: Stapleton, D. C., O'Day, B. L., Livermore, G. A., & Imparato, A. J. (2006). Dismantling the poverty trap; Organization for Economic Co-operation and Development (2010). *Sickness, Disability and Work.* Paris: Organization for Economic Co-operation and Development; Government Accountability Office (2005). *Federal Disability Assistance: Wide Array of Programs Needs to Be Examined in Light of 21st Century Challenges. GAO-05-626.* Washington, DC: Government Accountability Office; Government Accountability Office (2008). *Federal Disability Programs: More Strategic Coordination Could Help Overcome Challenges to Needed Transformation. GAO-08-635.* Washington, DC: Government Accountability Office; Social Security Advisory Board (2006). *A Disability System for the 21st Century.* Washington, DC: Social Security Advisory Board; Mashaw, J. L., & Reno, V. P. (Eds.) (1996). *Balancing Security and Opportunity: The Challenge of Disability Income Policy.* Washington, DC: National Academy of Social Insurance.

28. Reviews of evaluation efforts related to disability and employment initiatives appear in Wittenburg, D. C., Rangarajan, A., & Honeycutt, T. C. (2008). The United States Disability system and programs to promote employment for people with disabilities. *Revue Francaise Des Affaires Sociales 4,* 111–136; Livermore, G., & Goodman, N. (2009). *A Review of Recent Evaluation Efforts Associated with Programs and Policies Designed to Promote the Employment of Adults with Disabilities.* Ithaca, NY: Cornell University.

29. Government Accountability Office (2005), *Federal Disability Assistance.*

30. Further discussion of the welfare reforms and a comparison of the employment experience of unmarried mothers over this period with that of people with disabilities appear in Burkhauser, R. V., & Stapleton, D. C. (2004). Employing those not expected to work: the stunning changes in the employment of single mothers with children and people with disabilities in the United States in the

1990s. In B. Marin, C. Prinz, & M. Queisser (Eds.), *Disability Policy Under Review*, 331–332. Hants, United Kingdom: Ashgate.

31. Schmidt, L. & Sevak, P. (2004). AFDC, SSI, and Welfare reform aggressiveness: caseload reductions vs. caseload shifting. *Journal of Human Resources 39*(3), 792–812.

32. Pavetti, L., & Schott, L. (2011). *TANF's Inadequate Response to Recession Highlights Weakness of Block-Grant Structure*. Washington, DC: Center for Budget and Policy Priorities.

33. A review of the demonstrations preceding welfare reform appears in Moffitt, R. A. (2004). The role of randomized field trials in social science research: a perspective from evaluations of reforms of social welfare programs. *American Behavioral Scientist 47*(5), 506–540.

34. Pavetti, L., & Schott, L. (2011). *TANF's Inadequate Response*.

35. Mann, D. R., & Stapleton, D. C. (2011). *Fiscal Austerity and the Transition to Twenty-First Century Disability Policy: A Road Map. Working Paper*. Washington, DC: Mathematica Policy Research.

36. See Berkowitz, E. D. (1987). *Disabled Policy: America's Programs for the Handicapped*. New York: Cambridge University Press.

37. See Stapleton, D. C., & Wittenburg, D. C. (2011). *The SSDI Trust Fund: New Solutions to an Old Problem*. Issue Brief Report No. 11-02. Washington, DC: Center for Studying Disability Policy.

38. Mann, & Stapleton (2011). *Fiscal Austerity*

39. See Burkhauser, R. V., & Daly, M. C. (2011). *The Declining Work and Welfare of People with Disabilities*. Washington, DC: American Enterprise Institute.

40. See Moffitt, R. A. (2004). The role of randomized field trials in social science research: a perspective from evaluations of reforms of social welfare programs. *American Behavioral Scientist 47*(5), 506–540.

CHAPTER 14

Complementary Approaches

Japanese Disability and Employment Law

RYOKO SAKURABA

1. THE PRESENT SITUATION FOR PEOPLE WITH DISABILITIES IN JAPAN

In Japan today there are 3,663,000 people with physical disabilities, 547,000 people with intellectual disabilities and 3,233,000 people with mental disabilities (such as integration dysfunction syndrome or bipolar disorder).[1] The recognized population with disabilities comprises about 6% of the total population. By contrast, generally, disabled people represent around 15% of the world's population.[2] A precise international comparison would be difficult in this context, but if we think that the ratio of disabled people is similar from country to country, we can guess that the definition of disabilities is narrower in Japan than in other countries. This would mean only Japanese people with relatively severe disabilities are categorized as people with disabilities.

The employment rate of people with disabilities (the percentage of workers among the population aged 15–64) is high in Japan. It was 40.3% according to a 2006 survey (43.0% for people with physical disabilities, 52.6% for people with intellectual disabilities, and 17.3% for those with mental disabilities).[3] It is lower than that for nondisabled people (70.3%, 2011),[4] and thus in line with other countries. However, in light of the seemingly narrow coverage of disability as mentioned, the rate can be seen as relatively high.

Successful employment placements for disabled people at public employment security offices, which are local branches of the Ministry of Health, Labor and Welfare providing job placement services, have been increasing significantly. In 2004, there were 35,871 placements. In 2011, however, this figure rose to 59,367.[5] This reflects the fact that job applications at such offices also increased from 93,182 to 148,358 during the same period. Other causes of this increase would be the growth in popularity of the idea of corporate social responsibility and strengthened efforts on the part of the government, which are further explored later.

Yet problems persist in differences in working conditions between workers with and without disabilities. First, the percentage of regular workers is considerably lower for those with intellectual and mental disabilities: 18.8% and 32.5%, respectively.[6] Furthermore, it should be noted that among non-regular workers with disabilities, a considerable number work in employment facilities, which provide them with opportunities for employment and training with financial support from the government (59.1% of workers with intellectual disabilities and 37.7% of workers with mental disabilities).

In addition, wage levels are considerably lower for workers with disabilities than nondisabled workers.[7] The average monthly wage for regular, nondisabled workers is 270,000 yen (US $3,448), whereas that for people with physical disabilities it is 254,000 yen (US $3,244). For people with mental disabilities, the figure is even lower: 129,000 yen (US $1,647), and those with intellectual disabilities, average just 118,000 yen (US $1,507). The average monthly wage of physically disabled people working at welfare plants—one type of employment facility in which people with disabilities who are capable of working but experience difficulties finding employment at ordinary firms are offered opportunities for productive activity under the contract of employment, and receive training and other support from business operators—is 190,000 yen (US $2,426).[8] Those with intellectual disabilities fare considerably worse, averaging 85,000 yen (US $1,085), and the mentally disabled receive just 26,000 yen (US $332).

These average wage figures also serve to highlight the contrast between people with physical disabilities and those with intellectual or mental disabilities. This may reflect the differences in ratios of workers engaged in small or larger-sized establishments. Even compared with the general workforce, a greater proportion of workers with physical disabilities work in businesses employing 1,000 or more workers. On the other hand, 65.5% of people with mental disabilities work in businesses with between 5 and 29 workers.[9]

2. THE JAPANESE APPROACH

Looking at the relatively high employment rate of people with disabilities as described earlier, one could ask how it was accomplished. In reply to this question, it can be reasonably argued that Japanese laws promote the employment of people with disabilities quite efficiently. Although Japan's approach centers on the use of employment quotas, these would not be as effective without a system of complementary legislation and policy, including administrative

Table 14.1 DISTRIBUTION OF WORKERS WITH AND WITHOUT DISABILITIES, BY FIRM SIZE[10]

Firm Size (# of workers)	5–29	30–99	100–499	500–999	1,000+
Workers with physical disabilities	37.1	29.2	21.8	5.7	6.2
Workers with intellectual disabilities	34.2	41.8	18.0	3.9	2.1
Workers with mental disabilities	65.5	15.1	14.3	3.2	1.9
General Workforce	42.2	27.7	20.6	4.6	4.9
					(%)

guidance from the Japanese government, the use of a variety of subsidies for training and accommodation, and a solid public system of vocational rehabilitation. In addition, the quota system is complemented by a labor contracts doctrine, which in some ways functions as nondiscrimination legislation and mandates reassignments and reductions of workloads in response to disability onset while penalizing dismissal. Last, the quota system exists in an environment of social responsibility, in which both employers and government acknowledge the scale of the problem of employment for persons with disabilities and generally act in good faith to solve it.

2.1 Employment Quotas

Employment quotas require that employers hire and retain a certain number of persons with disabilities as a percentage of their regular employees, according to the Act on Employment Promotion of Persons with Disabilities.[11] This obligation applies to private sector employers with 56 employees or more, as well as to national and local public bodies. Currently, the rates for ordinary private employers are 1.8%, and for national and local government, 2.1% (2.0% for the Prefectural Board of Education).

The employment target for private sector employers is set in accordance with the following fraction. Underlying this is the idea that people with disabilities should have the same employment opportunities as nondisabled people.

> The total number of (full-time regular workers with physical disabilities + part-time regular workers with physical disabilities + unemployed people with physical disabilities + full-time regular workers with intellectual disabilities + part-time regular workers with intellectual disabilities + unemployed people with intellectual disabilities) / (The total number of full-time regular workers + 0.5 × the total number of part-time regular workers) × (1– the exclusion rate) + the total number of unemployed people

[362] *The Role of Government*

In certain categories of business, in which the universal application of employment quotas may not be compatible with the nature of the work, exclusion rates are set and applied. Through this, applicable employers in such industries are allowed to deduct a certain quantity from the total number of their actual employees, thus reducing the number of people with disabilities they are obliged to employ.[12]

In 2012, when the review was carried out, the preceding fraction was as follows:[13]

$$378,000 + 16,000 + 191,000 + 99,000 + 9,000 + 67,000 \ (=760,000)$$
$$/ \ \{(34,320,000 + 3,170,000 \times 0.5) \times (1 - 0.054) + 2,720,000\}$$
$$(=36,686,000) = 2.072\%$$

On the basis of this number, the employment targets for private employers will be raised to 2.0% from April 2013. Following this, the rates for national and local government will become 2.3% (2.2% for the Prefectural Board of Education).

2.2.1 Effect

These employment quotas can be assessed positively, to the extent that they do promote the employment with people with disabilities. Although the employment quota target (currently, 1.8%) has never been met, the actual employment rate of these employees has increased, especially in the last eight years; it rose from 1.52% in 2006 to 1.65% in 2011.[14] Part of this increase is attributed to the inclusion of certain categories of workers with disabilities in calculating the actual employment rates: These include part-time workers with physical or intellectual disabilities and workers with mental disabilities. However, by looking at the following table describing the increase in the numbers of full-time workers with physical or intellectual disabilities during the period from 2006 to 2010, and comparing this with the increase in the total number of regular workers, the increase in the employment of people with disabilities can be confirmed.

This seemingly good situation may be attributed to employment quotas, as the case of people with mental disabilities indicates.[15] In 2006, this group began to be included in the calculation of the actual employment rate of people with disabilities.[16] Accordingly, the number of them engaged in such enterprises reached 13,024 in 2011, 6.8 times the number engaged in 2006. Also, their proportion among workers with disabilities in those enterprises rose from 0.7% to 3.6% (workers with physical disabilities, 284,428 [77.7%] and those with intellectual disabilities, 68,747 [18.8%], respectively). This increase can be partly due to the increase in motivation of people with mental disabilities; in 2011, such job seekers registered at the

Table 14.2 EMPLOYMENT GROWTH FOR PERSONS WITH DISABILITIES[17]

	2006	2010	2010/2006
Number of full-time workers with severe physical or intellectual disabilities in firms covered by the quotas (A)	74,993	88,411	1.18
Number of full-time workers with physical or intellectual disabilities in firms covered by the quotas (B), not including (A)	127,800	149,274	1.17
Number of workers with physical or intellectual disabilities in firms covered by the quotas (C) = (A) + (B)	202,793	237,685	1.17
Number of regular workers × (1 – exclusion rate) (D)	18,652,344	20,356,456	1.09

Public Employment Security Offices reached 48,777 (2.6 times more than in 2006). Employers' changed attitudes also seem to have contributed to this. According to a 2011 survey, among 47 establishments that have newly employed those with mental disabilities, 20 replied that the main reason for their employment was that those with mental disabilities were included in calculating the quotas.[18]

Correspondingly, the next question to be asked about these changes, then, should be: How and why are employment quotas accepted and enforced in Japanese society?

2.2 Social Solidarity and Responsibility

The fundamental principles of the employment quotas are "normalization" and "social solidarity," as the Act for Employment Promotion etc. of Persons with Disabilities proclaimed.[19] According to these, workers with disabilities shall be given opportunities to utilize their abilities in vocational life as workers who are members of the economy and society. Based on this normalization policy, in order to advance the welfare of people with disabilities, they need to be able to work to support themselves. Here, vocational life embraces both self-employed workers as well as employees. However, most people in a modern economy have employers. Therefore, regarding the employment of people with disabilities, "all employers have the common responsibility to provide appropriate workplaces.... based on the principle of social solidarity."

Why, then, were employment quotas, and not the antidiscrimination approach, adopted to achieve this aim? The answer to this question can be explained historically.[20] Employment quotas were first introduced in 1960 with the enactment of the Act for Employment Promotion of People with

Physical Disabilities. This act was adopted to advance employment measures for people with physical disabilities, in light of poor employment opportunities and higher unemployment rates among this group. In doing this, references were made to the ILO Vocational Rehabilitation (Disabled) Recommendation, 1955 (No. 99) and to foreign countries' laws that existed at that time. In particular, it has been claimed that the employment quotas were inspired by the systems of European countries. In other words, the choice of the employment quota approach was made to meet what was then international standards; at the time it did not recognize, or disregard, the other possible option: antidiscrimination law. Actually, the Act included a provision that can be seen as a partial antidiscrimination approach. Article 3 of the then Act provides that, when a firm offers a job with limitations relating to a jobseeker's physical disabilities, and when these limitations are without justifiable reasons, the Public Employment Security Offices may reject such an offer (currently Article 10). They may also give guidance to such firms.

On the other hand, the choice of an employment quota approach can also be explained theoretically. The employment quotas are based on the theory that people with disabilities may face difficulties in a free competition because of their disabilities.[21] According to this, the abilities of people with disabilities may be utilized or even enhanced by employers' arrangements to accommodate them, such as, among others, suitable facilities and environments and the simplification of modus operandi. However, employers do not always fully understand the potential work-related needs of disabled employees. This is why several types of vocational rehabilitation are provided by national and public bodies. Even so, and in spite of these measures, in reality, in some cases, their abilities may not be always equal to those of nondisabled. Also, their employment entails costs for the establishment through necessary, appropriate improvements in facilities and working environment.

2.3 Administrative Guidance and Public Announcement

Administrative guidance is crucial in the quota system's enforcement. Private employers are required to report how many people with and without disabilities they are employing, as well as the employment rate of disabled people at their facilities. This information is submitted annually to the head of the Public Employment Security Office, which provides job placement services. The Public Employment Security Office may order an employer who has not met the required rate to formulate a hiring plan for disabled workers. The office can advise enterprises that are not satisfactorily implementing the plan. Company names may be made public.[22]

For instance, in March 2012, the Ministry of Health, Labor and Welfare announced that three firms did not meet the employment quotas.[23] The process leading to this was as follows. In June 2007, firms informed the Public Employment Security Offices of their employment situation regarding the number of their workers with and without disabilities. In response to this information, during the period from October to November 2007, 692 firms were ordered by the Public Employment Security Offices to make three-year plans for improving their rates of employment of people with disabilities.[24] These firms were picked up in accordance with the standard for administrative guidance. According to this, firms with 278 or more workers may be given guidance if the rates are below the average (currently, 1.65%) and the actual number of workers with disabilities are five or more short. The standard was strengthened relatively recently: before its 2007 amendment, only the firms whose actual employment rates were below 1.20% might have received such guidance. Enterprises with 277 or less workers that have no workers with disabilities may also be ordered to formulate such plans.

These plans were to be implemented by companies during the period from January 2008 to December 2010. Among these firms, 274 whose performance was poor received recommendations to carry out improvements to their employment practice during the period between October and December 2009.

After the three-year period of implementation passed, between April and December 2011, special guidance was given to 80 firms, including 20 firms with 1,000 employees and more, all of which were late in improving their employment numbers. During this period, the competent Public Employment Security Offices provided them with information about job seekers, and recommended them to take part in job fairs (joint job interviews), so that their employment rate of people with disabilities would be at least over the national average employment rate of 1.65%. As a result, 51 firms met the quota, and 22 others met the average rate. Among the remaining seven firms, the names of two were publicized by the Ministry as they did not meet even the standard for the postponement of public announcement. One of them was an airline company employing a total of 1,843 employees. They should have employed 11 more people with disabilities, and their actual employment rate of people with disabilities was 1.19%. Firms not fulfilling the quotas once again receive guidance the following year.

2.4 Levy-Grant System

Another enforcement system is found in the levy-grant system. If they fail to meet the specified employment rate, firms with more than 201 workers must pay levies for the employment of disabled people to the Japan Organization for Employment of the Elderly and Persons with Disabilities (JEED, an organization that was established to provide support to promote the employment of elderly and disabled persons).[25] This amounts to 50,000 yen (US $639) per person per month.[26] Conversely, when the employment rate exceeds the standard rate, they receive adjustment allowances of 27,000 yen (US $345) per person per month.[27] In addition, incentives to hire disabled people are given to the small-sized enterprises that are not covered by this sanction system. Rewards of 21,000 yen (US $268) per person per month are paid to the enterprises if either they employ six or more workers with disabilities or workers with disabilities constitute more than 4% of their workforce. Both of these allowances and rewards are financed by the levies paid by employers who fail to meet the employment rate. In the fiscal year 2010, 13,413 million yen (US $171 million) was collected in total levies; this amounts to 99.8% of the money that should have been received.

It can be deduced that this levy-grant system is significant in three main ways. First, it may alleviate dissatisfaction over inequality, a feeling that otherwise would be induced among firms complying with the employment quotas.[28] In fact, this system was created when the employment quota obligations were transformed from mere "efforts to endeavour" to a legal obligation with the 1976 amendment. The basic idea is for the preceding three amounts to be determined on the basis of the average monthly cost that employing a person with physical or intellectual disabilities normally entails. In order to calculate this additional cost, surveys are conducted, and businesses are visited and asked to provide information on the costs they bear during the period of one year, including: first, the costs of the provision or improvement of facilities or equipment to accommodate the needs of people with disabilities; second, the direct expense of the employment of people with disabilities, including special allowances, housing allowances, health benefits, expenditure for recreation activities or commutes, expenditure on education and training, and extra paid leave for people with disabilities; and third, the indirect expense of employing people with disabilities, including costs of assigning attendants or consultants, or those of educating other workers in facilitation.[29]

Taking these features into account, the "additional cost" is currently calculated at 42,000 yen per month. Based on this, the levy was set at 50,000 yen per month (42,000 × 1.282 = 53,840 ≒ 50,000); the adjustment allowance was set at 27,000 yen per month (42,000 × 0.655 = 27,510 ≒ 27,000). The levy is set at a higher amount than the allowance, because the additional cost is calculated to decrease in accordance with the increase in the number of workers with disabilities.[30]

Second, this system seems to function as a kind of sanction. This is indicated by the low profile of medium-sized firms.[31] Earlier, the obligation to pay levies had applied only to private sector employers with a workforce of 301 or more. This was because it was considered that the financial capacities of small- and medium-sized firms were lower than those of larger-sized firms. Also, their employment situation was taken into consideration—the total actual employment rate of people with disabilities among them was over the legal

Table 14.3 BREAKDOWN OF LEVY EXPENSES, 2004–2010[32]

	2004	2006	2008	2010
Collected levies	22,638	21,157	18,003	13,690
Total expenditures	21,082	22,650	23,251	23,645
Adjustment allowances	4,349	4,955	6,024	7,138
Rewards	4,680	4,631	4,729	4,742
Grants	6,871	7,423	7,631	7,879
Operating-costs, etc.	5,183	5,641	4,867	3,887

(million yen)

employment quotas, although the actual rate was low among major firms. Currently, this system is gradually being extended to medium-sized enterprises.[33] At the time of the discussion leading to these amendments, focused research found that there was a clear difference between enterprises with 278 to 300 workers and those with 301 to 333 workers. In the former, the proportion of those having no employees with disabilities was higher and their actual employment rate was lower. In addition, among enterprises with 301 workers or more, 80% or 90% of them maintained or aimed to employ a legally required or much higher number of people with disabilities, whereas this figure was only 40% among enterprises with 300 or less workers.

The third point relating to this is that the levies are also used to subsidize firms that promote the employment of people with disabilities. Their total amount is significant, as the breakdown of the expense of levies in 2004 to 2010 shows in table 14.3.

2.5 Subsidies

Grants are given for the establishment, installment, and lease of work/welfare facilities and equipment, and the appointment of attendants in cases in which the employment of people with disabilities would be difficult otherwise. Normally, employers who intend to receive the grants must submit application forms to the JEED, which examines their applications. Following this, approval is given by issuing a certificate of recipient qualification. After the facilities have been established, for instance, the request for payment of grants is made to the JEED. Then, if positive grant awards are made, these are paid to the employers. The amount of the grant depends on its category but, generally speaking, it is a certain rate of the actual costs that employers bear, up to a fixed maximum.

First, "Grants for the Provision of Workplace Facilities for Persons with Disabilities" may be given to employers who provide, for example, accessible bathrooms. The upper limit of payments to facilitate such modifications is 4.5 million yen (US $57,466) per disabled person. In a case of the totally blind person A, who was involved in checking Web accessibility and carrying out surveys targeted at visually impaired users, A's challenge was how to collect and save information. To overcome these obstacles, devices such as braille translation software and a braille printer were introduced. The employer owed 1,669,000 yen (US $21,314), and 1,113,000 yen (US $14,213) was subsidized to cover part of the cost.[34]

Second, the assignment of special support workers to help disabled workers is made possible by some grants. The "Grant for Workplace Attendants for Persons with Disabilities" is one of them. For instance, in the case of clerical workers with visual disabilities or with functional disabilities in both upper or lower limbs, the provision of attendants is supported by a grant of up to 150,000 yen (US $1,916) per month. In such instances, the term of payment should be less than 10 years. For example, in the case of person B, with disabilities related to movement, and who was assigned to sales for vending machines, one obstacle was that she was not able to move to and from her customers' offices on her own. To help her move, 126 hours of assistance were provided to her monthly, and the employer received 99,000 yen (US $1,264) per month, on average, to facilitate this need.[35]

Another facilitating grant is the "Grant for Job Coaches". Three types of support are possible. One is from the Local Vocational Center for Disabled People. Another is from welfare facilities, which are familiar with individual disabled people. The third type of coach is brought in at the employer's request, and is familiar with both job and workplace. In the latter two cases, subsidies are given to cover part of the costs. For instance, when employers have job coaches sent from social welfare facilities, the facilities can receive up to 14,200 yen (US $181) per day (for more than three hours' support per day); if less than three hours are required, 7,100 yen (US $91) comes from the JEED during the period across which the assistance program is provided, up to the maximum amount of 284,000 yen (US $3,627) per month and up to the maximum time limit of one year and eight months. As of March 2011, 1,142 job coaches were assigned. During that same year, 3,302 disabled employees were given support by them. Of those who received job coach services, 87.6% actually continued working for six months after the service terminated.[36]

Under this job coach system, employers are given advice about how to match the disabled worker's needs with their employment management. In addition, coworkers are advised on how to interact with and support their disabled colleague. Disabled people are given support to help them hone their work practice, communication skills, and health and life management skills. During the initial support period of about two to four months, issues around how to adapt the job and workplace to the disabled employee are analyzed, and improvements are attempted. During the next stage, experienced support is given; the key support person in the workplace is designated. Thus, the responsibility of this supporter is gradually moved from the job coach to the staff at the workplace.

Apart from the subsidies under the levy-grant system, several types of grants may be provided to employers under the employment insurance system. In particular, "Trial Employment for Disabled People" was introduced to help reduce employers' concerns over the employment of disabled people. Those who have employed disabled people through referrals from the Public Employment Offices, and maintained their employment for three months, are given 40,000 yen (US $511) per month per disabled worker. In 2010, 10,650 disabled people started working under this grant system; 86.4% of these workers moved onto regular employment.[37]

To date, this grant system seems to have been substantially utilized. The following figures shows the case numbers and grant amounts dealt with by the JEED during the fiscal year 2006.[38]

1 Grant for the provision of workplace facilities for persons with disabilities
   1,137 cases; 1,413,219 thousand yen

2 Grant for the provision of welfare facilities for persons with disabilities
   32 cases; 22,522 thousand yen

3 Grant for workplace attendants for persons with disabilities
   13,634 cases; 2,507,206 thousand yen

4 Grant for job coaches
   3,146 cases; 556,217 thousand yen

5 Grant for commuting measures for persons with severe disabilities
   3,128 cases; 799,643 thousand yen

6 Grant for the provision of facilities, in enterprises employing a large number of persons with severe disabilities
   31 cases; 528,719 thousand yen

2.6 Definition of People with Disabilities

In relation to the definition of physical disabilities, the identification of a person with a disability and its severity is based on official certificates that are issued to the individual by certain public bodies or designated doctors. To judge the possession and severity of disabilities, standards for certification, adopted for the purpose of welfare services, are utilized. These standards are set for each specific impairment relating to particular body parts. These include vision, hearing, speech, limbs, heart, kidneys, respiration, bladder, small intestine, HIV, or liver. According to this means of categorization, for instance, an individual with no fingers is treated as a person with severe disabilities. Distinctions are, however, in evidence among different—but apparently similar—cases. One individual, for instance, with whole fingers on one hand but with no fingers on the other can be classified as a person with mild disabilities. A person undergoing dialysis meets the standard—the extreme limitation of activity expected in normal daily life—to be categorized as a person with a severe disability.

In the case of intellectual disabilities, too, those with official booklets issued by certain public bodies or doctors are officially regarded as having disabilities. Whether they are severe or not depends on assessed levels of IQ and other diagnostic tests.

Such standards have been used since the employment quotas were made a legal obligation and the levy-grant system was introduced. This was because, to secure legal fairness and certainty, disabilities needed to be categorized in a nationally standardized way.[39] However, some argue that these means should be reformed to reflect the difficulty individual disabled people face in their vocational life.

2.6.1 People with Severe Disabilities

It should be noted that several mechanisms to promote the employment of people with severe disabilities are built into policy and legislation. First, under the employment quotas, the regular hiring of one person with severe disabilities counts as equal to the hiring of two disabled people; the hiring of one such person as a part-time worker, which is defined as a 20- to 30-hour working week, is equivalent to hiring one disabled person.[40] This system for those with severe disabilities was introduced because their employment was considered to bring employers an increased cost through necessarily improving and altering their facilities. The Japanese government conducted evaluation hearings on this measure in 2011–2012, and the Public Security Employment Office assessed this positively because it worked as an incentive for employers to hire people with severe disabilities.[41]

In addition, a great number of grants are offered specifically in order to achieve this goal. One action encouraged by grants involves setting up special subsidiaries and business establishments with a large number of workers with severe disabilities.[42] The value of the grant is dependent upon the number of employees with disabilities. If, for instance, there are between 10 and 14 employees, for the first year, 10 million yen (US $127,702) are paid. Subsequently, for the second and third years, 5 million yen (US $63,851) are paid. In addition, the "Grant for Commuting Measures for Persons with Severe Disabilities" is available. The most utilized ones were those for renting parking lots or accommodation. In order to lease a parking lot, up to 50,000 yen (US $639) per month, per person may be granted.

2.7 Special Subsidiaries

To increase the employment of people with disabilities in Japan, special subsidiaries seem to have played an important role. Parent companies can be deemed to have satisfied the quota by employing the required number of disabled people in special subsidiaries, even if the parent companies do not meet the rates by themselves.[43] In such cases, additional requirements have to be met. First, the total number of disabled employees in a special subsidiary must be five or more. Second, more than 20% of the employees in such companies must have a disability. And finally, more than 30% of the disabled employees must have a severe physical disability or an intellectual or mental disability.[44] Parent companies that have special subsidiary companies are allowed to calculate their actual employment rates across the group companies including subsidiary companies.[45]

This counting system seems to be positively viewed. According to the Japanese government's 2011–2012 hearing for evaluating opinions concerning this system, no clear negative views were shown by the organizations representing people with disabilities and the Public Employment Security Office.[46] Rather, they argued that special subsidiaries have played an important role in the promotion of the employment of people with disabilities, especially those with intellectual disabilities. During 2011, 319 special subsidiaries were set up by parent companies, and these subsidiaries employed a total of 10,883 disabled people. Of these workers, 46.2% were people with intellectual disabilities.[47]

The advantages of this system can be explained as follows. Employing disabled people in special subsidiaries enables employers to modify the work environment to match their different needs, and thus enable disabled people to fully utilize their abilities.[48] Employing disabled people at one workplace could also save on the outlay required for modifications to plants and equipment that are sometimes necessary precursors to employing disabled people. It also enables enterprises to provide different working conditions for disabled people compared with those for workers in parent companies and thus helps them to establish flexible employment management.

Certain special subsidiaries positively exploit opportunities that offer a close match of the disabled worker's skill to the type of work required. Parent companies take advantage of such chances for suitable employment matches. In the case of special subsidiary of an electronics parent company, the task of computer data imputing is farmed out by the parent company to the special subsidiary.[49] This company employs people with intellectual disabilities who, according to the company, have the ability to carry out accurate data input work.

In addition, it can be argued that, contrary to appearances, subsidiaries neither segregate people with disabilities in a separate place from nondisabled workers nor oppose the idea of normalization. According to a 1998 survey, their management philosophy embraced concepts of "normalization," and "social participation," among others.[50] Furthermore, they do not only hire people with disabilities. This survey shows that the number of firms with 40% of workers with disabilities was the highest, whereas those with 50% or 60% followed.

One real-life example is the famous Swan business, which operates a bakery that provides people with disabilities with opportunities to work. Swan is a special subsidiary of Yamato Unyu, a parcel delivery service company. In accordance with the philosophy of normalization, they strongly believe that people with and without disabilities should work together within the company, and thus they have applied this belief in practice.[51]

2.8 Corporate Social Responsibility

This idea of social solidarity seems to be strengthened by growing interest in the idea of Corporate Social Responsibility (CSR) since the early 2000s.[52] The employment rate of people with disabilities is listed as a factor to assess how seriously a firm is practicing CSR.[53] More than 60% of firms also referred to CSR as an explanation for their employment patterns.[54] Therefore, the increase in the number of workers with disabilities may, in part, be explained by this growing awareness of CSR.

On the other hand, in isolation, neither the shared idea of solidarity nor CSR would be enough to promote the employment of people with disabilities; the existence of the legal employment obligation seems to remain important. Actually, according to the survey cited earlier, many firms feel that employment quotas are needed to maintain the employment of people with disabilities.[55] In this regard, it should be noted that the employment quotas seem to be effectively enforced through the administrative guidance and levy-grant system, at least to some extent.

3. STRENGTHS AND LIMITATIONS OF DIFFERENT APPROACHES

There are some fundamental disadvantages to having employment quotas; some observers, for example, criticize employment policy for disabled people as potentially segregating and stigmatizing workers with disabilities. According to one article, special placement efforts are provided only when candidates register as disabled at the Public Employment Security Offices.[56] Such a label would not necessarily enhance the person's chance of finding a mainstream job with prospects of promotion. It has been suggested that employment quotas may also create an image of the disabled person as a burden that companies must bear. They may feel merely tolerated in the workplace due to the quota.

In addition, and most important, these approaches do not aim to achieve equality for people with disabilities. Therefore, employment quotas do not guarantee that people with disabilities can obtain jobs through which they can realize their aspirations and display their talents to their full extent. In fact, in a 2008 survey, one third of physically disabled employees consulted felt some improvements were needed in order to support their participation in their current work. They stated that evaluations and promotion based on workers' abilities, among other issues, were areas in need of further attention.[57] Also problematic is the fact that no regulations are in place to make the failure to hire disabled people on the grounds of their disability unlawful. This is a disadvantage inherent in the discussed employment policies because the purpose of the Act for Employment Promotion, etc., of Disabled Persons is to contribute to the occupational stability of the disabled (Article 1) rather than regulate discrimination.

On the other hand, under the Japanese employment quota system, employers are given clear numerical goals for the employment of people with disabilities. Quotas promote the employment of all people with disabilities, whether or not they are able to compete with nondisabled people, including those with severe or intellectual disabilities, even if they present greater challenges in integrating into mainstream jobs.

These clear numerical goals enable the effective enforcement of the quotas; both the administrative guidance and grant-levy system, which are crucial as sanctions as well as incentives, are made possible through employment quotas. It should be noted also that potential costs incurred from the employment of disabled people may be compensated by several different kinds of grants and allowances. Thus, the costs of accommodating the needs of disabled people are shared by enterprises.[58] Furthermore, without such goals, whether each firm fulfills their social responsibility or not would become less clear, and they would not be so concerned about societal monitoring.

As a result of such an enforcement system, the chances of disabled people obtaining employment can be improved without judicial relief. This strength is extremely important in a society like Japan, where informal resolution of disputes is preferred to lawsuits.[59] The infrequency of litigation is explained by institutional reasons, such as a low number of judges and attorneys, time-consuming and expensive legal processes, and limited remedial powers of judges, as well as cultural features, including deference to authority and the desire for harmony. Whatever the reasons, the field of labor disputes is not the exception. Rather, analysis shows that a party to labor disputes, in particular, tends to leave them without utilizing services from competent bodies.[60] Certainly, in recent years, the number of court cases relating to individual labor disputes has been increasing significantly: from 2,860 in 2006 to 6,593 in 2009. This reflects the surge in the number of such disputes and the popularity of the Labor Tribunal System, which was introduced to cope with those increasing disputes.[61] Despite this new trend, the number of caseloads remains relatively low as compared with other countries.

4. VOCATIONAL REHABILITATION

In addition, the Public Employment Security Office plays an important role in facilitating the employment of people with disabilities. They provide enterprises with information on job applications made by disabled people. But their function goes beyond this. They also play a more active role, including recommending that enterprises hire disabled people, matching offers of jobs to the abilities of disabled people, and providing information on various types of grants and subsidies. They set up joint job fairs to help employers and disabled people get together in one place.

Case working is also undertaken, which includes consultation on the disabled candidate's aptitude, skills, desired employment, and physical abilities. This also includes the provision of information on training, support, and grants. Staff members with special knowledge and experience are allocated to each Public Employment Security Office to support people with disabilities.

According to a 2006 survey of firms that have received some services from certain bodies in relation to hiring people with disabilities, Public Employment Security Offices were the most utilized. For people with physical disabilities, 90.9% of the firms did (the next most utilized bodies were schools, 18.8%); for people with intellectual disabilities, 78.8% (schools, 31.2%); those with mental disabilities, 85.1% (schools, 8.6%).[62]

In addition, as mentioned earlier, a considerable number of people with disabilities receive training at employment facilities, which provides them with employment opportunities as well.[63] These employment facilities are expected to facilitate the welfare-to-work transition, using employment measures such as trial employment and job coaches as outlined earlier.

5. REDUCTION OF MINIMUM WAGES

All the employment policies outlined in the preceding require or encourage positive discrimination toward people with disabilities. Alternatively, lower labor standards may be applied to them. That is, legal minimum wages,[64] upon application from employers, may be reduced for people "whose capabilities to work are considerably low because of their mental or physical disabilities."[65] Approval can be obtained, with a reduced rate specifically set for an individual worker with disabilities, from the director of the Prefectural Labor Bureau, a branch of the Ministry of Health, Labor and Welfare. Apart from the materials employers submit, on-the-spot investigation work is carried out by labor inspectors; this may include interviews with the worker with disabilities and with coworkers.

This special approval is granted only in cases in which the worker's disability apparently and considerably hinders performance of the work in which he or she shall engage, and their work efficiency is even lower than those engaging in the same or similar work. The reduction rate is set in accordance with the following process. First, the comparable worker is identified for purposes of comparison with the worker with disabilities. Second, the work efficiency of each is assessed, taking into consideration the results over two weeks. For instance, consideration is given to, in a case of manufacturing work, the number of products that pass a standard. In the case of the service industry, the amount of time needed to provide a certain level of service is a significant marker. Based on these evidences, when the efficiency of workers with disabilities is assessed as, for example, 60% of that of comparable workers, the maximum reduction rate is 40%. Up to this maximum, the applicable reduction rate is set considering the worker's job contents (including the level of difficulty and responsibility), job performance, the ability to work, and experience, among other factors.

This reduction is accepted because it is feared that, if minimum wages apply to them, employment opportunities could be lost; or, the level of minimum wages may be too low to protect the workers at large.[66] Therefore, this reduction system, which seemingly contravenes the other employment policies, actually shares the same aim, which is to create more employment opportunities for people with disabilities.

In particular, this reduction of the minimum wage is applied for workers with intellectual or severe disabilities.[67] According to a 2006 survey on welfare plants, 502 workers at welfare plants for people with intellectual disabilities (45.5% of such workers) were approved for exclusion from the coverage of minimum wages, whereas 99 workers at welfare plants for physical disabilities (8.5% of such workers) were treated likewise. Similarly, a 2005 survey on employers of people with severe disabilities showed that, of those employers, 37.6% had one or more workers with disabilities for whom the reduction of the minimum wage was approved. The reduction was less than or equal to 40% for more than 80% of these workers. For 25.8% of them (260/1,008), the amount of minimum wage was reduced by 30% to 40%.

6. CONCLUSION OF FIXED-TERM CONTRACTS

Similarly, there exists unfavorable treatment toward disabled people with regard to terms of employment. This was highlighted in a recent court case,[68] where the central issue rested on whether employers were allowed to hire disabled people on a fixed-term basis, whereas they hired able-bodied people on a permanent basis. In this case, a worker with a limb-related disability joined a job fair for disabled job seekers, which was held by the Public Employment Security Office. There, he was interviewed by a company manager who had joined the job fair. Following another interview, this disabled worker was hired, thus contributing to that company's employment quota for disabled people. According to the company, a six-month term of employment was fixed for any disabled employee, so that employers could ascertain whether the person had both the aptitude and the ability to perform necessary tasks.

After having allegedly involuntarily retired, the disabled worker demanded compensation for psychological injury under the law of tort, claiming that this employment system discriminated against disabled people without credible reason and, as such, was unlawful. According to the court, this system aimed to maintain and promote the employment of disabled people in the company. It enabled both the company and the disabled employee to conclude the employment contract. Disabled people could, therefore, expect to be hired, and, in practice, were usually hired in the same way as regular workers after a period of time unless insurmountable difficulties were found. Accordingly, this claim by the worker with the limb-related disability was not accepted by the court.

7. THE DEVELOPMENT OF LABOR CONTRACTS

People with disabilities who feel unfairly treated because of their disabilities seem to have no legal remedy. That is one of the disadvantages inherent in the employment policies as discussed earlier. However, legal protection may be given to those who acquire disabilities (or minor injuries or illnesses) during their course of employment through "Doctrines of Labor Contract."[69] Their legal basis was originally provided by certain parts of the Civil Code, including provisions on abuse of rights,[70] the principle of good faith,[71] and liabilities as torts;[72] based on these, they were shaped by case laws, and partially codified in the Labor Contract Act of 2007. The following describes the protection and accommodation these doctrines oblige employers to provide with regard to the employment of persons with illnesses or injuries.

7.1 Dismissals Against Disabled People

In cases of dismissals, first, the doctrine of abusive dismissals, one of the judge-formulated doctrines of employment contracts, offers protection.[73] One case involves the dismissal of a heavy machinery operator for sand-gathering with poor vision in one eye, which could not be corrected with eyeglasses.[74] The court nullified his dismissal on the grounds that the driver was qualified for the work because he had passed the skills test when, eight years ago, he had started working for that company. He had, ironically, just renewed his special driver's license at the time of the dismissal. He had some episodes of minor accidents with those machines, but they occurred only a few times. He was not so efficient as his coworkers; however, this was not accepted by the court as a proof of his incapacity.

It can also be said that the protection based on these doctrines is similar, in effect, to the concept of reasonable accommodation in disability anti-discrimination law. For instance, another case in Japan concerns a dental hygienist who visited many elementary schools but was dismissed on the grounds that she could no longer perform her job because, due to a spinal injury, she needed to use a wheelchair.[75] The dental hygienist argued that if pupils had also been seated in chairs, she would have been able to check their teeth from her wheelchair. The high court examined whether the employer had reasonable grounds to decline her request to use a wheelchair. Although the court held that this accommodation would be time consuming and would not be efficient for group dental checkups, and thus affirmed her dismissal, the reasonableness of the employer's decision was examined by them.

7.2 Redeployment for Workers

The protection conferred to people with some illnesses or injuries was strengthened during the last decade. This is shown by the cases in which employers must redeploy a worker who is not able fully to perform formerly assigned work because of his or her injury or illness, and assign them to lighter duty in order to enable them to continue working. Otherwise, such a worker may claim for wages that should have been paid during the time when the appropriate allocation was not carried out and, thus, the worker was not able to perform work.[76]

This was upheld by the Supreme Court in the Katayamagumi case.[77] In this case, the plaintiff, who worked for a construction firm and supervised construction as a foreman at a building site, became unable to work at such a site due to Basedow's disease, and made a request to be redeployed to indoor work. Because this request was declined by his employer, he had been absent from work for about four months, until his health recovered. The Supreme Court held that the worker may claim wages, even if unable to perform the assigned work, where the worker could do, and actually offered to do, another duty. This duty must be realistically possible, in light of the worker's ability, experience, and position as well as the company's size and type of industry, actual practice, and potential difficulties relating to redeployment of workers. In the Katayamagumi case, the remanded high court held that it was realistically possible to assign the foreman some office work, because supervisors at a building site in this firm, in practice, already carry out office work, during periods when they are off from their site-supervision duties.[78] Accordingly, the foreman won the right to claim wages.

7.3 The System of Suspension of Employment

As an example of voluntary reasonable accommodation, the system for suspending employment should be mentioned at this point. Many firms in Japan have a system for the suspension of employment, including for injury or sickness.[79] When employees cannot perform their work duties because of an injury or sickness, they can be kept from engaging in them for a certain fixed period of time. Typically, the employee recovers from the injury or illness during this period of time and, because he or she is able to resume work, the suspension will terminate, and the employee will be reinstated.

If, however, there is no recovery by the time the suspension expires, the suspension will be converted into a dismissal or an automatic termination of labor contracts. Accordingly, in many cases, the pressing issue is whether the required recovery has actually occurred. In this respect, the recovery cannot be said to have occurred unless the worker has recovered sufficiently well to work normally at the original duties. However, in some cases, employers are required to accommodate a worker's needs, even though he or she is unable, subsequently, to perform the former duty. These cases require employers to consider whether the employee has recovered to the point that he or she might be reinstated to lighter duty if not to the former job. Whether the employer is obliged to transfer the employee to a lighter job duty depends on some or all of the following factors: the employee's experiences and abilities, the employee's former employment position, the firm's size, and the realities and difficulties of transferring the employee. These rulings are affected by the Katayamagumi case.

In the J. R. Tokai case, a railway employee engaged in the inspection of vehicles had a brain hemorrhage.[80] After being absent from work for six months, he was suspended from work several times. Just before the three-year maximum period of suspension had elapsed, the company decided that the labor relationship with the worker would end. This was due to his medical certificate stating that his upper and lower right limbs were paralyzed, such that he was unable to perform precision work, unable to speak clearly, and was suffering from double vision. The court, however, invalidated the termination of his labor contract. This was because he had recovered enough to return to relatively light job duties, including tool maintenance jobs for which neither special skills nor speedy writing or walking were required. They also ruled that his intelligible language was sufficiently good to allow him to perform his work. Thus, we can say that the courts require employers to make reasonable accommodation for disabled people by arranging either transfer or reassignment.[81]

7.4 Reduction of Workloads

Furthermore, employers have an obligation to care for workers' security and health.[82] When they fail to provide such care for a worker with sickness or disability, and that failure results in any harm to that worker's life or body—for instance, death, injury, disease, or the aggravation of existing disease—that failure may constitute tort, or failure to perform an obligation. Thus, the employer shall pay damages.[83]

In this area, too, accommodation for people with injuries or illnesses is increasingly required in more cases than previously. The Dentsu case, decided by the Supreme Court, leads this trend.[84] This case involved the suicide by an employee with depression working in an advertising agency. His working hours had been very long for more than a year and sometimes he worked all night in order to meet clients' deadlines. His supervisor noticed physical signs of deterioration in his mental health but did not take any measures to lighten his workload. As a result, the Supreme Court ordered the company to pay around 90 million yen (US $1,149,320) to his family, under the provision of tort.[85]

8. EMPLOYEE COMMUNITY

All the case laws outlined in the preceding, which provide workers with security of employment, are thought to have been developed by reflecting social norms in Japan. They include long-term employment, which is considered as the most distinctive feature of Japanese employment relations.[86] It is likely that several factors contributed to the establishment of such an employment system. One is Japanese culture, including loyalty to the organization; others are social and economic contexts during the postwar period, including stable economic growth and bitter experiences that management and labor had through prolonged industrial action against dismissals.

In addition, it is said that corporate governance in Japanese corporations enables the development of this long-term employment system. Typically, major Japanese corporations hold each other's stocks, and, under such cross-stockholding, stockholders are not too interested in controlling a corporation. As a result, directors enjoy a wide discretion in considering the interests of the corporation's employees. This provides a basis on which a cooperative relationship between management and labor can be established, a so-called "employee community." One of the typical practices in such community is security in employment, which is accordingly reflected in the previously detailed case laws, and which provide legal protection for people with injuries or illnesses.

There are advantages to the implementation of the doctrines of labor contracts. They require employers to accommodate the needs of individual workers with injuries or illnesses, as antidiscrimination laws would do. In contrast to the employment quotas, each individual is given chances to exercise his or her rights by initiating lawsuits. In addition, judge-formulated doctrines of employment contracts might actually be more protective than disability antidiscrimination law or the employment quota system in that in these cases it is not necessary to define so narrowly who qualifies as a protected person. The protection through these doctrines is, in this sense, universal.

However, its limited coverage of workers should be noted: Such protection is only given to those who have obtained "membership" in the employee community. For instance, the doctrine for abuse of rights of dismissal applies only to workers on open-ended contracts.[87] Workers on fixed-term contracts do not enjoy universal coverage. Only in certain cases in which, for example, their contracts were repeatedly renewed, do these workers benefit.[88] Likewise, the transfer of workers with sickness or injury is required only in cases in which their types of jobs are not specified in their contracts. Another disadvantage lies in the basis of each worker's contract, because, since these doctrines are based on the contract relationship, failure to hire on the grounds of the applicant's disability would not be interpreted as unlawful act. Actually, the Japanese Supreme Court has shown an open attitude respecting the employer's freedom of contract in a case involving discrimination on the grounds of belief, considering the widespread practice of lifetime employment.[89] In short, protection through doctrines of labor contracts is only available to regular workers, who are already admitted to the employee community.

Furthermore, more fundamentally, current general employment practices based on employee community themselves may serve as hurdles for the integration of people with disabilities. In Japan, workers are generally required to work long hours, and are subject to frequent changes of places of work. Job contents may also be subject to regular alteration in many major companies. These working practices are prevalent, especially in large companies, and are considered a prerequisite for the employment and promotion of workers in the mainstream. In such a society, people with disabilities would be treated as having more need of accommodation than those in a different society.

9. ASSESSMENT OF EXISTING LAWS

To summarize what I have discussed, the advantages and disadvantages of the existing laws will be presented here. The Japanese approach, which mixes the aims and targets of employment quotas and the doctrines of labor contracts is, in some sense, adaptable. Employment quotas oblige employers to employ people with disabilities, including those who are not able to obtain jobs in free competition. They provide clear numerical goals, thus enabling their effective enforcement. Costs incurred through the employment of persons with disabilities can be shared through the levy-grant system. On the other hand, the doctrines of labor contract require employers to accommodate the needs of disabled people in a similar way to antidiscrimination law. For instance, employers are obliged to redeploy workers with injuries or illnesses at jobs with lighter duties. Thus, workers have chances to obtain legal remedies so that they can continue working at their workplaces. In such cases, it is not necessary to establish their qualification as disabled.

However, these approaches are not based on an ethical commitment to equality, and these aspects of employment have not, thus far, been sufficiently addressed. Especially, no regulations are in place that make the failure to hire disabled people on the grounds of their disability unlawful. Also, the doctrines of labor contracts limit their coverage to regular workers. These pluses and minuses can be considered as inherent in the existing two approaches, whose philosophies are social solidarity and employee community.

10. CHANGES IN LABOR LAWS AND PRACTICES

These weaknesses may be overcome by having disability antidiscrimination law simultaneously. The adoption of such law would have been in line with the overall trend toward normalization and independence of people with disabilities that Japanese laws have been facilitating. The employment quotas and vocational rehabilitation has been carried out for this purpose. In addition, new regulations have been introduced to attain these objectives during the last decade; the Act on Promotion of Smooth Transportation, etc., of Elderly Persons, Disabled Persons, etc. came into force in 2000; disqualifying standards for professional licensing for doctors or pharmacists also have been reexamined and amended since 1999.

Despite this trend, attempts to introduce disability antidiscrimination law had not been successful.[90] The Basic Act for Persons with Disabilities was amended in 2004 to include an antidiscrimination provision; Article 4 of the Act proclaims that any individual shall not discriminate against persons with disabilities on the grounds of their disabilities. It should be noted, however, that this provision is not interpreted to provide a firm legal basis on which persons with disabilities can obtain legal remedy. One might pose a question: Is Japanese society not aware of equality? Instead, it can be said that the late 2000s was the period when much advancement had been made in the area of employment discrimination law. The focus then, however, was on income inequality. To deal with this issue, in 2007, discrimination against part-time workers, and age discrimination in the context of hiring,[91] became subject to compulsory regulations for the first time. In this circumstance, politicians might not have been sufficient to put disability equality on top agendas— until the UN Convention, which had been signed by Japan, gave a decisive impetus to the adoption of such law.

Bearing this current situation in mind, this chapter concludes with an examination of possible changes and reforms to labor law.

There exists the potential for the protection of disabled people to be given a firm foundation. Because the doctrine of abuse of rights to dismiss is couched in general terms these terms may be relaxed if the economic downturn at the time of writing worsens in the future. However, even if protection from dismissal is generally relaxed, the prohibition of discrimination, and the requirement of accommodation of needs ought to remain. Moreover, there is a possibility that more accommodation of needs could be extended to disabled people.

In addition, an educational effect resulting from antidiscrimination legislation can be expected. Compared with existing laws and the current patchwork of case laws, such disability antidiscrimination legislation would raise people's awareness of the prejudices that exist against disabled people, and, correspondingly, raise awareness of how society needs to accommodate the needs of disabled people.

We may see discrimination, in relation to recruitment and hiring, prohibited. Obvious discrimination in relation to recruitment and hiring, at least, would be decreased. It should be noted in this respect, however, that it would not be easy to prove a firm's discriminatory intent. In particular, considering typical employment practices in Japan, disabled people might find it difficult to prove that they are qualified, since firms employ regular workers without job specifications. In addition, with mobility clauses integral to contracts, a specific place of work is not designated for each worker until the employer exercises their rights of personnel management. In such cases, difficulties might arise when deciding whether accommodation measures are required or not. Without knowing specific places of work, one would not be able to know whether accommodation would be available or not.

Similarly, we need to consider whether low wages for people with disabilities should be improved by the equal application of minimum wages and the application of the principle of equal wages for equal work. This issue has not been regarded as serious thus far because Japanese employment policy has mainly been aimed at the quantitative expansion of employment opportunities for disabled people. In this respect, the advantages and disadvantages of abolishment should be examined carefully, considering that people with disabilities are a diverse group depending on the type and severity of their disabilities.

Furthermore, if typical employment practices in Japan, including overtime work and transfer of workers, are modified in certain ways, the working environment and career prospects would be improved, not only for disabled people, but also for other workers, including women, who currently carry a disproportionate share of family responsibilities. Also, firms hiring workers for specified jobs and workplaces would be employing all workers on more equal footing, regardless of disability. However, because these flexible employment practices retain a protective function for workers who acquire disability whilst working (see, for example, the cases of suspension of employment referred to earlier), further analysis will be needed to resolve this complex issue.

In June 2013, the Act on Employment Promotion of Persons with Disabilities was amended to finally introduce anti-discrimination provisions. These include equal treatment with regard to the recruitment and employment (Article 34) and the wages and other matters (Article 35). Also, employers are obliged to accommodate the needs of disabled workers (Articles 36-2, 36-3 and 36-4). The amended act will come into force in years to come (from April 2016 for the former provisions; from April 2018 for the accommodation provisions).

NOTES

1. The data is based on 2005, 2006 and 2008 surveys. Naikakuhu [Cabinet Office] (2011). *Heisei 23 Nen Ban Shogaisha Hakusho [White Paper on Persons with Disabilities in 2011]*. Tokyo, Japan: Saeki Insatsu, 12.
2. World Health Organization & World Bank (2011). *World Report on Disability*. Geneva, Switzerland: WHO Press, 29.
3. Kosei Rodo Sho [Ministry of Health, Labor and Welfare] (2008). *Shintai Shogaisha, Chiteki Shogaisha oyobi Seishin Shogaisha Shugyo Jittai Chosa no Chosa Kekka ni tsuite [Result of the Survey of Actual Working Conditions for People with Physical, Intellectual and/or Mental Disabilities]*. Retrieved March 25, 2013, from http://www.mhlw.go.jp/houdou/2008/01/dl/h0118-2a.pdf.
4. Somu Sho [Ministry of Internal Affairs and Communications] (2011). *Heisei 23 Nen Rodo Ryoku Chosa Nenpou [An Annual Report on Labour Force Survey in 2011]*. Retrieved March 25, 2013, from http://www.stat.go.jp/data/roudou/report/2011/pdf/summary1.pdf.
5. Kosei Rodo Sho [Ministry of Health, Labor and Welfare] (2012). Press Release. Retrieved March 25, 2013, from http://www.mhlw.go.jp/stf/houdou/2r98520000029xr4-att/2r98520000029xuu.pdf.
6. Here, "regular workers" means those who are employed on open-ended contracts or are expected to continue working for one or more years.

7. The data is based on 2006 surveys and a 2008 survey. See Naikakuhu [Cabinet Office]. *Heisei 23 Nen Ban Shogaisha Hakusho [White Paper on Persons with Disabilities in 2011]*, 30.
8. They are now legally given the status of businesses "for support for continuous employment" under the Act for Supporting the Independence of Persons with Disabilities.
9. Kosei Rodo Sho [Ministry of Health, Labor and Welfare] (2008). *Heisei 20 Nendo Shogaisha Koyo Jittai Chosa Kekka no Gaiyo ni tsuite [A Summary Result of the Survey of Actual Working-Conditions of Employment for People with Disabilities in 2008]*. Retrieved March 25, 2013, from http://www.mhlw.go.jp/stf/houdou/2r98520000002fxj-img/2r98520000002fz1.pdf.
10. Ibid.
11. Articles 38 and 43. For details of quota system, see JEED (2011). *Supporting the Employment of Persons with Disabilities: Employment Guide for Employers and Persons with Disabilities*. Retrieved March 25, 2013, from http://www.jeed.or.jp/english/supporting.html.
12. This exclusionary system, which was abolished with the amendments of 2002, still remains as an interim measure. At the moment, its phased reduction is taking place. Among the different exclusion rates for several categories of industry, the highest one is 80% for seamen.
13. Kosei Rodo Sho [Ministry of Health, Labor and Welfare] (2012). *Shogaisha Koyo Ritsu no Settei no Kijun to naru Suchi no Chosa Kekka ni tsuite [A Result of the Investigation concerning Figures as the basis of setting Employment Quotas for People with Disabilities]*, Material No.2-1 distributed to the members of the People with the Disabilities and Employment Subcommittee, Labour Policy Council. Retrieved March 25, 2013, from http://www.mhlw.go.jp/stf/shingi/2r9852000002b5zs-att/2r9852000002b62z.pdf. Following this, the quota coverage will be also extended to enterprises with 50 workers or more.
14. Kosei Rodo Sho [Ministry of Health, Labor and Welfare] (2011). *Heisei 23 Nen Shogaisha Koyo Jyokyo no Shukei Kekka [Totaled Results of Conditions of Employment for People with Disabilities in 2011]*. Retrieved March 25, 2013, from www.mhlw.go.jp/stf/houdou/2r9852000001vuj6.html.
15. Regarding the following statistics and survey, see Shogaisha Koyo Sokushin Seido ni okeru Shogaisha no Hani to no Arikata ni kansuru Kenkyukai [the Expert Committee on the Coverage of People with Disabilities under the Employment Promotion Measures for People with Disabilities] (2012). *Shogaisha Koyo Sokushin Seido ni okeru Shogaisha no Hani to no Arikata ni kansuru Kenkyukai Hokokusho [Report of Expert Committee on Coverage of People with Disabilities under the Employment Promotion Measures for People with Disabilities]*. Retrieved March 25, 2013, from http://www.mhlw.go.jp/stf/houdou/2r9852000002gyh3-att/ 2r9852000002gyx7.pdf.
16. The target of the employment quota scheme was originally people with physical disabilities, but coverage has been extended over time. The 1987 revision also covered people with intellectual disabilities in calculating the actual employment rate of people with disabilities. Then, the 2005 revision enabled employers to include in their count employees with mental disabilities.
17. Kosei Rodo Sho [Ministry of Health, Labor and Welfare] (2006). Press Release. Retrieved March 25, 2013, from http://www.mhlw.go.jp/houdou/2006/12/dl/h1214-2a.pdf; Kosei Rodo Sho [Ministry of Health, Labor and Welfare] (2010). Press Release. Retrieved March 25, 2013, from http://www.mhlw.go.jp/stf/houdou/2r9852000000v2v6-img/2r9852000000v2wn.pdf (accessed #).

18. According to this survey, of 432 establishments, 62 establishments employed 116 workers with mental disabilities (36 establishments had employed those who have already had mental disabilities at the time of recruitment). In 2003, in contrast, of 415 establishments, 45 employed such workers, and only seven establishments had employed those who already had mental disabilities at the time of recruitment.
19. Articles 3, 5, and 37. See Soya, N (1998). *Shogaisha Koyo Taisaku no Riron to Kaisetsu [Theory and Commentary with regard to Employment Measures for People with Disabilities]*. Tokyo, Japan: Romugyosei Kenkyusho, 399–400.
20. Ibid., 55–60.
21. Ibid., 397–400.
22. When national and public bodies do not comply with the employment quota, they must make employment plans regarding the employment of people with disabilities. This plan and its implementation are to be provided for the Minister of the Health, Labor and Welfare (Articles 38 and 39). It should be noted here that the information on the actual employment rate of people with disabilities can be generally accessible under the Information Disclosure Act.
23. Kosei Rodo Sho [Ministry of Health, Labor and Welfare] (2012). Press Release. Retrieved March 25, 2013, from http://www.mhlw.go.jp/stf/houdou/2r98520000025uds-att/2r98520000025uf9.pdf.
24. This standard is currently revised; the hiring plan should be made for the following two years.
25. For public bodies, there are no similar requirements.
26. See Articles 53, 54 and 55, Ordinance 17.
27. See Article 50, Ordinance 15.
28. Soya (1998), *Shogaisha Koyo Taisaku no Riron to Kaisetsu [Theory and Commentary with regard to Employment Measures for People with Disabilities]*, 98–99.
29. Kosei Rodo Sho [Ministry of Health, Labor and Welfare] (2012). Material No.2 distributed to the members of the Rodo Koyo Bunya ni okeru Shogaisha Kenri Joyaku eno Taio no Arikata ni kansuru Kenkyukai [the Expert Committee on Handling of Labor and Employment Issues relating to the Convention on the Rights of Persons with Disabilities Treaty]. Retrieved March 25, 2013, from http://www.mhlw.go.jp/stf/shingi/2r9852000002daqh-att/2r9852000002db4o.pdf.
30. Kosei Rodo Sho [Ministry of Health, Labor and Welfare] (2012). *Shogaisha Koyo Ritsu no Settei no Kijun to naru Suchi no Chosa Kekka ni tsuite [A Result of the Investigation concerning Figures as the basis of setting Employment Quotas for People with Disabilities]*.
31. Chusho Kigyo ni okeru Syogaisha no Koyo no Sokushin ni kansuru Kenkyukai [the Expert Committee on the Promotion of the Employment of People with Disabilities in Small and Medium-Sized Enterprises] (2007). Chusho Kigyo ni okeru Syogaisha no Koyo no Sokushin ni kansuru Kenkyukai Hokokusho [Report of the Expert Committee on the Promotion of the Employment of People with Disabilities in Small and Medium-Sized Enterprises], 10–11.
32. Kosei Rodo Sho [Ministry of Health, Labor and Welfare] (2012). Reference Material No.1 distributed to the members of the Rodo Koyo Bunya ni okeru Shogaisha Kenri Joyaku eno Taio no Arikata ni kansuru Kenkyukai [the Expert Committee on Handling of Labor and Employment Issues relating to the Convention on the Rights of Persons with Disabilities Treaty]. Retrieved March 25, 2013, from http://www.mhlw.go.jp/stf/shingi/2r9852000002daqh-att/2r9852000002db5j.pdf.

33. Enterprises with 201-300 workers have been obliged to pay levies since July 2010. Smaller enterprises, with 101-200 workers, will be included from April 2015.

34. JEED (n.d.). *Shogaisha Koyo Jirei Refarensu Sabisu [Reference Service for Cases of the Employment of People with Disabilities]*. Retrieved March 25, 2013, from http://www.ref.jeed.or.jp/19/19445.html.

35. JEED (n.d.). *Shogaisha Koyo Jirei Refarensu Sabisu [Reference Service for Cases of the Employment of People with Disabilities]*. Retrieved March 25, 2013, from http://www.ref.jeed.or.jp/23/23704.html.

36. Kose Rodo Sho [Ministry of Health, Labor and Welfare] (2011). *Saikin no Shogaisha Koyo no Genjo to Kadai [The Current State of Affairs and Problems in the Employment of Disabled Persons]*, Reference Material No.3 distributed to the members of the People with the Disabilities and Employment Subcommittee, Labour Policy Council. Retrieved March 25, 2013, from http://www.mhlw.go.jp/stf/shingi/2r9852000001y5tn-att/2r9852000001y5yo.pdf

37. Ibid.

38. Kosei Rodo Sho [Ministry of Health, Labor and Welfare] (2007). Material No.1-4 distributed to the members of the Rodo Seisaku Shingikai Shogaisha Koyo Bunkakai [People with Disabilities and Employment Subcommittee, Labour Policy Council]. Retrieved March 25, 2013, from http://www.mhlw.go.jp/shingi/2007/10/dl/s1024-12d.pdf;

39. Soya (1998). *Shogaisha Koyo Taisaku no Riron to Kaisetsu [Theory and Commentary with regard to Employment Measures for People with Disabilities]*, 338.

40. Article 43, paragraphs 4 and 5; Ordinance 10; Enforcement Regulation 6-2.

41. Kosei Rodo Sho [Ministry of Health, Labor and Welfare] (2012). Reference Material No.4 distributed to the members of the Shogaisha Koyo Sokushin Seido ni okeru Shogaisha no Hani to no Arikata ni kansuru Kenkyukai [the Expert Committee on the Coverage of People with Disabilities under the Employment Promotion Measures for People with Disabilities]. Retrieved March 25, 2013, from http://www.mhlw.go.jp/stf/shingi/2r9852000002g2nt-att/2r9852000002g2t0.pdf.

42. To be recognized as business establishments with a large number of workers with severe disabilities, the following two conditions should be met: those with severe physical disabilities, intellectual disabilities, or mental disabilities, who are newly hired, total 10 or more; and those with such disabilities represent 20% or more of their workforce.

43. Articles 44, 45 and 45-2.

44. The other requirements are: first, the parent companies' control of the decision-making body of the special subsidiary companies; second, close relationships between the parent companies and the special subsidiary companies, shown by, for instance, the dispatch of executives to the subsidiaries; third, the subsidiary companies' ability to exercise the proper employment management of people with disabilities, with features such as improved facilities or special assistants and; fourth, their certain capability to promote and secure the employment of disabled people.

45. Likewise, medium-sized enterprises can establish cooperatives that hire disabled people (Article 45-3). This cooperative must employ one or more people with disabilities, and their employment rate must be over 20%. The medium-sized enterprise with 167-300 workers also must employ one such worker (or two for enterprises with 250-300 workers). Such medium-sized enterprises are allowed

to count their actual employment rates across them and the cooperative. This system entered into force in April 2009.

46. Kosei Rodo Sho [Ministry of Health, Labor and Welfare] (2012). Reference Material No.4 distributed to the members of the Shogaisha Koyo Sokushin Seido ni okeru Shogaisha no Hani to no Arikata ni kansuru Kenkyukai [the Expert Committee on the Coverage of People with Disabilities under the Employment Promotion Measures for People with Disabilities], Retrieved March 25, 2013, from http://www.mhlw.go.jp/stf/shingi/2r9852000002g2nt-att/2r9852000002g2t0.pdf

47. Kosei Rodo Sho [Ministry of Health, Labor and Welfare] (2012). Reference Material No.6 distributed to the members of the Shogaisha Koyo Sokushin Seido ni okeru Shogaisha no Hani to no Arikata ni kansuru Kenkyukai [the Expert Committee on the Coverage of People with Disabilities under the Employment Promotion Measures for People with Disabilities]. Retrieved March 25, 2013, from http://www.mhlw.go.jp/stf/shingi/2r9852000002bj5t-att/2r9852000002bja7.pdf. The increase in numbers of workers with intellectual disabilities is conspicuous during the period from 2003 to 2011. In 2003, there were 129 special subsidiaries employing 5,760 people with disabilities, including 1,335 people with intellectual disabilities. In 2011, 7594.5 people with intellectual disabilities were recorded, whilst 16,429.5 people with disabilities were employed by 319 special subsidiaries. The actual number of people with disabilities is less than these figures shown in this note, since it is calculated by counting those with severe disabilities twice.

48. Ibid.

49. Okada, S. (2007). *Shogaisha Koyo ni kakaru Jukyu no Ketsugo wo sokushin suru tameno Hosaku ni kansuru Kenkyu (sono3) [Research on Measures promoting the balanced Supply and Demand for the Employment of People with Disabilities (No.3)]*, Chiba, Japan: Shogaisha Shokugyo Sogo Senta 55.

50. Nihon Keieisha Dantai Renmei (1998). *Tokurei Kogaisha no Keiei ni kansuru Anketo Chosa Kekka Hokoku [A Report of the Result of the Survey of the Management of Special Subsidiaries]*, 12, 17–23. Japan: Nihon Keieisha Dantai Renmei.

51. Ogura, M. (2003). *Fukushi wo kaeru Keiei [Management as changing the Welfare]*. Tokyo, Japan: Nikkei BP.

52. According to the 2005 survey conducted by Keidanren, 75.2 % of the firms replied that they were aware of the CSR. See http://www.keidanren.or.jp/japanese/policy/2005/066.pdf.

53. For instance, see the website of CANPAN CSR Plus: https://csr.canpan.info/en/information/.

54. Shogaisha Shokugyo Sogo Senta [General Vocational Center for People with Disabilities] (2010). *Kigyo Keiei ni ataeru Shogaisha Koyo no Koka to ni kansuru Kenkyu [Research on the Effect of the Employment of People with Disabilities on Enterprise Management]*, 61–63.

55. Ibid., 51, 71.

56. Ison, T.G. (1992). Employment Quotas for Disabled People: The Japanese Experience. *Kobe University Law Review 26*, 15–19.

57. Kosei Rodo Sho [Ministry of Health, Labor and Welfare] (2008). *Heisei 20 Nendo Shogaisha Koyo Jittai Chosa Kekka no Gaiyo ni tsuite [A Summary Result of the Survey of Actual Conditions of Employment for People with Disabilities in 2008]*. Retrieved March 25, 2013, from http://www.mhlw.go.jp/stf/houdou/2r98520000002fxj.html.

58. Hasegawa, T. (2007). Equality of Opportunity or Employment Quotas? A Comparison of Japanese and American Employment Policies for the Disabled. *Social Science Japan Journal 10*(1), 53.

59. The infrequency of litigation in Japan was discussed first by Takeyoshi Kawashima in 1960s. See Kawashima, T. (1963). Dispute Resolution in Contemporary Japan. In A.T. von Mehren (Ed.). *Law in Japan: The Legal Order in a Changing Society* (Cambridge, MA: Harvard University Press), 41. Regarding the scholarly work which has been undertaken since then, see Feldman, E. (2007). Law, Culture, and Conflict: Dispute Resolution in Postwar Japan. In D. Foote (Ed.). *Law in Japan: A Turning Point* (Seattle, WA: University of Washington Press), 50–79.

60. Takahashi, H. (2009). Rodo wo meguru Funso wa donoyoni okiteirunoka [How Labor Disputes Arise]. In S. Ouchi (Ed.). *Hataraku Hito wo torimaku Horitsu Nyumon [An Introduction to Laws related to Workers]* (Kyoto, Japan: Mineruba shobo), 271–282.

61. Sato, I. (n.d.). Rodo Shinpan Riyosha Chosa no Nerai [Aims of the Survey of the Use of Labor Tribunals]. Retrieved March 25, 2013, from http://www.crs.or.jp/backno/No636/6361.htm; Sugeno, K. (2006). Judicial Reform and the Reform of the Labor Dispute Resolution System. *Japan Labor Review 3*(1), 4–12.

62. Kosei Rodo Sho [Ministry of Health, Labor and Welfare] (2008). *Heisei 20 Nendo Shogaisha Koyo Jittai Chosa Kekka no Gaiyo ni tsuite [A Summary Result of the Survey of Actual Conditions of Employment for People with Disabilities in 2008]*.

63. Counseling and training are also provided in collaboration with the Local Vocational Centre for Persons with Disabilities. Another body supporting the employment placement of disabled people is the Employment and Life Support Centre for Disabled Persons.

64. The Minimum Wage Act of 1959 currently provides for two systems of minimum wage. One is a regional minimum wage, which is set at prefecture level. The other is a specified minimum wage, the setting or amendment of which can be initiated by worker representatives or employer representatives of particular industries.

65. Article 7.

66. Kosei Rodo Sho [Ministry of Health, Labor and Welfare] (n.d.). *Saitei Chingin Ho Dai Nana Jo no Gengaku no Tokurei Kyoka Jimu Manyuaru [Staff Manual of Special Approval for the Reduction in accordance with Article 7 of the Minimum Wage Act]*, 1.

67. Shogaisha Shokugyo Sogo Senta [General Vocational Centre for Persons with Disabilities] (2010). *Syogaisha no Saitei Chingin no Gengaku Kyoka to Rodo Noryoku no Hyoka ni kansuru Kenkyu [Research concerning Approvals for the Reduction of Minimum Wages for People with Disabilities and the Assessment of their Job Performances]*, 30–34.

68. The Nihon Sodatsu Case, Rodo Hanrei [Labor Law Cases Reports] 924, 112 (Tokyo District Court, April 25, 2006).

69. Regarding the summary and analysis of the contract law in relation to disabled people, see Nakagawa, J., & Blanck, P. (2010). Future of Disability Law in Japan: Employment and Accommodation. *Loyola of Los Angeles, International & Comparative Law Review 33* (1), 182–193.

70. Article 1 Paragraph 3.

71. Article 1, Paragraph 2.

72. Articles 709 and 715.

73. The "abusive of dismissal rights" doctrine was codified in the Labor Contract Act (Article 16), in 2007.

74. The San Sekiyu Case, Rodo Hanrei [Labor Law Cases Reports] 938, 68 (Sapporo High Court, May 11, 2006).
75. The Yokohamashi Gakko Hokenkai Case, Rodo Hanrei [Labor Law Cases Reports] 890, 58 (Tokyo High Court, January 19, 2005).
76. In such a case, whether such a worker can successfully claim for wages or not depends on the application of Article 536, paragraph 2, according to which "an obligor (in the case of labor contracts, employees) shall not lose his/her right to receive performance in return (in such cases, wages), if the performance of any obligation (in such cases, work) has become impossible due to reasons attributable to the obligee (in the case of labor contracts, employers)." The key question here is whether the worker's tender of the performance is regarded as being consistent with the main purport of the obligation. If it is not, the reason why the performance of work duty was impossible is not attributable to employers. Thus workers lose their right to receive wages.
77. Rodo Hanrei [Labor Law Cases Reports] 736, 15 (Supreme Court, April 9, 1998).
78. Rodo Hanrei [Labor Law Cases Reports] 759, 15 (Tokyo High Court, April 27, 1999).
79. See Sugeno, K. (2002). *Japanese Employment and Labor Law*. Trans. L. Kanowitz (Durham, N.C.: Carolina Academic Press), 455–459.
80. The JR Tokai Case, Rodo Hanrei [Labor Law Cases Reports] 771, 25 (Osaka District Court, October 4, 1999).
81. The Canon Soft Joho System Case involves a computer programmer having contracted Cushing's Syndrome and autonomic dystonia. The court decided that she had recovered to the point where she would be able to work in a support department. There, she would not be required to work overtime, even if she might not have been able to perform the former job in the department of software development. Rodo Hanrei [Labor Law Cases Reports] 960, 49 (Osaka District Court, January 25, 2008).
82. This "duty to care" is codified in the Labor Contract Act: "an employer shall, in association with a labor contract, give the necessary consideration to allow a worker to work while securing the safety of his/her life, body and the like" (Article 5).
83. Civil Code, Articles 415, 709 and 715.
84. The Dentsu Case, Saiko Saibansho Minji Hanrei Shu [Supreme Court Reports (Civil Cases)] 54-3, 1155 (Supreme Court, March 24, 2000).
85. Civil Code, Article 715.
86. As to the following discussion, see Yamakawa, R. (2007). From Security to Mobility? Changing Aspects of Japanese Dismissal Law. In D. Foote (Ed.). *Law in Japan: A Turning Point* (Seattle, WA: University of Washington Press), 483–520.
87. See Nakagawa & Blanck (2010). Future of Disability Law in Japan.
88. The Toshiba Yanagicho Case, Saiko Saibansho Minji Hanrei Shu [Supreme Court Reports (Civil Cases)] 28-5, 927 (Supreme Court, July 22, 1974).
89. The Mitsubishi Jushi Case, Saiko Saibansho Minji Hanrei Shu [Supreme Court Reports (Civil Cases)] 27-11, 1536 (Supreme Court, December 12, 1973).
90. Regarding the movements for anti-disability discrimination law, see Nakagawa & Blanck (2010). Future of Disability Law in Japan.
91. Employment Measure Act, which was amended in 2007, Article 10. Regarding this provision, see Sakuraba, R. (2009). The Amendment of the Employment Measure Act: Japanese Anti-Age Discrimination Law. *Japan Labor Review* 6(2), 60–64.

CHAPTER 15

Disability and Employment in the European Union

Collective Strategies and Tools

ANNA LAWSON

1. INTRODUCTION

1.1 Disability and Employment in the European Union

Disabled people in Europe experience similar levels of exclusion and disadvantage in employment to those experienced by their counterparts elsewhere in the world and described in other chapters of this volume. Thus, in 2010 the European Commission, the principal executive organ of the European Union (EU), reported that the EU-wide employment rate for people with very severe degrees of disability was only 19.5% and, for people with severe degrees of disability, 44.1%.[1] There is evidence of significant gender differentiation in the employment rates of disabled people, the average employment rate for disabled women aged between 20 and 64 being 43% compared with 51.8% for disabled men.[2] There also appears to be considerable variation among countries. Thus, according to a 2009 report of the Academic network of European Disability Experts (ANED),[3] the employment rate for people who described themselves as "considerably restricted" was 58.6% in Belgium but only 7.4% in Slovakia. At least some of the disparity, however, seems likely to be caused by inconsistent data collection methods, different understandings of disability or restriction, and variations in willingness to identify oneself as being disabled or having a relevant restriction.[4]

The disproportionate exclusion of disabled people from employment has financial consequences, both for disabled people themselves and for the EU more generally. Limited employment opportunities for disabled people help to explain the statistics relating to poverty and standard of living. The incidence of poverty among disabled people is some 70% higher than for the population as a whole.[5] Further, according to a 2008 study,[6] reduced levels of employment and qualification among disabled people result in an annual loss to the EU of some €40.3 billion in GDP.[7]

1.2 Policymaking at the European Union Level

This chapter focuses on the efforts taken at the EU level to address concerns relating to disability and employment within the 28 EU Member States. It is important to stress at the outset, however, that the EU is a supranational organization that is not free to intervene in the domestic policy of its Member States to any greater extent than the powers (or "competences") transferred to it by them. The EU's founding treaties (the Treaty on the European Union (TEU) and the Treaty on the Functioning of the European Union (TFEU) lay down the broad framework of these competences, but their scope and exercise by the EU is "subject to continuous development."[8] Thus, as explained more fully in the next section, the EU does not have the freedom to prescribe details of the Member States' employment policies and is, in that respect, in a different position from the national governments dealt with in other chapters of this book.

Another point that should be made clear at the outset is that, despite some policy convergence resulting from obligations imposed by the EU (for example, the requirement that all Member States prohibit disability discrimination in employment) the policies relating to the employment of disabled people adopted by the 28 EU Member States remain far from homogenous.[9] For instance, a range of quota schemes, with different compliance rates and enforcement mechanisms,[10] operate in the majority of EU countries—including Austria, Belgium, Bulgaria, Cyprus, The Czech Republic, France, Germany, Greece, Hungary, Ireland, Italy, Lithuania, Luxemburg, Malta, Poland, Portugal, Romania, Slovakia, Slovenia, and Spain.[11] Disability employment quotas, however, do not operate in other countries—including Denmark, Estonia, Finland, the Netherlands, Sweden, and the United Kingdom.[12] Similarly, although sheltered (or segregated) employment continues to play a significant role in the disability employment policies and strategies of some countries (including Austria, Belgium, Finland, France, Germany, Italy, Luxemburg, Portugal, and Spain), there has been a decrease in the numbers of people in such employment in some other countries (including Poland, Sweden, and the United Kingdom).[13] In addition, there is considerable variation in guardianship schemes. Indeed, plenary guardianship systems continue to operate in some EU countries (including Latvia, Romania, and Bulgaria), with the result that people subjected to them may be prevented from working because they are deprived of the legal capacity to enter into an employment contract.[14]

This chapter is divided into four main sections. The first of these, section 2, provides a context for subsequent analyses by highlighting the key provisions of the EU's founding treaties. Section 3 then outlines relevant aspects of the three EU-level strategies that together set out EU disability employment policy. Section 4 provides an overview of three main types of tool or mechanism used by the EU to support this policy—hard law, or legislative intervention, requiring Member States to ensure that certain specified requirements or standards are achieved by their domestic law; experimentalist governance, in the form of the Open Method of Co-ordination; and direct funding. Finally, in the Conclusion, an attempt will be made to identify lessons that can be learned from the EU's experience of harnessing these three different tools to achieve its strategic objectives and to consider the extent to which they might have relevance to the world beyond the rather unique parameters of the EU.

2. TREATY PROVISIONS UNDERPINNING EUROPEAN UNION COMPETENCE IN DISABILITY POLICY

Alongside commitments to economic collaboration, principles of citizenship and human (or fundamental) rights are to be found at the heart of the EU.[15] According to Article 2 of the Treaty of the European Union:

> The Union is founded on the values of respect for human dignity, freedom, democracy, equality, the rule of law and respect for human rights, including the rights of persons belonging to minorities. These values are common to the Member States in a society in which pluralism, non-discrimination, tolerance, justice, solidarity and equality between women and men prevail.

Different types or levels of competence are conferred on the EU to pursue these goals—competence (which may be exclusive or shared with Member States) to legislate and enter into legally binding acts,[16] and competence to support, co-ordinate or supplement actions taken at Member-State level.[17] Even in policy domains in which there is competence to adopt laws that will bind Member States, EU legislation can be enacted only with the agreement of its elected body (the European Parliament) and its Council (which consists of representatives of Member State governments).[18] Although a qualified majority vote in the Council will generally suffice, for certain types of legislation (including legislation combating discrimination) the TFEU specifies that unanimous agreement is required.[19]

Title IX of the TFEU, originally inserted into the founding treaties by the 1998 Treaty of Amsterdam, requires Member States and the EU to "work towards developing a coordinated strategy for employment and.... promoting a skilled, trained and adaptable workforce and labour markets responsive to economic change."[20] It thus provides the basis for the European Employment Strategy, the content of which is considered more fully in section 3.2. Title IX also sets out a basic framework for the coordination of an employment strategy, including requirements for Member States to prepare annual reports and for the Council (on the basis of proposals from the Commission) to issue guidelines to be taken into account by national governments.[21] This represents a form of Open Method of Co-ordination, the operation of which is considered in more detail in section 4.2.

Employment-related provisions are also to be found in Title X of the TFEU on social policy. Within this title, Article 153(2) confers competence on the EU to adopt legislation laying down minimum standards on a variety of employment matters and also to take action designed to encourage cooperation between Member States on these issues.

Article 19 of the TFEU confers competence on the EU to introduce legislation combating discrimination on several grounds, one of which is disability. It was the predecessor of this provision that provided the legal basis for what remains the leading piece of EU legislation on disability—the 2000 Employment Equality Directive.[22] This requires Member States to prohibit disability (and other) discrimination in employment and occupation and is discussed further in section 4.1.

Various provisions of the founding treaties and the Charter of Fundamental Rights (which, by Article 6 of the TEU, is given the same legal standing as the founding treaties) require that disability rights considerations should be mainstreamed into the operation of the EU. Thus, Article 10 of The TFEU requires the EU to combat discrimination based on disability when it defines and implements its policies and activities. Article 21 of the Charter of Fundamental Rights prohibits the Union, and the Member States in their application of EU law, from discriminating on the basis of disability. In addition, Article 26 of the Charter provides that the EU "recognises and respects the right of persons with disabilities to benefit from measures designed to ensure their independence, social and occupational integration and participation in the life of the community."

In addition, the EU has now ratified (or "formally confirmed")[23] the United Nations Convention on the Rights of Persons with Disabilities (CRPD) and, in so doing, become party to an international human rights treaty for the first time. Novel questions therefore arise—about the extent of the obligations imposed on the EU and about the mechanisms and strategies that might be used to discharge them.[24] Despite these questions, as seen in section 3.3, the CRPD is explicitly placed at the forefront of the European Disability Strategy

2010–2020,[25] thereby laying down a firm human rights foundation for EU disability policy.

3. STRATEGIES: THE CONTENT OF EUROPEAN UNION DISABILITY EMPLOYMENT POLICY

The European Union's approach to disability and employment includes three channels of action: 1) the overall strategic approach to general EU issues, determined by leadership at the highest level; 2) a more specific approach to employment policy, as determined by the Council, the EU's steering body comprising the heads of state or government of its members; and 3) a similarly specific approach to disability, including disability and employment issues, as determined by the Commission, the EU's cabinet-like executive body.

3.1 Europe 2020

Europe 2020[26] sets out the overall strategic direction of the EU for the period 2010–2020. It is organized around three growth priorities that are described as "mutually reinforcing": smart, sustainable, and inclusive.[27]

The last of these has most obvious relevance to the employment of disabled people, as is demonstrated by the following explanation:

> Inclusive growth means empowering people through high levels of employment, investing in skills, fighting poverty and modernising labour markets, training and social protection systems so as to help people anticipate and manage change, and build a cohesive society..... It is about ensuring access and opportunities for all throughout the lifecycle. Europe needs to make full use of its labour potential to face the challenges of an ageing population and rising global competition.[28]

To support the Strategy, a number of headline targets (to be achieved by 2020) have been set. These include increasing the employment rate of people aged between 20 and 64 from 69% to at least 75%; reducing the percentage of early school leavers to less than 10% and increasing the percentage of people aged 30 to 34 with a tertiary education degree qualification to at least 40%; and reducing the number of people living below national poverty lines by 25%. Seven "flagship initiatives" designed to support EU and Member State efforts to move toward these targets, are outlined in the Strategy. Two of these have particular relevance to disability and employment—the agenda for new skills and jobs and the platform against poverty.

The EU-level actions set out under the agenda for new skills focus on supporting efforts to enhance the skills, adaptability, and flexibility of the workforce. The Strategy indicates that the steps that national governments might take to work toward the targets include reviewing tax and benefit systems to ensure that work pays.[29] The aim of the European platform against poverty is to "raise awareness and recognise the fundamental rights of people experiencing poverty and social exclusion" so as to enable them to "live in dignity and take an active part in society."[30] In line with this aim, the Commission pledges to support cooperation and the sharing of good practice and mutual learning between Member States; to provide financial support to promote "innovative education, training, and employment opportunities for deprived communities"; and to support efforts to fight discrimination.[31]

3.2 European Employment Strategy

3.2.1 Flexicurity and Active Labor Market Policies

The European Employment Strategy (EES) is closely aligned to Europe 2020 and works, in effect, to support its employment-related elements. The EES's content is articulated through the Employment Guidelines,[32] which are issued by the Council and must be taken into account by Member States when deciding on their employment policies.

The Employment Guidelines are organized around Europe 2020 objectives. They are divided into the four broad headings of "increasing labour market participation," "developing a skilled workforce," "improving education and training systems," and "promoting social inclusion and combating poverty." These Guidelines are underpinned by principles of "flexicurity"—a concept explained by the European Commission as follows:

> Flexicurity can be defined as an integrated strategy to enhance, at the same time, flexibility and security in the labour market. Flexibility, on the one hand, is about successful moves ("transitions") during one's life course: from school to work, from one job to another, between unemployment or inactivity and work, and from work to retirement. It is not limited to more freedom for companies to recruit or dismiss, and it does not imply that open-ended contracts are obsolete. It is about progress of workers into better jobs, "upward mobility" and optimal development of talent. Flexibility is also about flexible work organisations, capable of quickly and effectively mastering new productive needs and skills, and about facilitating the combination of work and private responsibilities. Security, on the other hand, is more than just the security to maintain one's job: it is about equipping people with the skills that enable them to progress in their working lives, and helping them find new employment. It is also about adequate

unemployment benefits to facilitate transitions. Finally, it encompasses training opportunities for all workers, especially the low skilled and older workers.[33]

This model thus seeks to generate flexibility by lifting unnecessary constraints on the freedom of employers to make recruitment and retention decisions and by enabling them to adopt flexible approaches to work patterns and arrangements (e.g., part-time work or working from home). It also seeks to enhance the adaptability of employees and other workers by supporting them, on an ongoing basis, to acquire and maintain relevant skills and training.

The EES also places weight on active labor market policies that seek to encourage people to become actively engaged in work or the pursuit of it. In relation to increasing labor market participation, the Employment Guidelines specify that "Member States must establish forward-looking measures to integrate young people and vulnerable groups into the labour market" and "make employment more attractive, particularly for the low-skilled." In relation to combating social exclusion, the Guidelines specify that "Member States should pay particular attention to the employment of those furthest away from the labour market" and that they must take measures that "empower people" and "combat in-work poverty" and foster "equal opportunities and [combat] discrimination."[34]

These policy objectives clearly have the potential to work strongly to the advantage of disabled people by enhancing their opportunities to develop work-relevant skills, to obtain good quality assistance and support in their efforts to find work, and to work in flexible arrangements appropriate to their particular circumstances. Evidence suggests that a wide range of disability-related supported employment and active labor market policies operate in EU countries;[35] according to a 2009 ANED report analyzing the information provided by Member States to the EU as part of the EES process,[36] several countries claimed to have wage subsidies for disabled employees and job seekers (e.g., Belgium, Finland, Malta, the Netherlands, and Romania). Liisberg has recently provided a helpful account of the way in which wage subsidy schemes operate in Denmark—where people with restricted work capacity may work on a part-time basis (generally one third of full-time hours) but be subsidized by the state to receive a full-time salary.[37] Other forms of financial incentives mentioned in the country reports analyzed by ANED took the form of employer tax or insurance concessions (e.g., Cyprus, the Czech Republic, Estonia, and Sweden). Although not highlighted in this 2009 report, a range of schemes exist in various EU countries (e.g., the Access to Work scheme in the United Kingdom) whereby the costs of employment-related reasonable accommodations are fully or partially paid by the State and not subject to an upper limit.[38]

Other measures identified focused on disabled people rather than on employers or workplaces. The Estonian ANED report referred to a scheme covering possible additional costs of employment associated with disability, including those related to transportation and personal assistance. Several countries described educational, vocational training, or rehabilitation schemes established to tackle employment barriers faced by disabled people with low educational qualifications (Austria, Estonia, Latvia, the Netherlands, Portugal, Slovakia, Slovenia, and the United Kingdom). Policies focusing on matching the skills of disabled people to available opportunities were also mentioned (e.g., by Belgium). So too were schemes to support disabled people's entrepreneurship and their setting up of small businesses (e.g., by Finland, Latvia, and Sweden). Efforts to address barriers to entering employment created by the disability benefit system were mentioned by countries including Germany and the United Kingdom.

3.2.2 Potential Drawbacks

Despite the potential advantages of flexicurity and active labor market policies for disabled people, there are also risks. In particular there is the risk that employers may take advantage of opportunities to make their practices more flexible (e.g., through temporary or zero-hour contracts) without employees being granted the benefits of enhanced security.[39] Liisberg, in a thought-provoking analysis, identifies some of these risks and calls for the modification of the EU flexicurity model to reduce them. She compares the employment regimes in Denmark, which she argues has adopted a flexicurity approach similar to that of the EU, and Sweden, which she describes as having greater employee protection on matters such as dismissal. Liisberg concludes that the lack of protection against dismissal in Denmark, integral to its flexicurity model, is a significant contributing factor to the startling disparity in the employment rates of disabled people in the two countries—26% in Denmark and 50% in Sweden. Disabled people, once dismissed and out of work, are likely to encounter more difficulty than nondisabled people in finding alternative employment. Liisberg therefore calls for the flexicurity model, operating in Denmark and promoted by the EU, to be modified so as to include explicit protection against dismissal on grounds of impairment-related reduced work capacity along the lines of the Swedish approach. This would prohibit employers from dismissing disabled people on grounds of reduced work capacity unless, after providing them with appropriate training and adjustments, the disabled employee could not perform work of value to the employer. Such an approach would be to the advantage of all employees, as nondisabled people may become disabled in the future. Strong protection against dismissal, however, may carry the risk (at least in some countries and contexts) of greater unwillingness on the part of employers to recruit people who are already disabled or at particular risk of becoming disabled in the future.[40]

Another risk is identified in the 2009 ANED report—the risk that active labor market policies may sometimes result in the "cherry picking" of the disabled people who are closest to the labor market, with the result that those regarded as more difficult to integrate into employment are ignored.[41] This may explain the tendency of educational and vocational training schemes to focus on younger disabled people, leaving the skill-development needs of older disabled people unaddressed.[42] "Cherry picking" might also result in less attention being given to the employment activation of people with more severe impairments or more expensive support costs. The EES and Europe 2020 explicitly direct Member States to have particular regard to integrating those furthest away from the labor market, but the extent to which this is occurring in practice is not apparent from the existing evidence.

Active labor market strategies may also risk attempting to make work attractive by reducing the level of benefits to such an extent as to push the standard of living of people outside work to the limits of what governments regard as acceptable.[43] This is a concern that is currently high on the agenda of disability organizations in Europe.[44] Although Europe 2020 and the EES emphasize the importance of social integration and reducing poverty, there is disturbing evidence that disabled people are being pushed deeper into poverty and further marginalized by austerity measures designed to encourage people into work.[45]

Another risk of a heavy focus on labor activation policies is that the lives and contributions of people who do not participate in paid work become socially devalued in a way that perpetuates and reinforces their marginalization from the mainstream. For this reason, disability activists have called for a reconfiguration of the notion of "work."[46] Instead of attaching value only to paid work, social value should also be attached to the unpaid work of disabled people. This might take the form of voluntary work or civic engagement, or the generation of employment for personal assistants, service providers and others.

In light of the risks associated with flexicurity and active labor market policies, there is a clear need for careful monitoring of the impact of the effect of such policies on disabled people in EU Member States. Such monitoring and data gathering feature prominently in the Disability Strategy, which is now considered.

3.3 The European Disability Strategy 2010–2020

3.3.1 Overview of the Employment-Related Content of the Disability Strategy

Current EU disability policy is to be found in the European Disability Strategy 2010–2020.[47] This has the "overall aim" of "empower[ing] people with disabilities so that they can enjoy their full rights, and benefit fully from participating in society and in the European economy." It identifies EU-level actions that, alongside national measures, are designed to achieve this goal and "ensure effective implementation of the UN Convention across the EU."[48] It focuses on the elimination of barriers under eight main "areas for action." One of these "areas for action" is employment and the others are accessibility, participation, equality, education and training, social protection, health, and external action.

In relation to employment, the key objective of the Commission is stated to be to "[e]nable many more people with disabilities to earn their living on the open labour market."[49] The commitments set out in connection with this area for action principally concern "providing Member States with analysis, political guidance, information exchange and other support"[50] relating to disabled people and employment, with a view to identifying challenges and proposing recommendations to support ongoing efforts to move toward Europe 2020 targets. Particular issues to be addressed include "improv[ing] knowledge of the employment situation of women and men with disabilities"; "pay[ing] particular attention to young people with disabilities in their transition from education to employment"; "address[ing] intra-job mobility on the open labour market and in sheltered workshops" and "self employment and quality jobs,"; and "step[ping] up its support for voluntary initiatives that promote diversity management at the workplace."[51] The Disability Strategy also states that the Commission will support and supplement relevant national efforts, including those concerning benefit traps, integration into the labor market, accessibility of workplaces, services for job placement, support structures and on-the-job training, active labor market policies, and analyses of the employment situation of disabled people.[52]

The approach revealed in the current Disability Strategy differs markedly in emphasis from early EU interventions relating to the employment of disabled people in the 1970s.[53] The focus of those early interventions was on the vocational rehabilitation and training of disabled individuals. Gradually, the focus has widened to reflect a growing emphasis on tackling the underemployment of disabled people, not simply through supporting measures principally targeting disabled individuals, but also by promoting measures aimed at employers—including principles of equality and nondiscrimination and of barrier removal and accessibility. "Accessibility" and "equality" constitute distinct areas for action within the Disability Strategy but, given their significance to employment, are also worthy of some attention here.

"Accessibility" is given a high priority in the Disability Strategy. The Strategy recognizes that accessibility is a "precondition for participation in society and in the economy" and indicates that the Commission will work toward proposing legislative and standardization measures that would constitute a European Accessibility Act that would build on existing EU accessibility laws[54] "to optimise the accessibility of the built environment, transport and ICT."[55]

"Equality" is another area for action of the Disability Strategy that has clear implications for the employment field. According to the Strategy, in order to combat disability discrimination, the Commission will adopt a two-pronged approach that seeks both to implement fully existing EU legislation prohibiting discrimination and also to ensure that EU policy more generally works to enhance disability equality.[56] As already mentioned, the principal instrument of existing EU disability nondiscrimination law is the Employment Equality Directive,[57] which requires Member States to prohibit discrimination in the contexts of employment, occupation, and vocational training on a number of grounds, including disability (as well as age, sexual orientation, and religion and belief). This piece of legislation thus sets out minimum standards that Member States must ensure are incorporated into their domestic law.

3.3.2 Content of the Employment Equality Directive

3.3.2.1 Whom the Directive Protects from Disability Discrimination

In an attempt to avoid the risk of generating litigation about whether or not claimants meet a statutory definition of disability (of the type that has blighted disability discrimination law in the United States and the United Kingdom),[58] no definition of disability was included in the Employment Equality Directive. However, responding to requests for clarification and guidance, the Court of Justice of the European Union (CJEU) ruled in 2008 that "disability" in the Directive means "a limitation which results in particular from physical, mental or psychological impairments and which hinders the participation of the person concerned in professional life."[59] It added that for a limitation to amount to a "disability," it must "be probable that it will last for a long time."[60]

This definition was criticized, with justification, for being unnecessarily restrictive and for being inconsistent with the social model[61] basis of modern EU disability policy.[62] It also fell short of the guidance as to the meaning of "disability" provided by Article 1 of the CRPD. This suggests that an actual hindrance of participation in society is not essential and recognizes that any such hindrance might result from the impairment "in interaction" with social barriers. In 2013, the CJEU reversed its previous approach in favor of a definition of disability consistent with Article 1 of the CRPD, explicitly because of the EU's commitment to that instrument.[63]

The CJEU has adopted a more expansive approach to the question of whether the Employment Equality Directive extends to cases in which a person experiences direct discrimination or harassment because of his or her association or relationship with a disabled person. In *Coleman*[64] it ruled that a mother would fall within the scope of the Directive if she were able to establish that her employer had treated her less favorably than other employees or subjected her to harassment on the ground that her son was disabled. This expansive interpretation of the Directive brings within its scope people who are subjected to direct discrimination and harassment because of disability, whether or not they are themselves disabled. It is thus in line with the guidance provided by the Committee on the Rights of Persons with Disabilities as regards the need to prohibit discrimination based on association and on perceived disability in order to comply with Article 5 of the CRPD.[65]

3.3.2.2 Extent of the Directive's Nondiscrimination Prohibition

The Employment Equality Directive requires Member States to prohibit direct discrimination,[66] indirect discrimination,[67] harassment[68] and instructions to discriminate[69] on grounds of disability. It also requires employers to make reasonable accommodations for disabled people[70] and to protect employees from any adverse treatment or victimization because of the making of a relevant complaint.[71]

3.3.2.3 Limitations of the Directive

The Employment Equality Directive has a number of weaknesses or limitations. First, as has already been mentioned, its scope is confined to the areas of employment, occupation, and vocational training.[72] This contrasts with the Racial Equality Directive,[73] also adopted in 2000, which extends beyond employment to cover discrimination in the fields of social protection, social advantages, education, and goods and services (including housing and transport).

It is evident that access to employment cannot be effectively tackled if discrimination is not also challenged in areas such as education, transport, and housing. Additional nondiscrimination legislation, the Equal Treatment Directive, was proposed by the Commission in 2008.[74] This would extend the obligation on Member States to prohibit discrimination on the grounds covered by the Employment Equality Directive to non-employment fields analogous to those falling within the scope of the Racial Equality Directive. At the time of writing, this proposed directive remains the subject of ongoing discussion in the Council, however, and cannot be adopted without unanimous agreement by all the Member States.[75]

Second, the Employment Equality Directive contains no proactive positive duties to promote disability equality.[76] It permits positive action,[77] but contains no duties to promote disability equality or remove disabling barriers in a proactive manner. The reasonable accommodation duty set out in Article 5 is a duty to react to the specific situation of the particular disabled individual in question. The proposed Equal Treatment Directive would represent an improvement because it would impose a duty to anticipate barriers for disabled people (in the non-employment fields to which it would apply) and take steps to remove them.[78] However, it would neither impose a general duty to promote equality nor provide for enforcement methods other than through individual litigation. It has therefore been criticized for failing to adopt a more dynamic, proactive approach to equality.[79]

Finally, unlike directives dealing with race[80] and gender,[81] the Employment Equality Directive imposes no obligation on Member States to establish independent equality bodies to promote and monitor their efforts to achieve equal treatment on the grounds of disability, age, sexual orientation, and religion or belief. This would be remedied by the proposed Equal Treatment Directive, which would require the establishment of equality bodies covering disability, age, sexual orientation, and religion or belief.[82]

3.3.3 Monitoring of Results

As indicated in section 3.2, the EU's Employment Strategy, with its heavy emphasis on flexicurity, carries potential risks as well as benefits for disabled people. Particular vigilance is therefore needed in order to ensure that it does not actually worsen the employment or social situation of disabled people generally or of particular groups of disabled people. The emphasis placed on the provision of analysis and information exchange in the employment area of action of the Disability Strategy is therefore to be welcomed.

In addition, the Commission identifies work on the development of "statistics, data collection and monitoring" as crucial to its work in all of the Strategy's areas for action.[83] The Strategy indicates that the Commission will "work to streamline information on disability collected through EU social surveys, ... develop a specific survey on barriers for social integration of disabled people and present a set of indicators to monitor their situation with reference to key Europe 2020 targets .... [and] establish a web-based tool giving an overview of the practical measures and legislation used to implement the UN Convention."[84] Progress in this regard is marked by the fact that the Web-based tool, promised in the Strategy, was released (in June 2012) under the name of the Disability Online Tool of the Commission, or DOTCOM.[85] This online database provides easy access to information about Member States' policies affecting disabled people in a number of areas, including employment. At present, however, it does not (yet) contain evaluations of the effectiveness of these policies or quantitative or qualitative data relating to impact.

4. TOOLS: THE IMPLEMENTATION OF EUROPEAN UNION DISABILITY EMPLOYMENT STRATEGY

For the implementation of the strategies described in the preceding, three types of tool or mechanism for implementing EU disability employment policy may be identified. Each of these is considered separately in the following. Although it is impossible to analyze the potential and the limitation of these tools without some reference to content, the primary focus of this section is on the mechanisms themselves and not on the content of the policies they seek to implement.

4.1 Binding Legislation Affecting Employment Law or Policy in Member States

As mentioned, the foremost piece of EU legislation on disability and employment is the Employment Equality Directive.[86] A detailed analysis of the content of this instrument is provided in the preceding. Further examination of the process of its transposition into domestic law, however, provides useful insights into its potential impact.

The Employment Equality Directive has undoubtedly played a highly influential role in driving legal change in Member States. Before it, only three EU Member States had enacted legislation prohibiting disability discrimination[87] and, even in those cases, considerable amendments were sometimes needed to ensure that domestic law met the higher standards required by the Directive. For instance, in Ireland, the preexisting limitation on the reasonable accommodation obligation, which protected employers from having to pay anything above a "nominal" cost, was removed in order to achieve consistency with the Directive;[88] and, in the United Kingdom, the preexisting exemption from the Disability Discrimination Act 1995 for employers with fewer than 20 employees was removed for the same reason.[89]

According to a 2009 report of the Network of Legal Experts in the Non-Discrimination Field (the Legal Network study),[90] two disability-related aspects of the Employment Equality Directive had proved particularly challenging for Member States to transpose into their domestic law. These were, first, the definition of disability and, second, the formulation of reasonable accommodation duties.

Because of the lack of guidance on the meaning of disability contained in the Directive itself, which lasted for some six years, it is unsurprising that a variety of approaches emerged at national level. The Legal Network study[91] identifies four main approaches.

First, a number of Member States (e.g., Austria, Malta, Portugal, Sweden, and the United Kingdom) include a specific definition of disability in their nondiscrimination legislation. In such cases, the definitions used generally appear to be in line with the guidance of the CJEU.[92] Second, in some countries (e.g., Belgium, Bulgaria, Greece, Italy, Poland, Romania, and Slovakia) there is no explicit definition of disability in the context of nondiscrimination measures. In these cases, as with the Directive itself, the concept is left to be interpreted by courts and there is a danger that such interpretations may be unnecessarily restrictive and even breach the Directive. Third, some countries (e.g., the Czech Republic and Slovenia) borrow the restrictive definitions of disability used in other fields of national law, such as the definitions of disability used for determining entitlement to social security or welfare benefits. These definitions tend to be more restrictive and thus fall short of what the Directive requires. Finally, a number of countries (e.g., France, Germany, Luxembourg, and Spain) have developed a twofold approach to the definition of disability in the context of nondiscrimination law. This generally entails applying a much stricter definition to the class of people to whom reasonable accommodation duties are owed than that used to define disability for other purposes connected with nondiscrimination. Again, this approach appears to breach the Directive, which does not restrict the reasonable accommodation duty to a particular subset of disabled people.

A further disability-related dimension of the Directive that, according to the Legal Experts study, has proved particularly challenging to transpose into domestic law is the reasonable accommodation obligation. This is unsurprising given that the Directive "brought the concept of reasonable accommodation to the attention of many European legislators, and indeed 'forced' the notion onto these legislators."[93] Difficulties have arisen both in connection with the domestic legislative provisions giving effect to reasonable accommodation duties and also with the operation of such duties in practice.

Both the Legal Experts study and a 2011 study by the EU Agency for Fundamental Rights (FRA) identify a considerable variety of approach to reasonable accommodation in Member States and a number of problematic cases in which national law appears to fall short of the Directive's requirements. These problematic cases fall into two broad categories. In the first are situations in which national law fails to include a clear and unambiguous reasonable accommodation duty applying to the full range of employment and occupation covered by the Directive. The Legal Network study gives Italy,

Slovenia, and Poland as examples of countries falling into this category.[94] In the second category of problematic cases are laws that restrict entitlement to reasonable accommodation to a subset of those people who are regarded as disabled (e.g., for purposes of direct and indirect disability discrimination), on the basis, for instance, of official registration as disabled or categorization as seriously disabled in some way. According to the FRA study, this approach is adopted in France, Germany, Hungary, and Spain.[95]

4.1.2 Implementation Challenges

As regards the practical operation of reasonable accommodation laws, there is also some evidence of difficulties.[96] Many of these appear to be linked to lack of awareness or understanding of the existence and nature of the reasonable accommodation obligation among employers, disabled people, trade unions, and even lawyers and judges. The need to provide additional guidance and information on this issue was included in the Committee on the Rights of Persons with Disabilities' concluding observations on Spain[97] and also features among the plans set out in the European Disability Strategy 2010–2020.[98] Among possible forms of guidance that have proved helpful in some countries (e.g., the United Kingdom)[99] are statutory codes of practice, authorized by parliament and to which judges must have regard when deciding relevant cases; these codes contain detailed explanations and practical examples. The European Commission has also funded an ongoing series of seminars designed to enhance understanding of concepts such as reasonable accommodation among lawyers, judges, NGOs, and academics.[100] The European Disability Forum has drawn attention to the crucial role played by disabled people's organizations in raising awareness about reasonable accommodation and other equality entitlements and also to the fact that, owing to austerity measures, many such organizations have experienced funding cuts with the result that they are now struggling to survive.[101]

In addition to enhancing awareness, research suggests that the effectiveness of reasonable accommodation duties could be considerably enhanced by the further development of facilitative policies (at national and EU level).[102] Such policies might include funding schemes to support employers with the costs of adjustments;[103] the development of schemes to provide expertise and advice as to technical devices and other forms of assistance that might be helpful to disabled employees; and the development of policies to encourage disability leave and flexible work. Liisberg, drawing on her comparative analysis of Denmark and Sweden, has argued that the concept of reasonable accommodation is likely to be interpreted and applied more expansively in countries that include strong protection for disabled people against dismissals.[104]

Another area in which the domestic law of a number of Member States appears to breach the Directive, but one that does not yet seem to have resulted in any enforcement action by the Commission, is that of legal capacity or guardianship. In a number of EU countries (including Latvia and Romania) people who are subjected to guardianship are deprived of legal capacity, and therefore prevented from entering into any form of contract, including an employment contract.[105] It is perhaps because such laws prevent people placed under guardianship from accessing so many rights other than the right to work that they do not appear to have been challenged as being in breach of the Directive to date. Although the Disability strategy 2010–2020 does not promise any such action, it does indicate that "EU action will support and supplement national policies and programmes to promote equality, for instance by promoting the conformity of Member State legislation on legal capacity with the [CRPD]."[106] In the action plan that accompanies the European Disability Strategy, promotion of the "exchange of good practices on legal capacity" is included as an action planned for 2010–2013.[107]

4.1.3 Overall Impact and Directions for the Future

It is clear from this discussion that despite some implementation challenges, the Employment Equality Directive has had a significant impact on the laws and policies of Member States. It has required changes, many of which are also required by the CRPD. An analysis of the implementation difficulties experienced by EU Member States is therefore likely to be of relevance to countries outside Europe that are now facing the challenges of implementing the CRPD's nondiscrimination obligations.

Given the power of EU legislation to bring about change in the laws and policies of Member States, it may be asked why more legislation has not been introduced—why, for instance, have the limitations of the Employment Equality Directive identified in the preceding not been addressed by the introduction of more legislative instruments? The ongoing difficulties in reaching agreement on the proposed Equal Treatment Directive (that would extend the disability discrimination prohibition beyond employment) illustrate some of the political challenges that may attend the enactment of new EU law, even where it clearly falls within the ambit of EU legislative competence. These challenges are exacerbated where the agreement of all the Member States is required, as it is for legislation based on Article 19 of the TFEU (which concerns the combating of discrimination).[108] Lisa Waddington has observed that, "all the signs are that, owing to the lack of enthusiasm among some Member States, and absolute opposition by others, the proposal will not be adopted."[109]

4.2 Experimentalist Governance

4.2.1 Open Method of Coordination

In relation to disability and employment, a number of EU-level mechanisms exist to support Member States in sharing and learning from mutual experience, with the aim of identifying and building on good practice and working toward the achievement of certain shared goals. Foremost among these is the concept of the Open Method of Co-ordination (OMC).

The OMC is a governance approach that, since the late 1990s, has been used by the EU in a number of policy fields. It is variously described as a type of "new" or "supple" or "experimentalist" governance and, indeed, is frequently presented as the "archetypal"[110] manifestation of such governance. The four key components of experimentalist governance, which characterize EU policy development in a range of domains, are identified by Sabel and Zenith as follows:

> ....framework goals (such as full employment, social inclusion,....) and measures for gauging their achievement are established by joint action of the Member States and EU institutions. Lower-level units (such as national ministries or regulatory authorities and the actors with whom they collaborate) are given the freedom to advance these ends as they see fit. Subsidiarity in this architecture implies that in writing framework rules the lower-level units should be given sufficient autonomy in implementing the rules to be able to propose changes to them. But in return for this autonomy, they must report regularly on their performance, especially as measured by the agreed indicators, and participate in a peer review in which their results are compared with those pursuing other means to the same general ends. Finally, the framework goals, metrics, and procedures themselves are periodically revised by the actors who initially established them, augmented by such new participants whose views come to be seen as indispensable to full and fair deliberation.[111]

Experimentalist governance thus represents a departure from more hierarchical forms of governance in which problems are identified and solutions are imposed in a top-down manner. Different stakeholders participate in a process that is based on mutual learning, reflection, and peer review. In the words of Sabel and Simon:

> ....instead of looking backward to a prior enactment and upward toward a central sovereign, [it] looks forward and sideways: forward to the on-going efforts at implementation, sideways to the efforts and views of peer institutions.
>
> Peer review is the answer of new governance to the inadequacies of principal-agent accountability. Peer review imposes on implementing 'agents'

the obligation to justify the exercise of discretion they have been granted by framework-making 'principals' in the light of pooled comparable experience. In peer review, the actors at all levels learn from and correct each other, thus undermining the hierarchical distinction between principals and agents and creating a form of dynamic accountability.[112]

For such systems to work effectively, however, certain structures and understandings, or background conditions, must be in place. These include incentives to encourage all actors to reflect on their own positions and, through a process of collective learning, be willing to alter their perceptions of the problem to be solved as well as their ideas about potential solutions.[113] Full engagement of relevant stakeholders (including civil society) has also been identified as crucial.[114]

In 2000, the Council of the EU described the elements of the OMC process as follows:

- fixing guidelines for the Union combined with specific timetables for achieving the goals that they set in the short, medium and long terms;
- establishing, where appropriate, quantitative and qualitative indicators and benchmarks against the best in the world and tailored to the needs of different Member States and sectors as a means of comparing best practice;
- translating these European guidelines into national and regional policies by setting specific targets and adopting measures, taking into account national and regional differences;
- periodic monitoring, evaluation and peer review, organized as mutual learning processes.[115]

The effectiveness of OMC processes is notoriously difficult to assess.[116] There is concern based on empirical work, however, that the employment OMC has not succeeded in effectively involving civil society and that it has not therefore managed to operate in the open, inclusive, and nonhierarchical manner to which it aspires.[117]

4.2.2 The Employment Open Method of Co-ordination and Disability

The framework for an employment OMC is laid down in the TFEU itself; article 148(2) provides that the Council (after relevant consultation and advice) will draw up regular employment guidelines and that these will be taken into account by Member States in their employment policies.[118] Further, in accordance with Article 148(3), Member States will provide reports to the Commission and the Council on their employment policies and the steps they have taken to achieve the guidelines and also specific national targets to which they have agreed. These reports are known as the national reform programmes (NRPs) and associated implementation reports. Importantly, although the overarching goals articulated in the guidelines are shared, this process allows Member States to adopt different policies and approaches.

After examining these reports, the Council may (according to Article 148(4)) issue recommendations to particular Member States and compile a report on the employment situation in Member States and on progress being made to implement the employment guidelines. The importance of engaging nongovernmental actors (in particular, social partners such as trade unions, civil society, and public authorities) in the process, both at national and EU level, has been stressed by the Council itself.[119]

Disability has undoubtedly had a presence within OMC processes relating to employment from the outset.[120] However, ongoing monitoring of the reports produced in connection with the employment OMC suggests that disability has not been sufficiently mainstreamed and included in the process. Since 2008, this monitoring has been carried out by the Academic Network of European Disability Experts (ANED), at the request of (and with funding from) the European Commission.[121]

According to the ANED analysis, the extent to which disability was addressed in the NRPs produced by different countries varied greatly. Further, the attention given to disability by the same countries varied over time—some of the countries that had given disability a relatively high profile in their 2008 report gave it a low profile in 2009. It is also clear from ANED's work that NRPs cover a wide range of other issues that inevitably will sometimes push disability into the corners—particularly when more pressing matters arise. Thus, the focus on the economic crisis in 2011 by those compiling the Joint Reports as well as the national reports appears to have left little room for the consideration of other issues, including disability.[122]

The wide variation in the treatment and coverage of disability in the NRPs makes it difficult to identify general patterns. However, Mark Priestley, the Scientific Director of ANED, notes that there was disappointingly little reference in the NRPs to the barriers that might prevent or hinder disabled people from participating in employment.[123] This lack of attention to the nature and extent of barriers would appear to fall short of the aspirations of both the European Disability Strategy and the CRPD. Another important issue that was frequently not included was statistical data relating to disability and employment. According to Priestley, in the majority of reports, there was no such data—employment rates were sometimes provided by reference to age and gender but not disability. In some cases, this appeared to reflect the absence of relevant data but, in other cases, data existed but had not been included.[124] Other shortcomings in the treatment of disability by the NRPs identified by Priestley include the failure of the majority of the NRPs to make references or links to national disability strategies or to supranational disability instruments influential on domestic policy.[125]

Also disappointing was the limited involvement that disabled people's organizations appeared to have had in the process of drafting the NRPs. Priestley notes that in this regard Denmark was an exception. The Danish NRP included, as an annex, a shadow report produced by Danish disabled people's organizations.[126]

The employment OMC thus offers a valuable opportunity to examine the steps being taken by the Member States to improve the employment opportunities of disabled people in line with the objectives of Europe 2020, the European Employment Strategy, and the Disability Strategy. Regrettably, ANED research reveals that, although some of the NRPs do provide useful information about the employment situation of disabled people, disability has not yet been effectively mainstreamed into the process.

4.2.3 Consolidating Experimentalist Governance in the Disability Field?

Clearly, questions arise about what should be done to ensure that disability policies receive the benefits of scrutiny, mutual learning, and ongoing monitoring of progress offered by the experimentalist governance structures of the EU. One possibility is to ensure that Member States are provided with guidance about mainstreaming disability into their NRPs—as was done by the Commission in 2005.[127] Such guidance, particularly if issued for OMCs in all policy fields, might well result in a significant improvement in the current situation. However, disability mainstreaming guidance was issued in connection with another OMC (the social protection and social inclusion OMC) before the 2008 cycle[128] and ANED's monitoring of the national reports submitted as part of that process provides little grounds for high hopes.[129]

Unsurprisingly, therefore, interest has developed in the establishment of a disability-specific governance structure, spanning the width of the European Disability Strategy and providing a mechanism for coordinating Member State and EU activities in line with their shared commitments to the CRPD. There have already been calls for moves to be made in this direction.[130]

The establishment of an OMC process to coordinate Member State and EU disability policy would carry considerable benefits. It would, as Priestley notes, "mark the coming of age of disability as a distinctive and transversal policy field in the EU."[131] It would provide an opportunity to develop disability-specific reporting structures. It would also enable these to be drawn up with regard to the reporting guidelines already issued by the Committee on the Rights of Persons with Disabilities, thereby facilitating OMC scrutiny of reports that will need to be developed, in any event, for that Committee. It would create an opportunity to consider disability in a more holistic way than is permitted by the current OMC approach and would also facilitate engagement by national and EU-level disability organizations.

Although no plans to develop a disability OMC have yet materialized, the past few years have witnessed the emergence of a number of mechanisms that appear to be building up the experimentalist architecture of EU disability policy.[132] For instance, the Disability High Level Group (DHLG), which consists of representatives of Member State governments, has begun to play a more active role. Since 2008, in collaboration with the Commission, it has prepared and published annual reports on the implementation of the CRPD in particular fields in the different EU countries and sought to identify areas in which further collaboration and exchange would be helpful. In addition, since 2010 the Commission has organized annual "Work Forum" meetings that are designed to support the implementation of Article 33 of the CRPD on national implementation and monitoring. These meetings bring together representatives of European government focal points and coordination mechanisms, independent monitoring mechanisms, and disability and human rights organizations.

Alongside these structures for bringing together relevant government representatives and other stakeholders, the Commission has developed its capacity to gather evidence and analysis from independent experts to support processes of mutual learning and peer review. Thus, at the end of 2007, it established the ANED. Other EU networks of experts, although not exclusively devoted to disability and not answerable to the Disability Unit of the Commission, also provide relevant monitoring and expertise. Notable among these are the Network of Legal Experts in the Non-Discrimination Field[133] and the Network of Legal Experts on Fundamental Rights (FRALEX).[134]

Thus, even though formal measures have not been taken to establish a disability OMC, elements of experimentalist, new, or supple governance are undoubtedly emerging around disability rights in the EU. The momentum behind these developments is strengthened by the CRPD and the EU's formal confirmation of it. Interestingly, Grainne de Burca has described the CRPD itself as having a "strikingly experimentalist architecture."[135] Elements of the CRPD that she identifies as contributing to this experimentalist character are: "the articulation of rights in broad and general terms"; "the existence of discretion on the part of state actors as to how to implement and elaborate on them"; "periodic reporting and monitoring"; "the central role accorded to stakeholders....mainly disability NGOs and national human rights institutions"; "a specific provision emphasising national implementation and monitoring, with a role for national institutions and stakeholders"; "an obligation on states to collect relevant research, data and statistics"; and "a provision for the holding of a substantive annual conference of the parties, to review all aspects of the operation of the Convention in practice."[136] It is perhaps ironic that the CRPD—an instrument of UN law—is proving a powerful catalyst for the construction of experimentalist architecture for disability rights in the EU given that, for the past 15 years, such architecture has been the signature piece of the EU. Definite progress has now been made in the construction of such architecture but more could still be done. In particular, the existing reporting processes of the DHLG could be enhanced to facilitate greater involvement of stakeholders, including, in particular, disabled people's organizations. Strong experimentalist governance structures, with the active involvement of disabled people's organizations, employers, and trade unions and the support of the Commission, have the potential to provide a powerful addition to the demands of binding EU legislation and thereby to hasten progress toward the realization of goals set out in Europe 2020 and in the CRPD.

4.3 Direct Funding

The third of the tools or mechanisms for implementing EU disability employment policy consists of funding made available for relevant projects, programs, and organizations within Member States. The technique of using the provision of funds to achieve policy objectives has been described, for example, by Clare Kilpatrick, as "government by *dominium*."[137] It may be contrasted with "government by *imperium*," which involves "attaining policy objectives through legal commands backed by sanctions"[138]—a method used by the Employment Equality Directive discussed in section 4.1.

Of particular importance to disability and employment is the European Social Fund (ESF) which, along with the European Regional Development Fund (ERDF), makes up the Structural Funds. Explicit reference is made to the role of these Funds at several points in the Disability Strategy. In the employment area for action, for instance, it is stated that EU action will be taken to support and supplement national efforts to integrate disabled people in the labor market by "making use of the European Social Fund."[139] In addition, the Strategy includes a specific section on the financial mechanisms that will be harnessed in order to implement its objectives. This acknowledges that "EU funding instruments, particularly the Structural Funds, need to be implemented in an accessible and non-discriminatory way" and indicates that "EU action will support and supplement national efforts to improve accessibility and combat discrimination through mainstream funding [and] proper application of Article 16 of the Structural Funds General Regulation."[140]

Subject to a number of exceptions in which projects are selected by the Commission, primary responsibility for selecting projects to be funded from these sources, and for their monitoring and evaluation, lies with Member States—which will have entered into partnership contracts with the Commission on the basis of which they will have drawn up operational plans.[141]

The ESF is particularly important in the context of disability employment policy as has been acknowledged by the Commission.[142] Its purpose is articulated in Article 162 of the TFEU, which reads:

In order to improve employment opportunities for workers in the internal market and to contribute thereby to raising the standard of living, a European Social Fund is hereby established ....; it shall aim to render the employment of workers easier and to increase their geographical and occupational mobility within the Union, and to facilitate their adaptation to industrial changes and to changes in production systems, in particular through vocational training and retraining. The ESF is intended, inter alia, to assist in: improving the adaptability of workers and enterprises, enhancing human capital and access to employment and participation in the labour market, reinforcing the social inclusion of disadvantaged people, combating discrimination, encouraging economically inactive persons to enter the labour market and promoting partnerships for reform.

The 2009 ANED report on employment and the NRPs[143] contains examples of ESF funding being used to support disability-related projects. According to it:

EU structural funds, particularly ESF, continue to be used to target employment-related initiatives for disabled people in several countries (e.g., Austria, Belgium, Greece, Ireland, Latvia, Malta and the United Kingdom).

There were good examples of mainstreaming initiatives, for example the Estonian report noted the extension of general employment assistance schemes to disabled people as opposed to the proliferation of 'special' schemes for vulnerable groups.[144]

Reference is also made to ESF-funded projects designed to increase the employment opportunities of people with specific impairments.[145] Details about other ESF-funded projects relating to disability and employment in the different EU countries can be found via the European Social Fund website.[146] However, although it is stated that the amount available for distribution through the European Social Funds for the period 2007–2013 will amount to some 75 billion euros, no EU-wide information is presented about how much of this has been devoted to disability-related projects and, within that, how spending has been allocated (e.g., on projects that are impairment-specific; on projects that focus on training of disabled people; on projects aimed at enhancing capacity among employment support services or employers; or on projects that support self-employment and entrepreneurship among disabled people).

Thus, although it is clear that many projects focusing on disability and employment have been and continue to be funded through the ESF, the overall impact of this funding on the employment of disabled people is difficult to ascertain. This issue has not received the high profile attention that has recently been given to the impact of the Structural Funds on opportunities for community living. A report, published by the European Coalition of Community Living in 2009, revealed that monies received by Member States through the Structural Funds were often used to renovate or even build institutions holding disabled people rather than to facilitate programs of deinstitutionalization and provide support for community living strategies.[147] Such revelations clearly raise concern and also questions as to whether more could be done, at the EU level, to ensure that EU monies are devoted to projects that are consistent with the objectives of EU disability policy and the CRPD.

The European Commission published its proposals for new regulations to govern the Structural Funds for the period of 2014–2020 in October 2011.[148] In addition to Articles requiring principles of nondiscrimination and accessibility to be factored into the operation of the funds,[149] the draft General Regulation proposes introducing a number of ex-ante conditions that Member States would need to satisfy in order to receive funding.[150] These ex-ante conditions include the establishment of services and structures relating to employment, education, and social inclusion,[151] which correspond to objectives of the Europe 2020 Strategy. They also include general thematic conditionalities, two of which are particularly relevant for purposes of this chapter: first, nondiscrimination and, second, the establishment of a mechanism "which ensures effective implementation and application" of the CRPD. These conditionalities have the potential to enhance considerably the focus of national authorities on issues of disability equality and human rights in their administration and monitoring of the Structural Funds. They have, however, met with considerable resistance from Member State governments and it is not at all clear whether they will survive into the final version of the new regulation.[152] Two powerful reports[153] have drawn attention to the fact that failure to include these ex-ante conditionalities would place "a question mark over Europe's commitment to principles" and to the EU's legal as well as moral obligations as a State Party to the CRPD.

5. CONCLUSION

This chapter has reflected upon EU disability employment policy—both in terms of its substantive content and also in terms of its implementation mechanisms. Both have stories to tell that may be of interest and value to those working to improve the employment opportunities of disabled people inside and outside the EU.

The content of EU disability employment policy emerges from the three overlapping EU strategies considered in section 3. There is an emphasis on employment activation, on flexicurity, on increasing the skills and adaptability of workers, and on nondiscrimination and accessibility. Although many of these policy objectives have the potential to benefit disabled people by enhancing their participation in the open labor market, there is also a serious risk that such policies may in practice prove unhelpful, or even harmful, to the employment opportunities of certain groups of disabled people.

There is a concern that employment activation policies may focus too much on trying to fit disabled people for work and not enough on measures aimed at employers and societal structures that place barriers (including ones that are physical, attitudinal, procedural, or even legal) in the way of disabled people's access to work. Unless such barriers to disabled people's employment are effectively removed, employment activation measures that entail reducing benefits will deepen the marginalization, dependence, and poverty of disabled people without enhancing their chances of finding work. Although the enactment of antidiscrimination law represents an important step in the direction of acknowledging the existence of these barriers, without dedicated and ongoing enforcement and implementation strategies it is likely to make little headway in dismantling them. Further, as Liisberg has argued, legislation granting specific protections for employees (e.g., against dismissal) may be needed.

European Union disability employment policy is implemented through a variety of tools, which have been divided into three categories for the purposes of this discussion—legislation binding on Member States, experimentalist governance, and direct funding. These three types of tools all have the potential to work together in a way that is mutually reinforcing. At present, important debates are underway about the future operation of the second and the third of these mechanisms in the disability context. The way in which these debates are resolved will undoubtedly have an impact on the combined effectiveness of the three implementation tools.

As regards the first of the tools, binding legislation underpins the nondiscrimination, and increasingly the accessibility, strands of EU disability employment policy. That legislation has resulted in significant change in national nondiscrimination laws. However, the transposition of elements of the Employment Equality Directive into domestic law has proved complex and, in some instances, required intervention from the EU. Interesting parallels may be drawn between this process and the implementation of the CRPD's nondiscrimination requirements by States Parties. In the EU context, particular difficulties have arisen in connection with defining disability for purposes of nondiscrimination law, and in the articulation and practical implementation of the reasonable accommodation obligation. A tendency to overlook the discriminatory impact of laws that deprive people of legal capacity, and thus the ability to enter into employment contracts, has also been noted.

The current employment OMC might appear to be the most obvious forum for entrenching monitoring systems, peer review processes, and mutual learning relating to the employment of disabled people. However, as has been argued, disability has not received consistent or detailed treatment in this process. Alternatives are therefore urgently needed and, as illustrated by the development of DOTCOM, the Disability High Level Group and the Work Forum, are beginning to emerge. Calls for further movement in this regard, however, are being made by the European Disability Forum and others.

Experimentalist governance mechanisms are also supported by the CRPD. This is likely to add weight to the movement toward greater experimentalist governance of disability rights in the EU. It may also prompt or support similar developments in other multinational structures[154] and even in national bodies or individual organizations.[155] Experimentalist governance in the context of disability rights, it is suggested, should not be regarded as a substitute for the translation of relevant rights into legally enforceable obligations.[156] The existence of obligations, such as those imposed by national law on employers or by CRPD ratification on governments, might provide useful incentives for engagement in processes of experimentalist governance.

Recent debates over the future of the Structural Funds draw attention to the power of funding and the importance that donors make every effort to ensure that monies granted are spent in a way that is supportive and not subversive of human rights. They also demonstrate the centrality of the CRPD to such debates. The extent to which the CRPD will lend support to arguments for further legal, practical, and financial change at the EU level, however, remains to be seen.

In conclusion, perhaps the most important lesson to be drawn from the EU experience is that the complex problem of the exclusion of disabled people from the labor market cannot be tackled without harnessing multiple tools and forms of policy intervention. The imposition of mandatory legal obligations is one extremely important tool. However, legal obligations not to discriminate against disabled people in employment need to be supplemented by nondiscrimination obligations in other areas of life (such as education and transport), as well as by accessibility requirements, if the barriers that keep disabled people out of work are to be tackled. Another important type of tool takes the form of measures designed to facilitate knowledge exchange and mutual learning. The EU's experience demonstrates that disability may well be sidelined if the focus of such exchange and mutual learning is employment generally. A structure that maintains a sharp focus on the employment of disabled people and facilitates the full participation of disabled people and their organizations is required. Funding programs to promote employment opportunities for marginalized groups also have an important role to play. However, as is highlighted by current debates in the EU, if we are to move toward a more inclusive accessible society in which disabling barriers to employment and other forms of societal participation are minimized, it is crucial that disability considerations are effectively mainstreamed into such schemes. Finally, as is recognized in the European Disability Strategy 2010–2020 as well as in the

CRPD, the importance of monitoring the social situation of disabled people and the impact of laws and policies upon them cannot be overstated.

ACKNOWLEDGMENT

The author is grateful to Professor Dagmar Schiek for her insightful comments on an earlier draft of this chapter.

NOTES

1. European Commission (2010), *Commission Staff Working Document to the European Disability Strategy 2010–2020*. Brussels, Belgium: European Commission.
2. Priestley, M. (2011). *Targeting and mainstreaming disability in the context of EU 2020 and the 2011 Annual Growth Survey*. Leeds, United Kingdom: Academic Network of European Disability Experts.
3. Greve, B. (2009). *The Labour Market Situation of Disabled People in European Countries and Implementation of Employment Policies: A Summary of Evidence from Country Reports and Research Studies*. Academic Network of European Disability Experts. Retrieved March 26, 2013, from http://www.disability-europe.net/ content/aned/media/ANED%20Task%206%20final%20report%20-%20final%20 version%2017-04-09.pdf
4. European Commission (2010), *Commission Staff Working Document to the European Disability Strategy 2010–2020*. Brussels: European Commission.
5. Ibid.
6. European Policy Evaluation Consortium (2008). *Study on Discrimination on Grounds of Religion and Belief, Age, Disability and Sexual Orientation Outside of Employment*. Brussels: EPEC.
7. European Commission (2010), *Commission Staff Working Document to the European Disability Strategy 2010–2020*. Brussels, Belgium: European Commission.
8. Council decision of 26 November 2009 concerning the conclusion, by the European Community, of the United Nations Convention on the Rights of Persons with Disabilities(2010/48/EC), [2010] OJ L 303/16, Annex II.
9. See further Greve, B. (2009). *The Labour Market Situation of Disabled People in European Countries*; Oorschot, W., & Hvinden, B. (Eds.) (2001). *Disability Policies in European Countries*. The Hague, The Netherlands: Kluwer Law International; Hvinden, B. (2003). The uncertain convergence of disability policies in Western Europe. *Social Policy and Administration, 37*(6), 609–624.
10. Zelderloo, L., & Reynaert, J. (2007). *An International Comparison of Methods of Financing Employment for Disadvantaged People*. Brussels, Belgium: European Association of Service Providers for Persons with Disabilities.
11. Greve, B. (2009). *The Labour Market Situation of Disabled People in European Countries*. Leeds, United Kingdom: Academic Network of European Disability Experts.
12. Ibid.

13. Ibid.
14. See further European Union Agency for Fundamental Rights (2013). *Legal Capacity of Persons with Intellectual Disabilities and Persons with Mental Health Problems*. Luxembourg: Publications Office of the EU; and also the Mental Disability Advocacy Centre guardianship reports, 2006–2008, available at http://www.mdac.info
15. See further, Alston, P. (Ed.) (1999). *The EU and Human Rights*. Oxford, United Kingdom: Oxford University Press, 1999; Craig, P., & de Burca, G. (Eds.) (1999). *The Evolution of EU Law*. Oxford, United Kingdom: Oxford University Press; McCrudden, C., & Kountouros, H. (2007). Human rights and European equality law. In H. Meenan (Ed.), *Equality Law in an Enlarged European Union: Understanding the Article 13 Directives*. Cambridge, United Kingdom: Cambridge University Press, 73–116; Leczykiewicz, D. (2010). "Effective judicial protection" of human rights after Lisbon: should national courts be empowered to review EU secondary law? *European Law Review 35*(3), 326–348; Williams, A. T. (2010). Promoting justice after Lisbon: groundwork for a new philosophy of EU law. *Oxford Journal of Legal Studies 30*(4), 663–693.
16. Which may take the form of a "regulation," a "directive" or a "decision"—the effects of all of which are explained in Consolidated Version of the Treaty on the Functioning of the European Union art. 288, 2008 O.J. C 115/47.
17. Consolidated Version of the Treaty on the Functioning of the European Union art. 2, 2008 O.J. C 115/47. Article 288.
18. Ibid., Article 294.
19. Ibid., Article 19.
20. Ibid., Article 145.
21. Ibid., Article 148.
22. Council Directive 2000/78/EC of 2 December 2000 establishing a general framework for equal treatment in employment and occupation, OJ L 303 16.
23. See UN General Assembly, *Convention on the Rights of Persons with Disabilities: resolution adopted by the General Assembly*, 24 January 2007, A/RES/61/106, Article 43.
24. See further Waddington, L. (2009). Breaking new ground: the implications of ratification of the United Nations convention on the rights of persons with disabilities for the European Community. In O. Arnardóttir, & G. Quinn (Eds.), *The UN Convention on the Rights of Persons with Disabilities: European and Scandinavian Perspectives*. Leiden, The Netherlands: Martinus Nijhoff, 111; Waddington, L.(2011). The European Union and the United Nations Convention on the Rights of Persons with Disabilities: a story of exclusive and shared competences. *Maastricht Journal 18*, 411; European Foundation Centre (2008). *Study on Challenges and Good Practice in the Implementation of the UN Convention on the Rights of Persons with Disabilities*. Brussels, Belgium: European Commission; Quinn, G., & Doyle, S. (2012). *Getting a Life—Living Independently and Being Included in the Community: A Legal Study of the Current Use and Future Potential of the European Structural Funds to Contribute to the Achievement of Article 19 of the United Nations Convention on the Rights of Persons with Disabilities*. Office of the High Commissioner for Human Rights European Region. Retrieved March 26, 2013, from http://europe.ohchr.org/Documents/Publications/Getting_a_Life.pdf
25. European Commission (2010). *European Disability Strategy 2010–2020: A Renewed Commitment to a Barrier-Free Europe*. Brussels, Belgium: European Commission.

26. European Commission (2010), *Europe 2020: A Strategy for Smart, Sustainable and Inclusive Growth. Communication from the Commission*. Brussels, Belgium: European Commission.

27. Ibid., 3. For arguments that the EU's strategic goals have prioritized competitiveness at the expense of social issues, see Magnusson, L. (2010). *After Lisbon— Social Europe at the Crossroads?* Brussels, Belgium: European Trade Union Institute, 18.

28. European Commission (2010), *Europe 2020*, 16.

29. Ibid, 17.

30. Ibid, 17.

31. Ibid, 18.

32. Council Decision 2010/707/EU of 21 October 2010 on guidelines for the employment policies of the Member States, OJ L 241.

33. European Commission (2007). *Towards Common Principles of Flexicurity: More and Better Jobs Through Flexibility and Security*. Brussels, Belgium: European Commission. See also European Foundation for the Improvement of Living and Working Conditions (2007). *Varieties of Flexicurity: Reflections on Key Elements of Flexibility and Security*. Dublin, Ireland: European Foundation for the Improvement of Living and Working Conditions; Schmidt, G. (2008). *Full Employment in Europe: Managing Labour Market Transitions and Risks* Cheltenham, United Kingdom: Edward Elgar.

34. Council Decision 2010/707/EU.

35. See, in particular, European Commission (2011). *Supported Employment for People with Disabilities in the EU and EFTA-EEA*. Luxembourg: Publications Office of the EU; Greve, B. (2009). *The Labour Market Situation of Disabled People in European Countries*; Priestley, M., & Roulstone, A. (2009). *Targeting and Mainstreaming Disability in the 2008–10 National Reform Programmes for Growth and Jobs*. Leeds, United Kingdom: Academic Network of European Disability Experts.

36. Priestley, M., & Roulstone, A. (2009). *Targeting and Mainstreaming Disability in the 2008–10 National Reform Programmes for Growth and Jobs*. Leeds, United Kingdom: Academic Network of European Disability Experts.

37. Ventegodt Liisberg, M. (2013). Flexicurity and Employment of Persons with Disability in Europe in a Contemporary Disability Human Rights Perspective. In L. Waddington, G. Quinn, & E. Flynn. *European Yearbook of Disability Law Vol 4*. Uitgevers, The Netherlands: Intersentia. 145–168.

38. Details on which are available at http://www.direct.gov.uk/en/DisabledPeople/Employmentsupport/WorkSchemesAndProgrammes/DG_4000347. For analysis of this scheme, see Lawson, A. (2008). *Disability and Equality Law in Britain: The Role of Reasonable Adjustment in Britain*. Oxford, United Kingdom: Hart Publishing, especially chapter 6. See also Department of Work and Pensions (2012). *Disability Employment Support: Fulfilling Potential*. London: Stationery Office.

39. See further Barnard, C. (2011). EU Social policy from employment law to labour market reform. In P. Craig, & G. de Burca (Eds.). *The Evolution of EU Law*. Oxford, United Kingdom: Oxford University Press, 678–681.

40. Ventegodt Liisberg, M. (2011). *Disability and Employment: A Contemporary Disability Human Rights Analysis applied to Danish, Swedish and EU Law*. Uitgevers, The Netherlands: Intersentia. See also Ventegodt Liisberg (2013). Flexicurity and Employment of Persons with Disability.

41. Priestley, M., & Roulstone, A. (2009). *Targeting and Mainstreaming Disability in the 2008–10 National Reform Programmes for Growth and Jobs*. Leeds, United Kingdom: Academic Network of European Disability Experts, 10.
42. Ibid.
43. This was a major concern emerging from the empirical evidence presented in: European Union Agency for Fundamental Rights (2012). *Choice and Control: The Right to Independent Living*. Luxembourg: Publications Office of the EU.
44. See e.g. European Disability Forum (2010). *EDF Resolution on the Economic Crisis in Europe*, and the European Disability Forum's Observatory on the Crisis. Retrieved March 26, 2013, from http://www.edf-feph.org/Page_Generale.asp?DocID=13854&thebloc=13856. See also Gomez Mugica, R. (2013). *Austerity Policies Affect People with Disabilities. Inclusion Europe*. Retrieved March 26, 2013, from http://www.e-include.eu/en/articles/1048-austerity-policies-effects-on-people-with-disabilities.
45. See the sources cited in the previous two notes.
46. See e.g. Barnes, C. (2000). A working social model? Disability, work and disability politics in the 21st century. *Critical Social Policy 20*(4), 441–57; Abberley, P. (2002). Work, disability and European social theory. In C. Barnes, M. Oliver, & L. Barton (Eds.). *Disability Studies Today*. Cambridge, United Kingdom: Polity Press, 120–138; Barnes, C., & Roulstone, A. (2005). Work is a four letter word: disability, work and welfare. In A. Roulstone, & C. Barnes (Eds.) (2005). *Working Futures? Disabled People, Policy and Social Inclusion*. Bristol, United Kingdom: Policy Press, 315–327.
47. European Commission (2010). *European Disability Strategy 2010–2020*.
48. Ibid, section 2.
49. Ibid, section 2.1.4.
50. Ibid.
51. Ibid.
52. Ibid.
53. See generally Waddington, L. (1995). *Disability, Employment and the European Community*. Apeldoorn Netherlands, MAKLU; Waddington, L. (2006). *From Rome to Nice in a Wheelchair*. Retrieved March 26, 2013, from http://ssrn.com/abstract=1026549; Mabbett, D. (2005). The development of rights-based social policy in the European Union. *Journal of Common Market Studies 43*, 97–120; Priestley, M. (2007). In search of European disability policy: between national and global. *European Journal of Disability Research 1*, 61–74; Waldschmidt, A. (2009). Disability policy of the European Union: The supranational level. *ALTER—European Journal of Disability Research 3*, 8–23.
54. European Commission (2010), *Commission Staff Working Document*, table 3; Waddington (2009). Breaking New Ground; Waddington, L. (2009). A disabled market: free movement of goods and services in the EU and disability accessibility. *European Law Journal 15*, 575–598.
55. European Commission (2010). *European Disability Strategy 2010–2020*, section 2.1.1.
56. Ibid, section 2.1.3.
57. Council Directive 2000/78/EC of 2 December 2000 establishing a general framework.
58. E.g., on the United States, Burgdorf, R. L. (1997). "Substantially limited" protection from disability discrimination: the special treatment model and

misconstructions of the definition of disability. *Villanova Law Review 42*, 409–426; Soifer, A. (2000). The disability term: dignity, default and negative capability. *University of California Los Angeles Law Review 47*, 1279–1331; Silvers, A., & Stein, M. A. (2002). Disability, equal protection, and the Supreme Court: standing at the crossroads of progressive and retrogressive logic in constitutional classification. *University of Michigan Journal of Law Reform 81*, 121–123; and, for an analysis of developments since the ADA Amendments Act 2008, Emens, E. F. (2012). Disabling attitudes: US disability law and the ADA Amendments Act. *American Journal of Comparative Law 60*, 205–234. For a recent discussion of the United Kingdom approach, see Lawson, A. (2011). Disability and employment in the Equality Act 2010: opportunities seized, lost and generated. *Industrial Law Journal 40*, 359–383.

59. *Chacón Navas v Eurest Colectividades SA* (Case C-13/05) [2006] ECR 1-6467, para 43.
60. Ibid, para 45.
61. Waddington, L. (2007). Case C-13/05, Chacón Navas v Eurest Colectividades SA, judgment of the Grand Chamber of 11 July 2006. *Common Market Law Review 44*(2) 487–499; Hosking, D. L. (2011). A high bar for EU disability rights. *Industrial Law Journal 36*, 228–237; and Perju,V. (2011). Impairment, discrimination, and the legal construction of disability in the European Union and the United States. *Cornell International Law Journal 44*, 279.
62. For a discussion of the social model of disability, see e.g. Oliver, M., & Barnes, C. (2012). *The New Politics of Disablement*. Basingstoke, United Kingdom: Palgrave Macmillan; Barnes, C., & Mercer, G. (2010). *Exploring Disability: A Sociological Introduction* (2nd Ed.). Cambridge, United Kingdom: Polity Press; Traustadóttir, R. (2009). Disability studies, the social model and legal developments. In O. Arnadóttir, & G. Quinn (Eds.). *The UN Convention on the Rights of Persons with Disabilities: European and Scandinavian Perspectives*. Leiden, The Netherlands: Martinus Nijhoff, 3–16.
63. *HK Danmark, acting on behalf of Jette Ring v. Dansk almennyttigt Boligselskab, and HK Danmark, acting on behalf of Lone Skouboe Werge v Dansk Arbejdsgiverforening, acting on behalf of Pro Disability A/S*. Joined cases C-335/11 and C-337/11, judgment of 11 April 2013.
64. *Coleman v Attridge Law and Steve Law*, Case C-303/06 Judgment of the Court (Grand Chamber) of 17 July 2008.
65. UN Committee on the Rights of Persons with Disabilities, Concluding Observations: Spain, 6th Session 19–23 September 2011, paras 19–20.
66. Council Directive 2000/78/EC of 2 December 2000 establishing a general framework, Article 2(1).
67. Ibid.
68. Ibid, Article 2(3).
69. Ibid, Article 2(4).
70. Ibid, Article 5.
71. Ibid, Article 11.
72. Defined more fully in Article 3(1) of the Directive.
73. Council Directive 2000/43/EC of 19 July 2000 implementing the principle of equal treatment between persons irrespective of racial or ethnic origin, OJ L180/22.
74. European Commission (2008). *Proposal for a Council Directive on Implementing the Principle of Equal Treatment Between Persons Irrespective of Religion or Belief, Disability, Age or Sexual Orientation*. Brussels, Belgium: European Commission.

75. This being specified by Article 19 of the Consolidated Version of the Treaty on the Functioning of the European Union.
76. See generally Waddington, L., & Bell, M. (2011). Exploring the boundaries of positive action under EU law: a search for conceptual clarity. *Common Market Law Review 48*(5), 1508–1526.
77. Council Directive 2000/78/EC of 2 December 2000 establishing a general framework, Article 7. For a thought-provoking analysis of this provision, see Quinn, G. (2007). Disability discrimination Law in the European Union. In H. Meenan (Ed.), *Equality Law in an Enlarged European Union: Understanding the Article 13 Directives*. Cambridge, United Kingdom: Cambridge University Press, 268–273.
78. European Commission (2008). *Proposal for a Council Directive*, Article 4.
79. Bell, M. (2009). Advancing EU anti-discrimination law: the European Commission's 2008 proposal for a new directive. *Equal Rights Review 3*, 7.
80. Directive 2000/43/EC, Article 13.
81. Council Directive 2004/113/EC of 21 December 2004 implementing the principle of equal treatment between women and men in the access to and supply of goods and services, OJ 2004 L 373, Article 12; and Council Directive 2006/54/EC of 5 July 2006 on the implementation of the principle of equal opportunities and equal treatment of men and women in matters of employment and occupation, OJ 2006 L 204/23, Article 20.
82. European Commission (2008). *Proposal for a Council Directive*, Article 12.
83. European Commission (2010). *European Disability Strategy 2010–2020*, section 2.2.3.
84. Ibid.
85. Available at http://www.disability-europe.net/dotcom. For analysis and discussion, see Lawson, A., & Priestley, M. (forthcoming, 2013). Multinational monitoring of disability rights in the European Union: potential, principle and pragmatism. *International Journal of Human Rights*.
86. Council Directive 2000/78/EC of 2 December 2000 establishing a general framework. For discussion of other EU employment legislation, see Barnard, C. (2007). *EC Employment Law* (3rd ed.). Oxford, United Kingdom: Oxford University Press; and, for analysis of its impact on disabled people, Ventegodt Liisberg (2011). *Disability and Employment*. Uitgevers, The Netherlands: Intersentia.
87. The United Kingdom's Disability Discrimination Act 1995, Ireland's Employment Equality Act 1998 and Sweden's Law Prohibiting Discrimination in Working Life on Grounds of Disability 1999.
88. The Employment Equality Act 1998 was amended so as to bring the reasonable accommodation duty into line with that contained in Article 5 of the Directive. See generally Quinn, G., & Quinlivan, S. (2003). Disability discrimination: the need to amend the Employment Equality Act 1998 in light of the EU Framework Directive on Employment. In C. Costello, & E. Barry (Eds.). *Quality in Diversity: The New Equality Directives*. Oxford, United Kingdom, and Dublin, Ireland: Irish Centre for European Law.
89. Disability Discrimination Act 1995 (Amendment) Regulations 2003.
90. Waddington, L., & Lawson, A. (2009). *Disability and Non-Discrimination Law in the European Union: Analysis of Disability Discrimination Law Within and Beyond the Employment Field*. Network of Legal Experts in the Non-Discrimination Field. Retrieved March 26, 2013, from www.ec.europa.eu/social/BlobServlet?docId=6154&langId=en.
91. Ibid.

92. *Chacón Navas* v *Eurest Colectividades SA.*
93. Waddington & Lawson (2009). *Disability and non-discrimination law*, section 2.3.3.
94. Ibid.
95. European Union Agency for Fundamental Rights (2012). *Choice and Control: The Right to Independent Living.* Luxembourg: Publications Office of the EU, section 2.2.1. See also UN Committee on the Rights of Persons with Disabilities, Concluding Observations, paragraph 19.
96. See generally European Disability Forum (2010). *Ten Years On: Practical Impact of the Employment Directive on Persons with Disabilities in Employment.* Brussels, Belgium: EDF; and also European Union Agency for Fundamental Rights (2012). *Choice and Control*—in which empirical evidence is presented which demonstrates that difficulties in accessing reasonable accommodations contributed to the exclusion from employment of many of the research participants.
97. UN Committee on the Rights of Persons with Disabilities, Concluding Observations, paragraphs 19 and 20.
98. European Commission (2010). *Initial plan to implement the European Disability Strategy 2010–2020, List of Actions 2010–2015.* Brussels, Belgium: European Commission, sections 1.3 and 1.4.
99. See, e.g., Equality and Human Rights Commission (n.d.). *Equality Act Codes of Practice and Technical Guidance.* Retrieved March 26, 2013, from http://www.equalityhumanrights.com/legal-and-policy/equality-act/equality-act-codes-of-practice/. For a discussion of earlier versions of these codes, see O'Brien, N. (2005). The GB Disability Rights Commission and strategic law enforcement: transcending the Common Law mind. In A. Lawson, & C. Gooding (Eds.). *Disability Rights in Europe: From Theory to Practice.* Oxford, United Kingdom: Hart Publishing, 249–263.
100. See e.g. the seminars on EU Equality Law and on the CRPD provided by the Academy of European Law, Trier, Germany and funded by the European Commission's Programme for Employment and Social Solidarity (PROGRESS) 2007–2013.
101. European Disability Forum (2010). *Ten Years On*, 3.
102. See e.g. KMU Forschung Austria (2008). *Providing Reasonable Accommodation for Persons with Disabilities in the Workplace in the EU—Good Practices and Financing Schemes.* Retrieved March 26, 2013, from www.ec.europa.eu/social/BlobServlet?docId=1961&langId=en. See also European Disability Forum (2010). *Ten Years On.*
103. Such as the United Kingdom Access to Work scheme. See also European Disability Forum (2010). *Ten Years On*, for descriptions of similar (but apparently more limited) schemes in Lithuania, Sweden, Finland, and Luxembourg.
104. Ventegodt Liisberg (2013). Flexicurity and Employment of Persons with Disability in Europe; Ventegodt Liisberg (2011). *Disability and Employment.*
105. See also European Disability Forum (2010). *Ten Years On*, 6-7—where reference is made to a 2010 decision of the Budapest Metropolitan Court (Hungary) allowing a person under plenary guardianship to enter into work but only if their guardian signed the employment contract.
106. European Commission (2010). *European Disability Strategy 2010–2020*, section 1.3.
107. European Commission (2010). *Initial plan*, section 1.3.
108. Consolidated Version of the Treaty on the Functioning of the European Union, Article 19.

109. Waddington, L. (2011). Future prospects for EU equality law: lessons to be learned from the proposed Equal Treatment Directive. *European Law Review 36*, 163–184.

110. A point noted by De Burca, G., & Scott, J. (2006). Introduction. In G. de Burca, & J. Scott (Eds.). *Law and New Governance in Europe and the US*. Oxford, United Kingdom: Hart, 3.

111. Sabel, C., & Zenith, J. (2008). Learning from difference: the new architecture of experimentalist governance in the EU. *European Law Journal 14*(3), 273–274.

112. Sabel, C., & Simon, W. (2006). Epilogue: accountability without sovereignty. In G. de Burca, & J. Scott (Eds.). *Law and New Governance in Europe and the US*. Oxford, United Kingdom: Hart Publishing, 400.

113. See further De Schutter, O., & Deakin, S. (2005). Introduction: reflexive governance and the dilemmas of social regulation. In O. De Schutter, & S. Deakin (Eds.). *Social Rights and Market Forces. Is the Open Co-ordination of Employment and Social Policies the Future of Social Europe?* Brussels, Belgium: Bruylant, 1–17.

114. See e.g. Smismans, S. (2005). Reflexive law in support of directly deliberative polyarchy: reflexive-deliberative polyarchy as a normative frame for the OMC. In O. De Schutter, & S. Deakin (Eds.). *Social Rights and Market Forces. Is the Open Co-ordination of Employment and Social Policies the Future of Social Europe?* Brussels, Belgium: Bruylant, 99–143.

115. Council of the European Union (2000). The on-going experience of the open method of co-ordination. *Presidency Note*, 13 June.

116. See e.g. Zeitlin, J. (2005). The open method of co-ordination in action: theoretical promise, empirical realities, reform strategy. In J. Zeitlin, & P. Pochet (Eds.). *The Open Method of Coordination in Action: the European Employment and Social Inclusion Strategies*. Brussels, Belgium: PIE-Peter Lang, 447–504.

117. For example, Zeitlin, J. (2005). The open method of co-ordination; Velluti, S. (2010). *New Governance and the European Employment Strategy*. London: Routledge; Heidenreich, M., & Bischoff, G. (2008). The open method of co-ordination: a way to the Europeanisation of social and employment policies? *Journal of Common Market Studies 46*, 497–532; Zeitlin, J. (2009). The open method of co-ordination and reform of national social and employment policies: influences, mechanisms, effects. In M. Heidenreich, & J. Zeitlin (Eds.). *Changing European Employment and Welfare Regimes: The Influence of the Open Method of Co-ordination on National Reforms*. London: Routledge, 2009, 214–245.

118. For an extremely thorough analysis of the history of the employment OMC, as well as analysis of its current effectiveness, see Velluti (2010). *New Governance*.

119. See eg Council Recommendation 2004/741/EC of 14 October 2004 on the implementation of Member States' employment policies (OJ L 326/49); and European Commission (2005). *Communication to the Spring European Council, "Working Together for Growth and Jobs: A New Start for the Lisbon Strategy."* Brussels, Belgium: European Commission.

120. European Commission (2005). *Disability Mainstreaming in the European Employment Strategy*. Brussels, Belgium: European Commission.

121. Reports detailing this work include: Greve, B. (2009). *The Labour Market Situation of Disabled People in European Countries*; Priestley, M., & Roulstone, A. (2009). *Targeting and Mainstreaming Disability in the 2008–10 National Reform Programmes for Growth and Jobs*. Leeds, United Kingdom: Academic Network of European Disability Experts; Priestley, M. (2011). *Targeting and Mainstreaming Disability*. They are helpfully analyzed in Priestley, M. (2009).

The Potential for Using OMC Instruments in the New European Disability Strategy. Leeds, United Kingdom: ANED; Priestley, M. (2012). Disability policies and the open method of co-ordination. In L. Waddington, G. Quinn, & E. Flynn (Eds.). *European Yearbook of Disability Law Volume 3*. Uitgevers, The Netherlands: Intersentia. 7–34.

122. Priestley, M. (2011). *Targeting and Mainstreaming Disability in the 2008–10 National Reform Programmes for Growth and Jobs*. Leeds, United Kingdom: Academic Network of European Disability Experts.

123. Priestley, M. (2012). Disability Policies and the Open Method of Co-ordination. 20.

124. Ibid, 21–22.

125. Ibid, 20–21.

126. Ibid, 21.

127. European Commission (2005). *Disability Mainstreaming*.

128. Disability High Level Group (2007). *Disability Mainstreaming in the New Streamlined European Social Protection and Social Inclusion Process*. Discussion Paper.

129. See generally Priestley, M. (2012). Disability Policies and the Open Method of Co-ordination.

130. See e.g. by delegates at the EU Summit of Ministers with responsibility for disability policies in Zaragoza in May 2010; European Economic and Social Committee, Opinion on "People with disabilities: employment and accessibility by stages for people with disabilities in the EU. Post-2010 Lisbon Strategy" of 17 March 2010, SOC/363, sections 3.1 and 3.3; and European Disability Forum (2010) *EDF Position Paper on the Future European Disability Strategy 2010–2020*. Brussels, Belgium: EDF.

131. Priestley, M. (2012). Disability Policies and the Open Method of Co-ordination,. 32.

132. See de Burca, G. (2012). Stumbling into experimentalism: the EU anti-discrimination regime. In C. Sabel, & J. Zeitlin (Eds.). *Experimentalist Governance in the European Union: Towards a New Architecture*. Oxford, United Kingdom: Oxford University Press, 215–236, for the argument that EU nondiscrimination law possesses a growing number of features of experimentalist governance, although it falls outside the ambit of formalized OMC processes.

133. See http://www.non-discrimination.net/

134. See http://fra.europa.eu/fraWebsite/partners_networks/research_partners/fralex/fralex_en.htm

135. de Burca, G. (2010). The European Union in the negotiation of the UN Disability Convention. *European Law Review 35*(2), 174.

136. Ibid., 177–179.

137. Kilpatrick, C. (2006). New EU employment governance and constitutionalism. In G. de Burca, & J. Scott (Eds.). *Law and New Governance in Europe and the US*. Oxford: Hart, 2006, 123.

138. Ibid.

139. European Commission (2010). *European Disability Strategy 2010–2020*, section 2.1.4.

140. Ibid, section 2.2.2.

141. For a lucid explanation of the operation of these funds, see Quinn, G., & Doyle, S. (2012). *Getting a Life—Living Independently and Being Included in the Community: A Legal Study of the Current Use and Future Potential of the European*

Structural Funds to Contribute to the Achievement of Article 19 of the United Nations Convention on the Rights of Persons with Disabilities, chapter 6. Office of the High Commissioner for Human Rights European Region. Retrieved March 26, 2013, from http://europe.ohchr.org/Documents/Publications/Getting_a_Life.pdf

142. European Commission (2009), *Ensuring Accessibility and Non-discrimination for People with Disabilities: Toolkit for Using Structural and Cohesion Funds*. Brussels, Belgium: European Commission,13, 15.

143. Priestley, M., & Roulstone, A. (2009). *Targeting and Mainstreaming Disability in the 2008–10 National Reform Programmes for Growth and Jobs*. Leeds, United Kingdom: Academic Network of European Disability Experts.

144. Ibid., 7.

145. Ibid.

146. See http://ec.europa.eu/esf/main.jsp?catId=31&langId=en

147. Parker, C., with Bulic, I. (2010). *Wasted Time, Wasted Money Wasted Lives: A Wasted Opportunity?* London, United Kingdom: ECCL.

148. Proposal for a Regulation of the European Parliament and of the Council laying down common provisions on the European Regional Development Fund, the European Social Fund, the Cohesion Fund, the European Agricultural Fund for Rural Development and the European Maritime and Fisheries Fund, covered by the Common Strategic Framework and laying down general provisions on the European Regional Development Fund, the European Social Fund and the Cohesion Fund and repealing Regulation (EC) No 1083/2006, Brussels, 6 October 2011 COM(2011).

149. Ibid., Articles 7 and 87(3)(ii).

150. For further details of the impact of these ex-ante conditions on Member States, see Article 17.

151. See, in particular, ex-ante conditions 8, 9 and 10.

152. On 24 April 2012, at the General Affairs Council meeting in Luxembourg, Member States adopted a compromise text which does not include the general ex ante conditionalities relating to non-discrimination, disability or gender equality.

153. Quinn, G., & Doyle, S. (2012). *Getting a Life—Living Independently and Being Included in the Community: A Legal Study of the Current Use and Future Potential of the European Structural Funds to Contribute to the Achievement of Article 19 of the United Nations Convention on the Rights of Persons with Disabilities*. Office of the High Commissioner for Human Rights European Region. Retrieved March 26, 2013, from http://europe.ohchr.org/Documents/Publications/Getting_a_Life. pdf; Parker, C., & Clements, L. (2012). *The European Union and the Right to Community Living: Structural Funds and the EU's Obligations under the Convention on the Rights of Persons with Disabilities*. New York: Open Society Foundations.

154. See e.g. Inter-American Human Rights Commission (2011). *Methodology and Parameters for Measuring Progress in the Implementation of the Inter-American Convention on the Elimination of All Forms of Discrimination against Persons with Disabilities, and the Program of Action for the Decade (PAD) of the Americas for the Rights and Dignity of Persons with Disabilities*. San Salvador, El Salvador: CEDDIS.

155. For a discussion of the importance of encouraging experimentalism (in the context of positive action measures) among employers, see Barmes, L. (2009). Equality law and experimentation: the positive action challenge. *Cambridge Law Journal 68*, 623–654.

156. For suggestions along these lines, see Sturm, S. (2001). Second generation employment discrimination: a structural approach. *Columbia Law Review 101*, 458–568; and, for criticism of this position, see Somek, A. (2011). *Engineering Equality: An Essay on European Anti-Discrimination Law.* Oxford, United Kingdom: Oxford University Press.

INDEX

Pages in *italics* indicate tables.

Android TalkBack, 153
ANED. *See* Academic Network of
    European Disability Experts
antidiscrimination laws, 27- 28,
    214–215, 230–231, 252–253, 288,
    364, 401
apps, mobile, 151–153, 165
APPT. *See* Alleviating Poverty through
    Peer Training
Argentina, 99, 216, 299n64, 315
assistive technology
    accessibility, 7, 139, 156–157
    barriers to switching, 163–164
    braille-based technology, 143–144
    Braille displays, 150–151
    Braille embossers, 149–150
    Braille keyboards, 144
    Braille printer, 368
    Braille translator, 143–144
    employability in low-/middle-income
        countries and, 153–164
    employment engineering and,
        158–159
    forms, 139
    framework technologies, 141–147
    general obligations, 138–139
    hardware technologies, 147–153
    hiring attitudes and, 154–155
    implicit roles, 138
    international law and, 137–140
    Internet, 60–61
    job search constraints and, 290
    Kurzweil Reading Machine, 142
    language support, 145–147
    magnification apps, 151–152
    mobile phones, 152–153
    OCR tools, 141–143
    open source tools, 145
    peer groups, 159–160
    personal mobility, 139
    piracy, 161
    rehabilitation, 140
    roles, 138
    screen modifier, 151–152
    screen readers, 144–147, 162
    smartphones, 151–152
    social networks, 159–160
    software accessibility, 139, 161
    speech recognition, 143
    speech synthesizers, 148–149

telemarketing jobs, 159
transcription jobs, 159
translation software, 368
United Nations Convention on the
    Rights of Persons with Disabilities
    and, 136
web applications, 60–61
workplace access to, 160–161
Association of Microfinance
    Institutions of Uganda
    (AMFIU), 179
A Trabajar, 316
audio output technology, 148–149
Australia, 3, 8, 13, 46, 95, 99, *245,
    246,* 252
Austria, 59, *245, 246, 246,* 392, 398
awareness-raising, employment. *See*
    disability awareness

BABD. *See* Business Advisory Board on
    Disability
Banco D-MIRO, 187
Bangladesh, 5, 177, *270, 273*
BBC World Service Trust, 289
BDF. *See* Business Disability Forum
Belgium, 14, *245, 246,* 250, *251,*
    391, 392
benefits, disability
    cash benefits, 26
    characteristics, *350*
    chronic disease and, 261
    dependency on, 245–246, *246*
    dependency reform, 254–259
    mental health disorders and, 244, 261
    outflow to job market and, 11–12
    schemes, 253–254
    short-term work incapacity,
        249–251, 260
    wage subsidies, 29
    work disincentives, 26
Blue Ribbon Employment Council
    (BREC), 35
Braille-based technology, 143–144
Braille displays, 150–151
Braille embossers, 149–150
Braille keyboards, 144
Braille printer, 368
Braille translator, 143–144
Brazil, 10, 99, 106–108, *271,* 315. *See
    also* Serasa Experian

public assistance programs, 217–218
public awareness campaigns, 123
Public Employment Security Office,
    364–365
Public Sector Equality Duty (United
    Kingdom), 72, 78–79
public works programs, 287–288, 319

quotas
    administrative guidance to, 364
    benefits of, 373–374
    in Brazil, 107–108
    disadvantages to, 372–373
    employer discrimination, 288–289
    enforcement systems, 365
    in Japan, 13, 361–364
    job retention and, 253
    legislation, 27, 59, 107–108
    in Peru, 318–319
    public employment and, 318–319

Racial Equality Directive, 402
reasonable accommodations, 228–229,
    284, 377
Red-CIL, 316
Redemptorist Center, 30
redeployment of workers, 377–378
regulations. *See* policies/policymakers
rehabilitation, 140
Rehabilitation Act (United States,
    1973), 339–340, 344
reintegration policies, 247
reservation, 289. *See also* quotas
retention. *See* job retention; school
    retention
Romania, 59, 392–393, 407
rotating savings and credit associations
    (ROSCA), 179–180, 192n41
Russia, 35–36, 99
Rwanda, 269, 275–276

SAMHSA. *See* Substance Abuse
    and Mental Health Services
    Administration
savings, importance of, 184–185
Sayce Review, 72
school-based job training, 204
school retention, 202–203
school-to-work programs, 215
screen modifiers, 151–152

screen readers, 144–147, 162
segregation, 122–123
self-employment
    access to credit, 10–11, 32, 174
        (*See also* microfinance)
    borrowing activities, 183–184
    constraints, 280
    employment strategy, 38
    financial disincentives, 217–218
    in low- and middle-income countries,
        272
    public assistance programs, 217–218
    rates, *273–274*
self-esteem. *See also* self-exclusion
    credit access and, 175–176, 289–290
    exclusion and, 175–176
    training programs and, 113, 121
self-exclusion, 176, 188
self-help groups (SHGs), 33
sensitization training, 118, 124–125
Serasa Experian
    diversity and reputation, 123–124
    employee fit, 113
    impact on employees with disabilities,
        119–122
    lack of promotional opportunities,
        126–127
    program strategies, 109–111
    sharing knowledge, 118–119
    training program, 111–115
    "two-way street" framework, 109–110
severe disabilities, 370–371
sheltered employment, 29, 253
SHG. *See* self-help groups
short-term work incapacity,
    249–251, 260
sickness absence, 249–251, *251*,
    258, 260
sickness and disability policies,
    248–251
Singapore, 99
skills constraints, 277
Slovakia, 59, 391, 392, 398
Slovenia, 392, 398, 405–406
smartphones, 151–152
social-democratic disability policy
    model, 251–252
social inclusion, 257
social model of disability, 73, 114, 248,
    401n62